Blood Farm

Blood Farm

The Explosive Big Pharma Scandal

That Altered the AIDS Crisis

CARA McGOOGAN

DIVERSION
BOOKS

For more information, email info@diversionbooks.com.

Diversion Books

A division of Diversion Publishing Corp.
www.diversionbooks.com

First Diversion Books Edition: October 2023
Hardcover ISBN: 9781635768886
eBook ISBN: 9781635769548

Printed in the United States of America
10 9 8 7 6 5 4 3 2 1

For everyone who lost their lives
and the survivors who keep fighting

Things fall apart; the centre cannot hold;
Mere anarchy is loosed upon the world,
The blood-dimmed tide is loosed, and everywhere
The ceremony of innocence is drowned

    W. B. Yeats, 'The Second Coming'

Contents

Prologue: The Farm

At the northern edge of Louisiana, the state line cuts a sharp turn south and follows the shape of the Mississippi River, meandering left and right with the flow of the water. Two hundred and fifty kilometers pass from Lake Providence to Lettsworth before the border heads eastwards at a right angle, drawing the state into a fat L-shape. In the corner of that L is a penned-in plot of land. On one side, the slow-moving hulk of the river; on the other, barbed-wire fences. It is here that Isaac Franklin, co-founder of the largest slave trading company in the United States, created seven plantations in the 1830s. Franklin brought in enslaved people to work the fields overlooking the river, harvesting sugarcane, cotton and corn. From the break of day until nightfall they toiled under the blistering Southern sun. The sub-tropical climate in this region can be erratic: periods of biting heat and overpowering mugginess are swept away by frenzied storms. Winter is a respite.

With slavery, Franklin imported a new name to the area: Angola, after the country where he had stolen his lucrative trade. Following the abolition of slavery in 1865, Angola adapted but failed to outgrow its roots. What was once a plantation became land farmed by leased convicts. Prisoners, many of them descendants of enslaved people, had to work for little or no recompense. By 1901 this arrangement was formalized and Angola took on its contemporary form: barbed-wire fences were erected along with a sprawling complex of imposing buildings. Angola was now Louisiana State Penitentiary. All the while, it retained its singular history of exploitation and brutality. Angola became the largest maximum-security prison in America, with more than five thousand inmates and nearly two thousand members of staff. Those serving time have committed the most violent crimes, including murder, rape and armed robbery. Many have a life sentence with hard labor. And so it came to be that the fields surrounding Angola are lined with rows and rows of white crosses, marking the graves of the inmates who never escape its grounds, even in death.

In the late months of 1997 a lawyer arrived at Angola. Tom Mull had driven up from New Orleans in his soft-top Checker car, trundling a hundred miles along a winding two-lane road through Louisiana's swampy bayou. It was becoming less sweaty in America's South, but the air was thick and muggy. Louisiana's Route 66 was a far cry from the famous artery that connects Chicago to Los Angeles; this Route 66 had big cracks running through it like veins. It carved through an American backwater known for its alligators, crawfish and slow pace of life. As a public defender, Tom had represented a number of Angola's inmates accused of violent crimes and was accustomed to visiting them in prison. He wasn't scared of those who had committed murders, nor of the brutality of life behind its walls. He believed that made him an unusual person. These prisoners were some of the most interesting people Tom had ever met. He was intrigued by the lifestyle and culture they had developed within Angola's eighteen thousand acres.

Then, as now, Angola was known for its annual rodeo. Every year, thousands of people travel down that narrow road with tickets to the prison's arena, where they are presented with an incongruous spectacle. Inmates cling to raging bulls, hoping that even if they don't win the competition they will at least earn some time in the prison's hospital wing and away from their cells. There is an array of entertainment: prisoners wrestle a bulldog out of a chute in one event and try to mount wild horses as they charge around the arena in another. As a light reprieve, monkeys wearing sparkly waistcoats ride sheepdogs in front of the hooting crowd. The rodeo isn't the only tourist attraction at Angola. It also has a museum that documents its lethal history: the traveling electric chair from the 1940s, descriptions of a great flood that washed disease and fear into the prison walls, and the story of the group of inmates who slashed their Achilles tendons in protest against forced labor. It was a slice of this culture Tom was there to investigate. On this particular day in 1997 he wasn't thinking about his criminal clients. He had a new mission: he had been tipped off about a secret industry inside the prison walls.

The greatest horrors tend to linger in the imagination, spawning further myths. That is perhaps why Louisiana State Penitentiary has so many nicknames. To some, it is still Angola. Others call it The Farm, because inmates are forced to work the land. Every morning, they rise at a scheduled time and leave their cells for work. One group of prisoners harvests the fields, another waters the Prison View Golf Course and looks after the animals. Some have been known to make their own coffins in the prison workshop. It is also called the Alcatraz of the South, after riots and assaults became so common-place in the 1950s that its reputation grew as notorious as that of the island fortress in San Francisco Bay. But there is another description of Louisiana State Penitentiary, one that Tom suspected could be its most fitting: America's bloodiest prison.

Tom knew what to expect as he approached. There were the white barriers that suddenly cut the road short and the sign warning visitors they could have their 'body cavities searched' if they went farther. He had heard the rumors of wolf-dog hybrids patrolling the grounds and seen the armed guards on horseback, but that would not deter him. He passed smoothly through the layers of security. As guards checked his identity and rifled through his possessions, he thought about his time in the US Air Force and the checkpoints he would go through to enter the Pentagon. He pushed down the memories, trying to block the trauma from surfacing. Tom liked to think of himself as a modern-day Don Quixote on a chivalrous quest to help people, alongside him his wife, Lorraine, with her analytical brain, and their band of small-town lawyer colleagues. Their lives were an organized chaos, traveling back and forth between Louisiana, where their law practice was based, and Hawaii, where they later moved. They needed the mental break afforded by their second home. After all, they had spent the best part of the 1990s investigating the needless deaths of thousands of American children, an investigation that had now brought him to Angola.

The first family to approach the Mulls came from outside Baton Rouge, the state capital that lies between New Orleans and Angola.

Karen and Gary Cross were terrified for their son, Darren Bradley, known as Brad, who was fifteen at the time and had a terminal illness. Since that first meeting, more and more families had approached them until they had hundreds of clients.

The guards were Tom's first port of call. He knew some of them from his many visits to the prison, so he approached them with confidence. He wasn't fazed by the guns that hung from their torsos. He didn't feel the need for protection; when the inmates discovered the truth, he was sure they would want to help him. A guard took Tom to a private room. He said he knew a hunter had recently come across a trove of evidence buried in the land outside Angola – needles and medical equipment that Tom believed were proof of the secret industry in the prison. He had spoken to a former inmate and the editor of the prison newspaper, *The Angolite*, both of whom were scared to testify because of the repercussions they could face. The guards were initially reticent, too. If they gave Tom information on the record, they could lose their jobs. Tom conceded that they could talk privately to begin with. He just needed to get more information. With that, they started to open up.

What the guards were about to tell Tom would prove his theory about how his young clients had come to be infected. Diseases that were rife within the prison walls had started to seep out. Not only across America, but around the world. They were hiding in sanitary medical vials that pharmaceutical companies were billing as a miracle treatment.

'It blew my mind,' says Tom. The discovery would help unravel a mystery that had haunted people for over fifteen years. Eventually, it would give victims the weapon they needed to fight for justice.

A quarter of a century later, Tom tells me, 'You are someone I have been hoping would come along for over thirty years.'

PART ONE

The Fall

1. Schoolboy Games

The school day began with a cooked English breakfast. Pupils lined up – some walking, a few on crutches, others in wheelchairs – to find a seat at the refectory tables, where teal-colored plates were waiting for them. Stainless steel dishes laden with food were placed in the middle of the tables. They were an active group of children, in spite of their differing physical abilities, and would devour the breakfast before heading to assembly: lower-school children would have theirs in Newton-Davis Hall and upper school in Florence Treloar Hall.

Headmaster Alec Macpherson would address the pupils and they would sing a couple of hymns from red bibles before heading to the first lessons of the day. Some would have to report to the medical center for routine treatment before joining their peers in class. All were dressed the same, in dark blue uniforms with emerald green ties that were embroidered with a pattern of red overlapping initials: LMTC, for Lord Mayor Treloar College. The T was larger than the other three letters, indicative of the shorthand everyone used for the school: Treloar's.

Ten-year-old Richard Warwick was slowly getting used to this new world that had been thrust upon him in September 1976. He was nearly three hundred miles and a six-hour drive from his parents – the school was in Hampshire while they were up in Scarborough – and he was homesick. He had soft nut-brown hair and hazel eyes, with a smile that revealed delicate teeth. Just a few weeks earlier, his mother's arms had been around him as she said goodbye while he lay in a hospital bed in the unfamiliar medical center at Treloar's – or 'sickbay,' as the pupils called it. Since then, he had phoned home every week and begged to come back through sobs. His mum, at the other end of the line, would be crying as well. Richard often found himself in tears during those early weeks. He wanted to be with his parents and younger sister for his mum's Sunday lunches; to greet his dad as he came home from work. Treloar's was wildly different from anything he had known before. Richard had never worn a tie, never spent much time away from his parents and never had proper friends. His parents had wrapped him up in cotton wool throughout his early childhood and now, with the protective blanket gone, he had to fend for himself. He wasn't coping. He missed home terribly.

Richard's first week at the new boarding school hadn't gone to plan. The problems started on the journey from Scarborough, when he was squeezed into the back of his family's Austin Maxi. They were somewhere on the M1 when he felt a familiar tickle in his left knee. He had been twisted into an uncomfortable position for a couple of hours when it suddenly gave way. Richard could feel warm liquid seeping into his knee. At first, there was relief from the ache he usually felt in the joint, but before long it became excruciating. He had a bleed coming on – and the timing couldn't have been worse. Blood was pooling into the joint, causing his knee to swell and swell, until his skin couldn't stretch any farther. To Richard, it looked like his knee had grown to the size of a small football. Adding to his parents' problems, the car's brakes had locked on. They pulled into the next service station and hurriedly tried to decide on their next move. They hadn't brought any treatment with them for Richard – what could they do? Richard started to cry out in pain.

Richard's parents, John and Denise, were thirty-two years old. His dad was part of Britain's Cold War effort, working as a telecoms engineer at GCHQ's Scarborough office, while his mum stayed at home to look after Richard and his sister full-time. They had struggled with Richard's health throughout his life, taking him back and forth to hospital on many occasions. The smallest accident would leave him with terrible injuries: he was forever having his limbs encased in plaster casts and his joints bound with splints. Doctors looked for infections, abscesses and broken bones. They became concerned and brought in social services amid suspicions of abuse; the police were informed. John and Denise were appalled, and fretful about what could be wrong with their son. Denise would cry at the smallest of things because of the stress caused by Richard's condition; John regularly missed days at work. When Richard was two, their daughter was born, but their attention remained squarely focused on their eldest child. A few months later, Richard's thumb swelled to the size of a small plum. This time, John and Denise took him to the hospital in Hull for a second opinion, and he was finally given a diagnosis. Richard had severe hemophilia A, a rare genetic condition that makes the body deficient in a protein needed to form blood clots. It could have been identified when he was a baby.

In Hull, after diagnosing Richard with hemophilia, doctors gave him his first treatment for the bleeding disorder. In those days, that meant cryoprecipitate, or 'cryo' for short, which was made from fresh frozen plasma and administered in hospital. The plastic bag of yellow-ish liquid was thawed in a bath of warm water. While he waited an hour or two for it to be ready, the bleed that had taken the Warwicks to Hull continued, becoming ever more painful as blood pooled beneath his skin. Once the bag of cryo was defrosted, the doctor hung it onto a drip and infused it into Richard's arm. He cried and then shuddered as the cold fluid entered his veins, feeling it crawl up his arm and over his shoulders. 'Mum, make it stop,' he whimpered. Richard sat in bed sniffling for the hour and a half it took to infuse two bags. In addition to hemophilia, he had an allergic reaction to the one treatment that would help his blood to clot. To stave off severe anaphylactic shock subsequently, doctors had to give him preemptive injections of antihistamine while they waited for the cryo to thaw.

Richard's soft baby skin became a pincushion. Throughout his childhood, he needed cryo several times a week. Each dose required another hospital trip. Childhood passed in a blur of medical scrubs and endless days lying prone on the sofa. His parents banned him from going farther than the end of the front garden. When he was well, he would sit on the wall and watch the other children run up and down the cul-de-sac, but he wasn't allowed to join them. By the time he was ten, Richard had lost months of school and fallen behind his peers. It came as no surprise to the family that a new approach would be needed if Richard was to have a chance of developing into a 'happy, well-rounded' teenager. The advice came from the hospital and local authority that John and Denise should send him to Lord

Mayor Treloar College for secondary schooling. Denise initially balked at her son being so far from home. But the school had a dedicated hemophilia center; Richard would be safe there and have a chance to meet boys just like him.

At the service station on the M1 on their way down to Treloar's, Richard's parents had to make a decision. They were miles from home and with every second more blood was draining into Richard's swollen knee. He was in agony. They could return home, where they had supplies of his medicine in the fridge, but the journey back to Scarborough would take hours. They could detour to a nearby hospital, but that offered a new set of problems: Would it have Richard's medication? What if he was kept in for monitoring? . . . No, neither of those options would work. The best choice was to get to Hampshire as quickly as possible.

When the Warwicks arrived at Treloar's in the early afternoon, Richard went straight to sick bay. For the rest of the week, the aluminium traveling trunk containing the brand-new uniform with his name stitched into it remained unpacked in his dorm room. The other three boys he would be sharing a room with in Burnham House settled in and got to know one another while Richard recovered in sick bay. Unruly schoolkids explored their new playground; Richard wallowed in a fog of homesickness.

After he left sick bay and got used to being away from his family, Richard saw just how utopian and liberating his new school was. Treloar's was a specialist institution for children with physical disabilities, and there were hundreds of other pupils there who were just like him. The campus was centered around a Jacobean mansion, a grand building with gabled roofs and ivy crawling up its limestone exterior. Inside, there were decorative ceilings and wood-paneled walls. The lower school, Froyle, was in the central mansion, while the upper school, Holybourne, was in a newer, purpose-made building. A blue minibus shuttled children back and forth between the two sites, three miles apart. Altogether, Treloar's covered dozens of acres of English countryside. There were tennis courts, ponds, woodland and a riding stables. The lawns were always neatly trimmed. Everything about it was designed to be accessible for the two hundred and fifty or so pupils, aged nine to eighteen, who had a range of conditions including spina bifida, muscular dystrophy and cerebral palsy. Some had been paralyzed after being infected with polio when they were younger and there were children born with disabilities after their mothers had been prescribed thalidomide for morning sickness. But the largest group was Richard's – those with hemophilia.

Sir William Purdie Treloar, the lord mayor of the City of London, had the idea for a school next to a children's hospital in 1907. He wanted to help children with non-pulmonary tuberculosis and he had the support of Queen Alexandra, wife of King Edward VII, who dedicated her summer fete to his fund. Within a year, he had raised enough money to open the Lord Mayor Treloar College. The combination of fees and additional funding from companies in the City of London meant Treloar's had better resources than most specialist schools in Britain, with an indoor swimming pool, a hydrotherapy pool and accessible housing. Although Treloar's was for children with physical disabilities, its ethos was to let pupils live as active and normal lives as possible, whether that meant learning to swim or preparing for university.

As those early weeks passed, Richard started to feel more comfortable and soon came to think of Treloar's as a wonderland. He compared notes with other pupils about his unconventional childhood, which became blessedly normal in this new environment. Other boys knew the pain of a joint bleed, and the unique embarrassment of seeing their peers be told they can't hit you because it could kill you. It was a revelation to feel like everyone else. He could live in the way all children should: making friends spontaneously, without judgment, being fearless in the playground. With the nearby hemophilia center, pupils no longer had to miss days of school when they had a bleed. When students felt the familiar tickle in the joint that came before debilitating pain, they would report to sick bay in the lower school Froyle and wait to be driven to the Holybourne end for treatment at the hemophilia center. If a child was in a wheelchair recovering from a bleed, their peers would help push them around.

Richard went from being a boy who had known little more than the confines of his living room and hospital ward, to a teenager who relished the activities Treloar's had to offer: archery, shooting, boating and fishing. When summer arrived, with its long evenings and warmer weather, some children went camping in the grounds. Richard soon learned his limits, testing the boundaries with his new friends. Late at night, they would have water fights in their dorm. This was risky for children with hemophilia, but knowledge that doctors were nearby empowered them, freed them. It was a drastic change from the years he had spent watching other children from his garden wall, lying on the sofa in agony and blowing out his birthday candles in a hospital bed.

But it wasn't just Treloar's and its on-site hemophilia center that had given Richard a shot at a normal childhood; a revolutionary new treatment for hemophilia had recently come onto the market.

Hemophilia affects the body's ability to clot its blood effectively. Blood continues to flow when someone with the condition is injured, either internally or externally. Normally when a person cuts themselves, proteins in their blood called clotting factors link together one by one in a cascade to create a sticky mesh known as a fibrin clot. Richard had severe hemophilia A, meaning his blood was deficient in a clotting protein called factor VIII. Hemophilia A is caused by a recessive gene carried on the X chromosome, so it passes from mothers to sons, skipping generations of families and lying dormant for the next son. As a result, the condition mostly affects men, but some women who are carriers can be deficient in factor VIII. The symptoms include skin that bruises easily, excessive bleeding from wounds and nosebleeds that continue for hours. Other forms of the bleeding condition include hemophilia B, which is caused by a deficiency in the protein factor IX, and von Willebrand disease, a lack of a factor with the same name, which affects men and women.

There is a common misconception that people with hemophilia are at risk of death from loss of blood after a minor injury like a paper cut. In fact, it is internal bleeding that causes the most damage. When a blood vessel bursts inside the body, people with hemophilia get what is known as a bleed. In around twenty minutes, the joint or muscle fills with blood, becoming solid and permanently damaged.

The pain is equivalent to breaking a bone. Any surgery carries a high risk because patients could bleed profusely without clotting medication. The most life-threatening bleeds are those in the brain. Today, more than eight thousand people in the United Kingdom have hemophilia A.

By far the best known cases of hemophilia from the nineteenth and twentieth centuries were in the British royal family. Queen Victoria was a carrier of hemophilia B, which she passed down to three of her nine children. Her son Leopold had a lethal brain hemorrhage after falling and hitting his head in the South of France when he was thirty, leaving behind his pregnant wife. Two of Queen Victoria's daughters, Alice and Beatrice, inherited the faulty gene from their mother, becoming hemophilia carriers and in turn passing it on to their children. Alice's daughter Alexandra married Russia's Tsar Nicholas II, and in 1904 gave birth to their first son, Alexei. The newborn was swaddled tight as per Russian tradition – so tight that the cloth grated on his newly cut umbilical cord and caused him to bleed. Blood seeped out of his naval without letup. Doctors said the baby had hemophilia and would be lucky to live to the age of sixteen. To prevent anything from happening to their firstborn son, the heir to the Russian throne, Tsar Nicholas II ruled that Alexei must be protected. The young prince spent his childhood lying down, with ice intermittently applied to various parts of his body. Tsar Nicholas and Alexandra brought in a mystic with healing powers to help their son, Rasputin. Alexei's condition was a state secret until 1912. For three generations, descendants of Queen Victoria in England, Russia, Germany and Spain were born with hemophilia. The condition eventually vanished from royal bloodlines, but not without leaving a legacy: throughout the twentieth century, hemophilia was often called 'the royal disease.'

Even for non-royals, hemophilia could twist the lines of a family tree. Identical twins Simon and Nigel Hamilton came from a long line of hemophiliacs. Their grandfather had the bleeding disorder, as did many of their cousins. Regardless, they were energetic young boys from Belfast who would quickly seek out whatever sport they could take up as the more popular ones were ruled out: rugby was too dangerous, so they became rowers instead. Still, they were accident prone so would often end up needing treatment. Simon once bit his tongue and it swelled up so badly he couldn't close his mouth. The mishap earned him two weeks in hospital. At the dentist, they would both bleed profusely from a regular tooth extraction. With the metallic taste of blood sloshing around their mouths, dark memories resurfaced. Both their grandfather and his brother had bled to death in the 1960s after having their wisdom teeth pulled out.

For people with hemophilia, *when* in history they were born has dictated what kind of life they will lead. In the same decade that Simon and Nigel's forebears died from routine dental work, researchers made a discovery that would completely overhaul life for people with the condition. The early 1960s were 'heady years in the history of hemophilia treatment,' according to Dr Carol Kasper, former director of a Los Angeles hemophilia center, which culminated in a breakthrough in 1964. Dr Judith Graham Pool, a researcher at Stanford University, found that by freezing plasma and thawing it slowly she could isolate its constituent parts. At the bottom of the thawed plasma was a fibrous-looking paste that remained partly frozen. Dr Pool tested the paste and discovered it was made up of the factor proteins needed for clotting. With that, she had a new treatment for people with hemophilia: cryo, the translucent yellow frozen substance that made Richard shudder as it crawled through his veins. In each treatment, children would be given two bags, while adults could receive four to six bags.

Dr Pool's findings laid the foundation for a revolutionary new treatment. In the late 1960s, she shared her research with Dr Edward Shanbrom, medical director at Hyland Therapeutics, a division of pharmaceutical company Baxter Healthcare. He pooled hundreds of donations of plasma together to make a large batch of cryo, then extracted the factor VIII proteins and freeze-dried them to create a white powder. This concentrated form of factor VIII could be bottled and stored in a fridge, rather than in freezers. People with hemophilia could simply dilute it with sterile distilled water and infuse themselves. The new concentrate made by Hyland was called Factor VIII and it was licensed in the US in 1969. The American

Red Cross, which supplied most of the country's blood and blood products, decided it would be too expensive to make its own not-for-profit version and instead started shipping its plasma to Hyland so it could supply this revolutionary treatment. To treat patients with severe hemophilia cost tens of thousands of dollars a year. Before long, realizing how much profit stood to be made, other pharma companies released their own versions of Factor VIII, and a multi-billion-dollar industry was born.

The treatment was licensed in the UK in 1973 and started to make its way into the arms of people with hemophilia. Centers like the one at Treloar's quickly transitioned from cryo to Factor VIII, which was pitched to doctors and patients as a miracle treatment that would change lives. It took just fifteen minutes to administer, rather than the multiple hours cryo needed to thaw and transfuse via a drip. With cryo, patients often had to stay in hospital for a week to complete treatment and recovery. Factor VIII could be administered at home – or even on the move. No more did patients need to go to the hemophilia center whenever they had a bleed; they could go to their kitchens and retrieve Factor VIII straight from the fridge. Added to that, the new treatment was far less uncomfortable and caused fewer reactions, such as allergies or inhibitors (when the body thinks it is under attack from a foreign substance and tries to destroy the invader). For Richard, that meant no more antihistamines. Life for people with hemophilia became easier and patients around the world felt liberated. 'Passport to freedom for hemophiliacs,' said one early advert for Factor VIII.

Gary Webster had his inaugural treatment of Factor VIII aged ten, during his first year at Treloar's in the Easter term of 1976. Having spent three or four days a month being infused with cryo and waiting hours for it to take effect, Gary was thrilled with Factor VIII. He had hated not being able to play football or ride a bike, so he quickly embraced his newfound freedom: running amok at night, sneaking into girls' dormitories and enjoying the inter-house rivalries. The teachers were more relaxed, too. They watched balls ricochet off the boys' legs without panicking that it could bring on debilitating bleeds. As at most British schools in the 1970s, life at Treloar's could be harsh at times. If a child got carried away and was being particularly disruptive, a teacher might throw a wooden board rubber at them or hit them with a ruler (corporal punishment existed even for children with disabilities). But if the boys with hemophilia had a bleed after being hit with a hard object, they could go to the hemophilia center for Factor VIII. They were free from the hospital's handcuffs.

Every year, Headmaster Macpherson would invite some boys to join him on his Moody 36 yacht to race around the Isle of Wight, off the southern coast of England. Gary had a gift for sailing and was invited to help crew the boat in the race. Salt water sprayed their faces as they curved around the island. When he was older, Gary would skip going home at the weekend and instead travel to London in secret to watch concerts. He saw David Bowie live at Wembley Stadium.

One of the regular Treloar's trips was to Churchtown Farm, an outdoor pursuits center in Cornwall for children with disabilities. From one countryside haven to another, they went climbing, abseiling and helped out on the working farm. Doctors as well as teachers would accompany them in case they had a bleed. Gary had recently hit his teens and was on a visit to Churchtown Farm when he bonded with the boy who would become his best friend, Stephen. They were both fans of motor racing and saw themselves as adrenaline-fueled go-getters. Stephen, whose father was a pig farmer in Norfolk, had a thick country accent and a dry sense of humor. In the same form class, the pair spent all of their time together.

Every era has its fad toys. For Gary and Stephen it was Citizen's Band radio, a boxy, metallic precursor to the modern handheld radio. They would thread an aerial out of their dorm room window late at night to pick up signals and talk to people from the local area over the airwaves. They each had a handle: Gary's was Buttonhole because he was studying tailoring and Stephen's was Black Panther. With Stephen by his side, Gary had a comrade in arms. They went abroad on one another's family holidays and became as close as brothers, bound by their hemophilia and the unconventional childhood it necessitated.

★

Quality of life was improving for people with hemophilia across Britain – and the world. In London in 1978 Dr Edward Tuddenham joined the Royal Free Hospital as co-director of the hemophilia center, making him one of the country's leading hemophilia doctors. He was a ruminative man in his thirties, born in South Wales during the Second World War, who spoke with a careful, soft voice. His father, a physicist, had run the local munitions factory during the conflict, after which his family had moved to Dorking in Surrey, and he went through the punishment of public school before studying medicine in London. In hematology, the branch of medicine that specializes in blood disorders, Dr Tuddenham found an intimate combination of laboratory and clinical work. He had an interest in pathology, the study of disease, and thought he might want to specialize in malignant hematology, but he changed his mind when he was training. During a stint in adult acute leukemia, he discovered the psychological toll of looking after patients with a death sentence hanging over them was unbearable.

Dr Tuddenham moved towards benign hematology and narrowed his interest down to hemophilia. The reason for his devotion to the bleeding disorder was twofold: he cared for the patients he was looking after, but he was also fascinated by the factor VIII protein itself. Unlike other clotting proteins, which the body makes in the liver, factor VIII is created in the endothelial cells – those which line every blood vessel like a pavement. Dr Tuddenham became so fascinated by factor VIII that he would dedicate more than fifty years of his life to researching it.

His office at the Royal Free was in a brand-new building that towered over Hampstead in north London, the grey love child of a 1970s housing estate and the brutalism of the Barbican. He was in charge of research, with a senior lectureship, while his colleague Dr Peter Kernoff managed the center on a daily basis. They had two hundred and fifty patients, most of whom were young boys. And he was excited to oversee their transition from cryo to Factor VIII.

It was an unhappy reality that before treatment with cryo began in the 1960s few people with hemophilia had lived into adulthood. With each development, life expectancy had slowly inched up. In the

1940s, someone with severe hemophilia was expected to live until their mid-teens. After the advent of treatment with fresh frozen plasma, that increased to around twenty years old. When cryo became the main treatment, that jumped to fifty-seven years, close to that of the general population. By the 1970s, with Factor VIII widely available, the median age of death was around sixty.

As the months passed, Dr Tuddenham developed close ties with his patients and their families. Hemophilia care was unique in medicine because of its longevity and the frequency with which patients needed treatment. A year into his new job, Dr Tuddenham invited some of the boys from the center to attend a week-long church youth camp with him and his two sons, who were six and eight. He later linked up with a doctor who ran the hemophilia center in Bangor, North Wales, and they started taking patients on adventure holidays to Snowdonia National Park. Together they ran an annual summer camp. In the shadow of the highest mountain in England and Wales, the doctors would go climbing and kayaking with the boys. They carried doses of Factor VIII with them in a rucksack. If one of his patients had a bleed halfway up the mountain, Dr Tuddenham would inject them so they could continue their hike. It was thrilling to be able to expand the boys' horizons and introduce them to invigorating outdoor pursuits. Gaining in confidence, Dr Tuddenham took half a dozen teenage patients on a challenging climb along the Grand Randonnée 10 in the Pyrenees, which runs along the border between France and Spain. The boys carried their own treatment and injected themselves regularly to prevent mountaineering-induced bleeds. On the cusp of a new decade, patients finally had the chance to grab life and run with it.

In the laboratory back in London in 1979, Dr Tuddenham was having some research success. Along with his colleague Dr Frances Rotblat, also a hematologist, he was close to retrieving a pure sample of the factor VIII protein. In the long term, if researchers could sequence its gene, they could clone it and create a synthetic version of the Factor VIII treatment, which would be safer and cheaper because it wasn't made with human plasma. They worked long hours in the labs above the hemophilia center, sometimes staying through the night sealed off by heavy fire doors, their shoes squeaking against the plastic of the hospital floors. They had blocks of frozen cryo rich in factor VIII, which they thawed in a stainless steel bin, before using chemical reactions called precipitation and chromatography to isolate a sample of the protein. To prevent it from breaking down, they used nerve gas. Extreme caution was advised, given they had enough nerve gas in the lab to kill half the population of Hampstead. Biohazard stickers on the door to the lab warned of the dangers.

After an initial grant from the Medical Research Council, British pharmaceutical company Speywood, which also supplied the hospital with Factor VIII, provided around £300,000 for the research.

'Frances, if this succeeds you are going to be rich and famous,' said Victor Hoffbrand, head of hematology at the Royal Free.

'No,' Dr Rotblat replied. '[Speywood founder] David Heath will be rich, Ted will be famous, and I'll be out of work.'

Dr Tuddenham and his team managed to extract a pure sample of factor VIII using monoclonal antibodies and sent it from the laboratory in Hampstead to an American biotechnology company. Dr Tuddenham popped the cork on a bottle of champagne to celebrate. It took Genentech eighteen months to sequence the genetic code of the factor VIII protein, but it would be another thirteen years before the first-version synthetic treatment, known as recombinant Factor VIII, became available to patients in 1992.

Clair was seventeen when she fell in love for the first time. She was a quiet and diminutive teenager, not least because she was painfully shy, often speaking so quietly that her voice was almost a whisper. People used to cruelly joke that she should, 'Shut up, Clair,' because they struggled to hear her. Sometimes, it was easier not to speak at all. Clair found other ways to express herself through art, using her hands and materials to bring her deepest thoughts into the world.

It was the end of the decade and the 1980s were about to dawn with a heavy rasp of synthesizer and a streak of eyeliner. James Callaghan was in power with a minority Labour government and the Winter of Discontent was drawing in. Shops had recently been forced to ration bread because of panic buying and strikes were about to cause uncollected rubbish to pile up in the streets of London. But those were alien problems to teenage Clair, who was part of the local biker scene in Leamington Spa and spent her weekends clad in leathers, listening to Led Zeppelin.

On November 21, 1978, the sun struggled to break through the clouds all day and the air was cool. Rain peppered with grains of snow fell steadily on the white Regency terraces of Leamington Spa high street. That evening, Clair was going to a local nightclub called Chimes. It was out of character – clubs were for 'straights,' or non-bikers at least – but she was excited, because she was going with a guy she had recently met. After school, she changed into her leather jacket and jeans. She knew the bouncers would look her up and down in judgment before granting her entry – the dress code was 'smart' – but she was determined to be herself. Bryan arrived in the same clothes, leathers and jeans. Three years older than her at twenty, Bryan had a zest for life that made him raucous at times. Part of the same scene as Clair, he was into vintage sports cars and rock music. Inside, with a drink in hand and Rod Stewart's 'Da Ya Think I'm Sexy?' prickling through the speakers. Clair looked at Bryan with his thick brown hair and beard; there was a strange kind of magnetism to him.

From that night, Clair and Bryan were firmly together. They would talk into the small hours, confessing and learning all they could about one another. Bryan told her how he had left school when he was sixteen and was now working in a petrol station. One day, he wanted to run his own station, or a chain of them; she dreamt of going to art school and becoming an artist. Into adulthood, he harbored a lifelong ambition to tour the wild plains of Iceland.

The couple basked in the warm haze of early love, spending long evenings together at the pub drinking lager dashes. When Bryan had the day off, he would drive Clair into the countryside so they could explore the Warwickshire hills. The days were innocent as they got to know one another in the final months of the decade.

But Clair noticed Bryan had an edge to his ambition. He walked with a limp, which he initially brushed off when she asked him about it. As they got to know one another more intimately, Bryan trusted her with the truth. He had severe hemophilia A, a genetic condition which meant his blood couldn't clot properly without medication. As a child, he had gone to a specialist boarding school called Treloar's. But Bryan refused to be defined by the condition and the prejudice that came with having a disability in the 1970s. The last thing he wanted was for people to think of him as a victim. Hemophilia was precisely the reason he was a vintage car fanatic. The risks of riding a motorbike were serious, but behind the wheel of a car, he existed without hemophilia.

As Clair approached the end of her time at school in the summer of 1979, she decided to stay in Leamington Spa and train as an archive conservator rather than doing an art foundation course, so she could begin her life with Bryan. They were young enough to know exactly what they wanted in life. Theirs were modest ambitions – save money, buy a house, move across the country, drive classic cars and have children – but they desired more for their future than the three-day weeks and candlelit evenings of 1970s Britain. They started lining their bank account with savings to go towards their own home.

Clair soon learned exactly what it meant for Bryan to live with hemophilia. Every so often his mood would slowly change and he would become taciturn, the opposite of his usual gregarious self. Bleeds were a game of endurance and he refused to let them strip him of his independence. When the pain became excruciating, he would retreat to the kitchen to get his Factor VIII from the fridge. It looked like the white crumbling powder of a dishwasher tablet and was stored in a box that could just as easily have contained acetaminophen as Factor VIII. For him, it was a mundane household object. Bryan would mix distilled water into the little glass vial that contained the powder, extract the solution through a syringe and inject it into a vein. The bleeding would ease and he could relax. The treatment enabled him to be active and carefree, at least to a degree, but if he overexerted himself he could still trigger a bleed. At other times, they came on spontaneously.

Bryan was used to missing out when he had a bleed, so if Clair wanted to be with him she was going to have to come to terms with sometimes doing the same. But when he was feeling well – which was most of the time – Bryan was outside making the most of life. Clair had one of those profound realizations that come to people in the early stages of love: she was happy to arrange her life around Bryan.

It was a cold afternoon in the late 1970s and Richard Warwick had been at Treloar's for a couple of years. He and his fellow pupils filed into the dining hall for dinner and were met with an uncommon scene. The hall was filled with large wooden refectory tables as always, but as they came through the door there was a member of staff waiting for them. The teacher was selecting certain pupils and directing them to a table away from their peers. Instead of following his normal route, Richard was one of the pupils who was sent in the opposite direction. He did as he was told. Sitting down, he noticed his usual teal-colored plate had a red sticker on it. In fact, all the plates and cutlery on the table were marked with little red dots. The boys sitting around him looked at one another with confusion. They all had hemophilia.

Without explanation, they were given their food separately. The catering staff brought the usual stainless-steel serving dishes to their tables, piled with food as on any other day, but these, too, were marked with red stickers. The next day, the pattern was repeated: the boys with hemophilia were directed to sit on their own table and use the crockery marked with red stickers. Richard was disturbed by the change. Something strange was happening within the school, and he wondered if it had anything to do with the illness some of them had recently had.

2. Outbreak

Ten-year-old Ade Goodyear was hopping with excitement when he returned to Treloar's after the Easter holidays in 1981. He was still in his first year at the school, but the experience had already been transformative. Coming from the grey maritime city of Portsmouth, he was struck by the beautiful green hills around Treloar's, and the views that went on for miles and miles. Ade was an active boy who liked riding his bike, skateboarding and climbing trees. If the winter term had been fun, he was expecting the latter months of the school year to be even better. He wanted to get out on the river and into the grounds with the coming warm weather.

But as soon as Ade put his bag down in his dorm room he noticed a piece of paper on his bed. 'Adrian, report to the medical centre,' it said. There was no signature, just the instruction.

Without saying hello to any of his friends, Ade turned and made his way to sick bay, taking his small, still-packed tartan suitcase with him.

Ade was an inquisitive but sheltered boy who was loving towards his peers and shied away from conflict. Adults always remarked on how precious looking he was, with his strikingly blue oval eyes and mop of dark brown hair. He had been adopted after an early life that was complicated by illness. When he was six months old he was diagnosed with severe hemophilia A, around the same time that his mother developed kidney disease. The former would have been manageable if not for the latter: she didn't have the energy to get herself better while looking after Ade. So the local authority in Portsmouth put him into foster care with Bernard and Margaret Goodyear, who formally adopted him when he was six. Ade became one more fragment of a splintered family, each person making their own individual way in the world. He lost touch with his two half brothers from his mother's first marriage, Gary and Jason, who also had hemophilia A and who went to live with their father.

On his third day at Purbrook Infant School in Portsmouth's outer suburbs, Ade had felt humiliated when the headmaster brought him to the front of the assembly hall and told his fellow pupils he couldn't be harmed in any way because of his hemophilia. Teachers were told not to hit him with a slipper. Children were told not to hurt him. The bullying started that very day and continued throughout his time at Purbrook. When he was nine, a child smacked him on the elbow with an iron bar to see what would happen. Ade's bone shattered. His adoptive dad, Bernard, pulled him out of the school and he never went back.

At the Treloar's sick bay with his tartan suitcase, Ade was ushered into an isolation room and told to wait. There were two beds, but it was otherwise empty. A nurse came in and asked him to sit on the edge of one of the beds for an examination. She pulled down the lower lids of his eyes and nodded grimly. They had a yellow tinge.

'You need to stay in this room for two weeks,' she told him.

Ade began to feel ill; there were aches and exhaustion, then he lost his appetite. His body would convulse intermittently and vomit green bile. He was the sickest he had ever been. For a fortnight he remained in the isolation room, the starkness of its white walls broken only by a single painting of a toy boat. Hours passed as he oscillated between feeling terrible and staring at the small picture of the boat for some kind of solace, some escape. There was no television, just the murmur of a radio to keep him company.

A small moment of respite came when his adoptive mum phoned the school. She was concerned that she hadn't received her usual weekly call home.

'I've gone yellow again,' he told her.

After they ended the call, he wondered why he wasn't at the hospital – that was how dreadful he felt. As he stared at the picture on the wall, he felt frighteningly unwell.

A week into his stay, a new boy joined him. The two of them lay in separate beds, unable to speak. When Ade had recovered, he found out they were two of ten boys who had been taken down by a bout of hepatitis. That word wasn't new to his ten-year-old ears, because Ade had, in fact, had hepatitis twice already.

The first came just a few hours after his inaugural dose of Factor VIII. He was seven and had a bleed in his right ankle. The doctor at St Mary's Hospital, Portsmouth, mixed the white powder with distilled water, drew it into a syringe and injected it into Ade's arm. Ade's skin blistered around the puncture wound and up his arm. He later turned yellow, then started to vomit. Bernard Goodyear recognized hepatitis in his adopted son straight away; he had served in the British Navy, which had a history of outbreaks of the virus. Bernard was furious that his boy could have contracted an infection like that while in hospital.

'What have you done to my son?' he demanded from the doctor. 'Why does he look like that?'

The doctor told Bernard he didn't need to worry. This was a normal reaction to Factor VIII, a treatment so revolutionary it would change Ade's life. Hepatitis was always a risk with blood products, but it didn't outweigh the benefits and the illness would eventually pass. From that day, Bernard was suspicious about the treatment that doctors were giving Ade. He wanted to know what they were injecting his son with. He would ask Ade to recount every word the doctor had said to him. Then he insisted on leaving work to come to every appointment. After one bleed, Bernard took Ade out of hospital early against a doctor's advice. But that was one of his last protective acts, because when Ade was nine Bernard had a heart attack and died unexpectedly. Ade's early months at Treloar's were tainted by grief. Slowly, he started to feel safe and happy there, but when he contracted hepatitis, he didn't have his former protector to act for him.

Ade left isolation at Treloar's after a fortnight, but the hangover from his symptoms continued throughout the term. He couldn't concentrate in lessons and was put on 'lighter learning' for six weeks. All the promise that summer term had to offer went unrealized – and the memory of how unwell he was stayed with him.

Over successive years, Ade himself grew more suspicious of the hemophilia treatment and began to echo his dad, asking his mum if there was something wrong with Factor VIII. But having been a nurse herself, Margaret was certain of one thing: doctors cured people, they didn't harm them.

★

Dr Tony Aronstam had become director of the Treloar's hemophilia center in autumn 1977. He was a burly man with salt-and-pepper hair, a thick grey moustache and eyes that were heavy-lidded but kind. He wore the smart clothes of a 1970s medical professional: a shirt, tie and heavy tweed jacket. Originally from South Africa, he spoke with short, rounded vowels. On the wall of his transfusion room hung a picture of Queen Victoria and Leopold to remind the children that theirs was the royal disease – and they were aligned with some of the great makers of history.

In his role, Dr Aronstam was responsible for the care of fifty-five children with severe hemophilia, including Richard Warwick; Gary Webster; Gary's best friend, Stephen; and, later, Ade Goodyear. From his first days in the vast grounds it was clear to Dr Aronstam that he was going to need to be more than just a doctor to these boys, many of whom were living far from home. With their parents not around to discuss their care on a regular basis, he had to be a blend of doctor and guardian. The work was all-consuming. It required long hours and a kind of emotional investment that was new to Dr Aronstam. Ade and the other children looked up to him as an almost heroic figure: unlike teachers, he never had reason to discipline them and he made their bleeds go away. He was lucky that his own three children were uncomplaining about having to share their father's time with his patients.

Dr Aronstam set about devising a treatment strategy, first poring over the notes of his predecessor, which included information about five and a half thousand bleeds treated at Treloar's over four years – an average of nearly four per day. In the year Dr Aronstam joined, pupils would have nearly one thousand four hundred bleeds and the hemophilia center would administer almost two thousand transfusions of Factor VIII and cryo. As well as reacting quickly when patients had bleeds, he had to assess their joints for damage and make sure their condition wasn't worsening. His wife, Gill, helped him as a research assistant, processing the piles of clinical information that amassed in the hemophilia center.

Dr Aronstam had an open-door policy: children could come and see him whenever they wanted. He attended daily treatment appointments in the center, which had ten beds, a surgery, consulting rooms and physio space. His colleague Dr Mounir Wassef lived in the grounds of Treloar's with his wife, so he could look after children when they had bleeds in the middle of the night. There was a collegiate atmosphere between the staff and pupils, who had a playful rapport. One of the nurses, Annie Kelly, would call the patients her 'Golden Boys,' because cryo had been yellow and sometimes it and Factor VIII would turn them the same color.

Once a week, Dr Aronstam would go to Headmaster Macpherson's office to drink coffee and discuss how the boys with hemophilia were getting on: who was in pain, who hadn't been feeling well. The news would filter down to teachers so they could make adjustments for those who were having a tough time. Dr Aronstam didn't have to answer to Macpherson – he was employed by the National Health Service, not the school, and the headmaster trusted him to give the pupils with hemophilia the best treatment available. Macpherson didn't question the other healthcare professionals working across the needs of children at the school either. He took for granted that everyone was doing their utmost to give the children a bright future.

Dr Aronstam wasn't going to waste the privilege of his position at Treloar's. With dozens of pupils living next door to the hemophilia center, he had the opportunity to improve care not just for his patients, but for many more. Like his predecessors, he started collecting information after every bleed so he could review and update the practices of the hemophilia center according to hard data. He conducted controlled clinical studies to see if there were improvements to be made. Some research was paid for by pharma companies who made Factor VIII, and much of it contributed to scientific papers he wrote. First, there was the question of how to make the most of Factor VIII and its transformative properties. Dr Aronstam followed his peers across the country and started to prescribe the concentrate in a new way: to actually prevent bleeds rather than merely reacting to them. This preventative method, known as prophylaxis, was being promoted by pharmaceutical companies and pioneered by doctors as a way to treat hemophilia. The idea was that by giving patients regular doses of Factor VIII, they might maintain a high enough level of the protein in their blood to stop bleeds altogether.

The young pupils at Treloar's didn't know the intricacies of their treatment, but they noticed it change over time. In Hampshire, at the opposite end of the country to Scarborough, Richard's parents no longer had control over their son's treatment. John and Denise didn't know when Richard had a bleed, or what the doctors at the Treloar's hemophilia center were prescribing him. Even Richard's specialist doctor back home, Dr Layinka Swinburne, lost influence over her young patient's care. In the month before Richard went to Treloar's, Dr Swinburne had written to the school's hemophilia center to ask them to restrict Richard's treatment to one brand of Factor VIII, Kryobulin, which was made by the Austrian company Immuno in Europe. He could be allergic to others, she said, like he had been to cryo. Dr Peter Kirk, who worked alongside Dr Aronstam, replied that he would ensure Richard's treatment would remain the same at the school.

In the first weeks following his traumatic arrival at Treloar's in 1976, Richard had had multiple bleeds in his left knee and right elbow. He had gone to the hemophilia center on September 27, then again on consecutive days in October. Each time, he was given Kryobulin. But then on October 12, after a bleed in his left knee, Richard was given Hemofil, which was made in America by Baxter Hyland. For the next year, almost every time Richard went to the hemophilia center with a bleed, he was treated with Kryobulin. Most of his bleeds were in his left knee or right elbow, but occasionally he had them elsewhere: a right-hand finger or left thumb. But the stability in his treatment didn't last. By October 1977 Treloar's doctors were treating him with whatever Factor VIII product they had to hand. They had fifty-five patients with severe hemophilia in their care and they chose to prioritize convenience for their center over the requests of their patients' home doctors. In his first two and a half years at Treloar's, Richard received more than two hundred transfusions of Factor VIII. These included eighty doses of Kryobulin and seventy-three of Lister, which was made by the NHS at Blood Products Laboratory in Elstree, near London. The rest came from America: twenty-four of Factorate by Armour Pharmaceutical, sixteen of Hemofil and fifteen of Koate by Bayer's Cutter Laboratories. Dr Aronstam wrote in Richard's medical notes that his treatment had been so changeable because of the 'difficulties that we experience in supplying' Factor VIII for all the boys.

In the early 1980s, the boys were on a constant hamster wheel of injections. New treatments were being pumped into their veins and blood was taken to be tested. Dr Aronstam and his colleagues took samples from the pupils once a month, sometimes every fortnight. The children would stretch out their arms for the test without knowing what it was for. When they were having prophylactic treatment, they could be given Factor VIII every day. They would have breakfast, then go to the hemophilia center, where the treatment would be laid out for them to inject themselves with. Richard went through multiple phases of having prophylaxis at Treloar's, receiving Factor VIII every other day for more than a month. He didn't understand why he was having to inject himself day after day – and no one explained it to him.

Gary's friend Stephen, along with a handful of the older boys at Treloar's, asked medical staff why they were being given Factor VIII when they hadn't had a bleed.

'I'm sure they're bloody experimenting on us,' Stephen said to Gary, concerned about the number of injections they were being given.

But Stephen's questions about why the doctors were plying them with so much treatment fell on deaf ears. Doctors Aronstam and Wassef were in charge and they didn't feel the need to explain every decision to their young patients. As doctors, they had the authority, and they expected the boys to defer to them.

As he moved through the lower school at Treloar's into the upper school, Gary noticed that his medical program was changing, and he wasn't happy about it. He began having prophylaxis to prevent bleeds during physio to loosen his joints. Gary only had bleeds once or twice a month, but to stop him from causing further damage in physio, doctors told him to inject himself beforehand. In 1981 he was prescribed Factor VIII three times a week – Monday, Wednesday, Friday – to cover him during a weekly fitness class at the Alton Sports Centre. Even though he had grown up with hemophilia, Gary hated sticking needles into himself. He didn't understand why he needed to have so many injections of Factor VIII when he wasn't bleeding much anyway. He protested more strongly: 'Can I go to the gym without Factor VIII?' With that, his stint of prophylaxis came to an end.

A more pressing piece of research for Dr Aronstam concerned the side effects of Factor VIII. Ade's bout of hepatitis in 1981 had come as no surprise to him; there had already been multiple outbreaks of the virus at the school, each one bringing with it concern from pupils, parents and staff. Dr Aronstam could see details of previous outbreaks in the notes he had inherited from Dr Kirk. And the pupils were all aware – in their 'home training guide,' Dr Aronstam instructed them to dispose of the needle, syringe and other equipment they had used by putting them into a sharps bin, the front of which was marked 'hepatitis risk.'

Hepatitis is an inflammation of the liver, which can arise as the result of infection by a number of different viruses or by damage through drinking excess alcohol. Symptoms can include a high temperature, sickness, body aches and jaundice. Today we know of five viruses that cause hepatitis – A, B, C, D and E – but in the early 1980s only three had been identified: hepatitis A, B and D. Doctors were aware of other strains of the virus, which they called non-A, non-B hepatitis. They knew hepatitis B could be transmitted through blood and, given Factor VIII was made with human plasma, it was an inevitable risk. Many of those in hemophilia care believed hepatitis was a relatively mild, short-lived condition that was unavoidable when treating patients with blood products. After all, there was always a chance of donors having viruses. Compared to the revolutionary upsides of Factor VIII, it was deemed an acceptable risk.

With the first outbreak of hepatitis at Treloar's in the mid-1970s, Macpherson realized there was a need to address the entire school. The head told the children there was an illness going around. He said there were two types of hepatitis: one that can be fatal and another less severe strain. Those infected at Treloar's had the second type – hepatitis that wasn't fatal. They shouldn't be worried.

Dr John Craske, a virologist at Withington Hospital in Manchester and director of the Public Health Laboratory Service, was charged with monitoring national outbreaks of viruses like hepatitis. He asked Dr Aronstam if he would help find out how much of a hepatitis risk there was in different brands of Factor VIII, and the long-term effects of the virus on patients. Dr Aronstam had dozens of pupils under his care whom he could monitor every day, and his predecessor had helped with similar research, so he agreed to help. But there was one part of Dr Craske's research that Dr Aronstam didn't want to be involved in. Dr Craske suggested that next time some of Dr Aronstam's milder hemophiliacs came to the center for a non-urgent procedure like a tooth removal, he could treat them with Factor VIII rather than cryo to see if they developed hepatitis.

'We have found from observations at Oxford that this is the best way of finding out whether the material is associated with cases of hepatitis,' Dr Craske wrote to him. 'It would provide valuable information if you could use some of the material issued in the way I have suggested.'

Dr Aronstam wasn't at all comfortable with the idea of intentionally giving his patients a more risky product for the purpose of this research. He didn't like to see the young boys becoming jaundiced and unwell with a disease more commonly seen in adults. Instead, he would continue treating those patients with cryo, which was less likely to contain hepatitis because it was made with plasma from one donor. He wrote back to Dr Craske with a firm rejection. 'As far as your suggestion about transfusing mild haemophiliacs with this material is concerned, I totally disagree with this concept,' he said. 'I do not wish any of my mild haemophiliacs to develop hepatitis in any form.'

But for his patients with severe hemophilia, Dr Aronstam was less cautious. He believed sticking to cryo wasn't an option for them: the higher concentration offered by Factor VIII would help them have more normal childhoods, and with so many boys to look after, it was far easier to have them inject themselves with Factor VIII than to spend hours defrosting and infusing cryo for every bleed. As head of the hemophilia center, Dr Aronstam made this decision on behalf of his patients without consulting them or their parents.

Dr Aronstam kept his concerns to himself, but hepatitis continued to niggle at him. In 1978 he wrote to one patient's home doctor and said, 'I am increasingly wary of the indiscriminate use of blood products in our boys.' Most of his patients had signs of liver inflammation, indicative of chronic hepatitis, which 'several authorities have recently reported increased incidences of.' But he still believed prophylaxis would help the boys have a better quality of life, so he kept up with his treatment program regardless. For his hemophilia center to remain one of the leading facilities for care in the UK, he would have to keep innovating.

In the background, Dr Aronstam followed the latest research on hepatitis and Factor VIII. After hearing about a new version of the treatment in Germany that had been heated to kill hepatitis, he started to experiment with his own ways of making Factor VIII safer. He would take the bottles and heat them up in a bath of warm water, their labels peeling off, to try to kill the virus.

'Don't worry, boys, we're going to warm it up,' he would say. 'There will be no more yellow.'

Ade's friends at Treloar's taught him a dictionary's worth of new words. There were the swear words that came via his peers, which he would look up in an actual dictionary in the library at break time. Then there were sophisticated adult words connected to hemophilia that he found impossible to spell. One of these was 'paraphernalia.' He liked how it sounded. Paraphernalia was the name for the stash of goods in the hemophilia center that the pupils would scramble for. There were notebooks, stationery kits, towels and rucksacks in boxes next to the fridges containing Factor VIII. All the items were branded with the logo or name of an American pharmaceutical company. Familiar names, because they were also on the vials of the medicine the boys would inject themselves with.

The hemophilia nurses would use these pharma wares as gifts for the children: if they were well behaved and reported their bleeds to the center in good time, they would be rewarded with a branded product. Children went to lessons with backpacks emblazoned with ALPHA and pulled out pencil cases that contained stationery from ARMOUR. Ade once looked down at his pencil case and noticed every pen inside it had the name of a pharma company on it. Elsewhere in the country, Armour teamed up with another brand that was popular with children: Mr Men. Some of the more exciting items included kites, a bat and ball, and a Beanie Baby with BAXTER written across its chest. The Treloar's pupils became competitive about who got what. The ultimate prize was a chronograph watch.

Ade coveted the watch, with its deep navy-blue sheen and brown leather strap. The rim around the face was bronze and it had silver stopwatch dials. It was heavy for a young boy – Ade wouldn't have been able to wear it after a bleed. And he would never consider wearing it on his wrist outside in Portsmouth; it was too precious. But he wanted one nevertheless. It would be his prized possession, kept safely in its soft leather box with velvet lining. The watch face was inscribed BAXTER. There were nine of them on offer and Ade went into battle against his dorm-mate Ray to get one. He tried sweet-talking one of the nurses: he would be forever grateful if he could have a watch, he said. Ade won the competition and got the first watch. When Ray saw it on Ade's wrist at homework club later that day, he looked so crestfallen that Ade immediately felt guilty. Ray wasn't a fighter at heart, so Ade decided that he would have to secure a watch for his friend.

'Is Ray going to get one, too?' he asked the nurse when he next saw her.

'Don't worry, Ade,' she replied, promising to sort it out.

The next day, Ray had his own watch.

Britain was teetering on the edge of depression at the beginning of summer in 1981. Inflation was climbing as unemployment approached three million people, or 10 percent of the workforce. Bobby Sands had become the first hunger striker to die as violence ripped through Northern Ireland. London was threatening to erupt as well, with tensions between the police and West Indian communities heating up in

Brixton. In that very British way, Prime Minister Margaret Thatcher and her government were pinning their hopes on a big event to mask the growing unrest – the royal wedding between Prince Charles and Lady Diana Spencer.

But Treloar's had its own problem to contend with: more sickness. Almost immediately after Ade and nine other boys had recovered from hepatitis, around a dozen pupils contracted an infection that looked like an illness common in teenagers, glandular fever. Richard was fifteen and had never been in a relationship, but he was struck down with the classic symptoms of the 'kissing disease' over the summer holidays, when he was back in Scarborough. He had a painful throat, swollen lymph nodes and a temperature.

The year had been difficult for Richard. In the Easter holidays, he had been drifting off to sleep when his parents came into his bedroom to say goodnight. He suddenly felt dizzy, then his body locked up and he started to tremble. John and Denise panicked as they watched their son lie rigid and convulsing. A few minutes later, he fell into a deep sleep. When he woke up, he had no memory of having had a fit.

Speaking to a neurologist at Leeds Hospital a week later, Richard recounted a few incidents from the past six months when his parents and the staff at Treloar's had told him he had behaved in a strange way during his sleep. One evening, the night sister at Treloar's woke him up with a torch soon after he had fallen asleep and said, 'You shocked me.' The neurologist concluded that Richard had developed a mild form of nocturnal epilepsy, of which there was no family history. He was prescribed phenytoin to prevent seizures.

At the end of July, his doctor tested him for the Epstein-Barr virus that causes glandular fever. When the result came back, it only added to the unsolved puzzle that was his health.

'Paul-Bunnell Negative,' wrote Richard's doctor, citing the name of the test. 'Looks very like glandular fever to me despite the negative PB. This is clinically recognized.'

Despite the certainty of Richard's notes, his doctor was perplexed. He also had oral thrush and was having difficulty swallowing. A week later, at the beginning of August, the doctor tested Richard for glandular fever a second time. Again, the test came back negative. His doctor ignored the result and recorded a diagnosis regardless: 'Looks like glandular fever to me.'

Like many children, the boys at Treloar's were always coming down with various bugs. They weren't preoccupied by them, even if they were different from the customary coughs and colds that most children suffered from. In addition to hepatitis and glandular fever, they had shingles, cold sores, oral thrush, warts and parvovirus.

Back in the summer term of 1978 a group of boys had all come down with the symptoms of glandular fever at the same time. Among them was Gary Webster, who was laid up in sick bay for a fortnight. One day, while he was still feeling under the weather, a member of staff dragged him out of bed for the school photo. He hid himself in the middle of the back row, masking all but his head behind his peers. Everyone else was in school uniform, emerald green ties embossed with LMTC and navy jackets, while he was in the uniform of a sick child, a tracksuit. Years later this photo – showing rows of children beaming into the camera – would become unbearably poignant, marking the moment before everything turned.

Joe lived to the extreme – and then some. Raised in a small town in Warwickshire, Joe was always on two wheels from a young age despite his hemophilia. First bicycles, then scooters. He had a small frame, but was fiercely independent, forever defying his parents' attempts to coddle him as an only child. When a teacher suggested he wear a rugby helmet at school he said, 'No way.' And when someone at Birmingham Children's Hospital said he should go to Treloar's for secondary school, he refused. He started to plan how he would escape if his parents did force him to go. But thankfully they decided the local comprehensive would work just fine for their son.

Joe was one of the few children with hemophilia of his generation whose parents had treated him with cryo at home, giving him a freer life. They would collect bags of cryo from the hospital in a polystyrene box and transfuse it into Joe's arm. When they went on holiday to Benidorm, the cryo went with them. As the family disembarked from the plane, there was a photographer waiting to take their picture and sell it to them – a common hustle of the time. Next to Joe and his parents was the bright orange coolbox that contained his treatment. Throughout the trip, the cryo lived in their hotel's freezer, beside the ice cream. Joe was always disconcerted by how changeable the color of the cryo was: sometimes clear, at other times bright orange, like the coolbox. So Factor VIII came as a revelation. It was far less cumbersome and Joe was relieved to have a treatment that no longer took his breath away with the cold.

Joe wanted to join the army's tank regiment when he turned sixteen. In the face of his career's adviser saying he wouldn't be accepted, he tried to sign up anyway, but the service rejected him. He watched with envy as friends went to fight in the Falklands War, while he got a mundane job in the agricultural engineering factory where his father worked.

Pushing on, Joe found the 1980s subculture that ended up forming his identity. He combined Levi 501s with button-down shirts, bought a Vesper 50 and became a mod. On more than one occasion, he had to have his jeans cut off because a bleed in his right knee caused it to swell, but that didn't deter him. He would tear down the West Midlands country roads on his scooter, hang out with friends and talk to girls. In December 1981 he met a girl called Frankie. Fifteen to his seventeen, she agreed to go out with him.

Frankie had grown up on a council estate in a market town in Warwickshire. She was the second youngest of five children, and the only girl. She and her four brothers were troublemakers; if they hadn't grown up in such a small town, where there was only so much opportunity for trouble, she believes they could have easily ended up in jail. But she always balked at her dad's description of the working class as 'cannon fodder.' Her parents worked hard – her father on the assembly line making car parts and her mother as a capstan-lathe operator in a factory – so Frankie's brothers were often left to look after her. On days when they weren't in school, they would play outside from dawn until nightfall, coming home only for a quick sandwich filled with sugar or tomato ketchup. When her dad was home, he was known to turn the electricity off at the mains if her brother played 'My Way' by the Sex Pistols because he couldn't bear to hear Frank

Sinatra bastardized. From the age of thirteen, Frankie had caught the twopenny bus to Coventry to watch The Specials performing at a local club. She had a lot of freedom, which meant she matured before her time.

Frankie dressed androgynously in washed-out jeans, and never wore makeup. She would model at the hairdressers for free cuts, which meant she always had one of the latest alternative styles. When she met Joe, she had a short blonde mullet. Later, a red-and-black side bob. They bonded over their shared love of mod music: two-tone and northern soul. Both equally outgoing, they fell for one another fast.

Frankie and Joe were children of the 1980s, fueled by a spirit of aspiration. Thatcher had swept into power with a promise to lift Britain out of recession, telling the public they could be whatever they wanted to be, as long as they remained steadfast and worked hard. 'I came to office with one deliberate intent: to change Britain from a dependent to a self-reliant society, from a give-it-to-me to a do-it-yourself nation,' she said. With that ethos, Frankie and Joe started hitting their goals almost as soon as they got together. After just a year, when Frankie was sixteen, she asked Joe to marry her. He said yes and she bought herself an engagement ring – gold with a tiny diamond – with a Provident check from her mum.

The young couple wanted to leave their working-class roots behind, making plans to buy a house and get married as soon as Frankie turned eighteen. Her dad couldn't understand where her drive had come from – he thought there was nothing wrong with their council estate and working-class life – but she was determined to own her future, and Joe was her route out. When she told her dad they were engaged, he didn't speak to her for six months. She was his only daughter and he believed she was making a terrible mistake by making such a commitment. Joe's parents were wary about them getting married, too, knowing what a burden hemophilia could be.

Soon after their engagement, Frankie and Joe bought their first house for £16,500. They were both working in factories and got a 100 percent mortgage. Frankie was still sixteen and she chose a burgundy color for the bathroom. They also bought a Lambretta scooter with a sidecar for their dog, and a pair of goggles for it to wear. They rode up to Skegness and down to Yarmouth on the Isle of Wight to attend rallies with thousands of other people.

For their wedding, Frankie bought a second hand dress. Her mum picked up an extra pot-washing job to cover the £500 cost of the church and party, while her friend's father was busy making brides-maids' dresses.

But there was a hitch in their well-made plan. A few months before their big day, Joe came down with a fever. He felt worse than hemophilia had ever made him feel. Frankie was surprised to see her usu-ally energetic partner taken out by something as innocuous as a throat infection. The village doctor came to see him and diagnosed glandu-lar fever. But the doctor also advised Joe's parents to take him to the hemophilia center; the virus could be connected to something out-side their experience.

'You need to read about what's happening in America,' the doctor said. Those words weren't revealing in themselves, but the tone made it feel like they were holding something back.

It would be another year before Joe understood what his doctor had meant with that veiled reference to America. Happily, before that happened, he recovered in time to marry Frankie.

Every year, Treloar's ran an exchange program with a group of chil-dren with disabilities from a Canadian school. When Gary went to Canada on the exchange, he spent a fortnight staying in hospitals and schools, traveling through the Rocky Mountains to Calgary and Edmonton, as well as completing his Duke of Edinburgh Award.

Ade's family couldn't afford for him to go on the trip to Canada, but he loved it when the exchange students came to England. He thought these boys from across the Atlantic were the height of cool. He liked their accents and the red hockey jackets they wore. But by 1983 they were starting to bring ominous news with them, too.

'Have you heard about the AIDS?' one of the boys asked Ade.

That word was new to Ade. He and his classmates brushed the question away at first – most of them hadn't heard about it and weren't particularly interested. But the Canadian boys kept bringing it up.

They wanted Ade and his classmates to know about this new illness. Eventually, there was one terrifying story that penetrated Ade's consciousness.

'My friend at home died of AIDS last week,' said one of the exchange students. 'Something went wrong with his brain.'

A distant fear began to creep into the vernacular of Treloar's. The staff fielded anxious questions from pupils with hemophilia about why they kept falling ill. Could it have something to do with this new disease? The doctors said there was nothing to worry about – just like hepatitis, these illnesses would pass. But one of the nurses succumbed under questioning and disclosed that the reason some of them had become ill with hepatitis was because their treatment came from America, and it was made with the blood of lots of people, some of whom might be ill. Those unidentified diseases had made it into their treatment.

Ade checked his pulse. His heart was still beating normally. He was healthy; he didn't need to worry. But that was the last time he saw the boys from Canada at Treloar's.

3. Do No Harm

Boxing Day had come and gone in the South Wales Valleys in 1982 when Kevin Slater developed a strange set of medical symptoms. Around him, people were relaxing into a post-Christmas stupor, plans for the new year just starting to take shape in the backs of their minds. There was hope the coming January would prove to be milder than the previous year, which had brought sixty centimeters of snowfall in thirty-six hours. Drifts had reached six meters high and the army had been drafted in to dig people out of their homes. Livestock had been decimated and people had queued to buy milk from the backs of lorries. This winter was holding up, so far.

But Kevin was feeling out of sorts. He was twenty years old, with the fair skin of the mining valleys, and he lived in a bungalow in a new town called Cwmbran, which had been built after the Second World War to serve the workers in nearby coalfields. Kevin hadn't gone to work in the mines himself, but instead trained as a precision-tool engineer. Usually an ebullient young man who liked to drink half a pint in the evenings, Kevin had become unnaturally tired, sleeping much longer than usual and lacking energy when he was awake. Ever since Christmas he had been suffering from bad acid reflux and indigestion. Whenever he ate food or bent over, he felt a burning pain through his chest and stomach. Antacid tablets only partially eased the discomfort. He might have written the symptoms off as a side effect of festive overindulgence, but as New Year's Eve passed and 1983 began, they only got worse. His indigestion became so uncomfortable that he developed anorexia, losing a stone in weight. He was already slight for a twenty-year-old, so the drop was noticeable. Kevin tried to maintain his cheery disposition and take the pain in stride, but beneath the surface, his body was beginning to struggle.

On March 14, 1983, Kevin traveled sixteen miles to University Hospital of Wales in Cardiff. The doctor put a stethoscope to his chest, then took his pulse. All normal and clear. The doctor pressed on his stomach, which was tender, and checked his lymph nodes, which were swollen in his groin. Kevin gave a sample of his urine and held his arm out for a blood test. When he opened his mouth wide, the doctor discovered another problem: the inside was carpeted with white spots. They swabbed his throat for further testing.

The initial assessment wasn't encouraging. Kevin listened as the doctor reeled off numerous problems that were ailing him. He had reflux esophagitis, a painful inflammation that causes the contents of the stomach to rise back up into the esophagus. He also had a severe case of oral thrush, or candida, which was giving him a sore, itchy mouth and problems when eating. It was no wonder he had lost weight.

Kevin was told to wait for the results of his tests. He didn't think the problems were connected to his hemophilia, which he treated fairly easily by injecting himself with Factor VIII once a week, so he was at a loss about what could be wrong. But he took the assessment in stride, hoping the hospital would be able to locate the problem. There was no point in worrying until he knew more.

The first sign that something dark was cresting the horizon had come from the US Centers for Disease Control. On July 16, 1982, the CDC announced in its weekly bulletin that three people with hemophilia had been diagnosed with Pneumocystis carinii pneumonia (PCP), a rare and often fatal fungal infection in the lungs. Their symptoms included rapid weight loss, a recurring fever and nausea, among other problems. Two had died and the third was critically ill. Their conditions bore resemblance to a severe immune dysfunction seen in some gay men, which had been puzzling researchers in America and had become known as gay-related immune deficiency, or GRID. It was identified by an ever-expanding array of symptoms, including PCP, Kaposi's sarcoma (a type of skin cancer that manifests as dark spots across the body), other cancers such as non-Hodgkin's lymphoma, and swollen lymph nodes. The symptoms appeared to wax and wane, leading some researchers to think there could be mild and severe forms of GRID.

The three hemophilia patients with PCP had evidence of severe immune dysfunction in their T-cell counts. An important part of the immune system, T-cells are a type of white blood cell that activate when they come into contact with foreign organisms in the body. There are two types of T-cells, known as helper and suppressor cells, or CD4 T lymphocytes and CD8 T lymphocytes. Early research had shown a drop in the number of helper T-cells compared to suppressors in patients who had this perplexing condition. The drop in T-cell count was evident in the three hemophilia cases, which added to a slowly emerging picture that GRID wasn't restricted to gay men. Although the cause was unknown, the CDC said the cases in three patients with hemophilia suggested 'the possible transmission of an agent through blood products.'

Dr Tuddenham kept up to date with medical developments by reading international journals and bulletins. He saw the report from the CDC as soon as it was published, and found it unsettling. Being a doctor, he knew it wouldn't be wise to speculate about the mystery illness before more was known, but he kept an eye on developments.

A couple of months after the CDC report, Dr Tuddenham traveled to Manchester with his Royal Free colleague Dr Kernoff for a meeting with sixty-four other doctors. Dr Kernoff was a reserved man, most often seen in a suit and tie with a laboratory coat over the top, but he had a good sense of humor once he warmed up to people. He and Dr Tuddenham were both part of the UK Hemophilia Centre Directors Organization (UKHCDO), a professional group that met regularly to share data and discuss new treatment policies. Dr Aronstam came from Treloar's and Dr Swinburne from Leeds.

On a warm Monday morning at a university building in Manchester, they mentioned this new syndrome for the first time. It was low on their agenda, following items about how much Factor VIII they were using and hepatitis in hemophilia patients. Dr Craske, the virologist who was leading the hepatitis research, had looked into the CDC report and said there appeared to be a 'remote possibility' that Factor VIII made in America could somehow have caused the illness in three people with hemophilia there. But they shouldn't be overly concerned, there being so few cases. Dr Tuddenham and the others agreed to look out for any signs of PCP in their patients and Dr Craske said he would consider the implications further.

Within a fortnight, on September 24 1982, the CDC deployed a new official name for the disparate threat: acquired immunodeficiency syndrome, or AIDS. That summer, it said, nearly six hundred people in the US had come down with PCP, Kaposi's sarcoma and other opportunistic infections, which occur when a person's immune system is severely weakened. Cases of AIDS in America had doubled every six months since the middle of 1979, when it was first identified. Three-quarters of those affected were gay and bisexual men.

The news from America trickled over to the UK. In January 1983 Dr Tuddenham read a concerning article in the *New England Journal of Medicine*. 'We are becoming aware that treating haemophiliacs with Factor VIII preparations may exact a high cost,' wrote Dr Jane Desforges, the journal's associate editor and a renowned hematologist from Massachusetts. 'The fact that haemophiliacs are at risk for AIDS is becoming clear.' By then, ten people with hemophilia had contracted AIDS in the US and five had died. She had a message for doctors: they 'must now be alert to this risk.'

Dr Desforges had a possible solution. She had found that patients treated with cryo were less likely to have abnormal T-cell readings – the closest thing they had to a test – than those who had received Factor VIII. She speculated this could be because each bag of cryo was made from the blood of one donor compared with the thousands of pooled donations that went into Factor VIII. 'In view of this finding, current modes of treatment must be scrutinized,' she wrote. Dr Desforges admitted that it could be difficult to meet the demand if all patients immediately switched to cryo and that it could hamper home treatment, which had been 'extremely successful and would be given up by physicians and patients only with great reluctance. Yet, it is time to consider doing so, even though we may not have enough evidence to demand such a radical change.' Ultimately, Dr Desforges concluded, the consideration of the risk of AIDS 'may have to take precedence over preventing the complications of hemophilia itself.'

The matter wasn't so clear cut for Dr Tuddenham and his colleagues in the UK, where there had been very few cases of AIDS in the general population. The first British person known to have contracted AIDS had traveled regularly to Florida and died of PCP at the end of 1981. In the summer of 1982 barman and DJ Terrence Higgins had collapsed at gay nightclub Heaven in London and later died from AIDS-related illness, including PCP. He, too, had spent a lot of time in the US. The developing epidemic didn't feel like a British problem.

A few days after Dr Desforges's piece, Christine Doyle wrote in the *Observer* about the 'mystery disease threat' to people with hemophilia. She said there could be an 'impending epidemic' caused by imported American blood products. Pharmaceutical companies had withdrawn two batches of Factor VIII after a donor who contributed to them had later developed AIDS. Doctors in Britain were just waking up to the possibility that hemophilia medication could transmit AIDS, she said, but for most it still felt like a remote possibility. Dr Kernoff told Doyle, 'Assessing the risk is not a straightforward matter: we need much more hard evidence. Factor VIII is a very valuable product and the advantages far outweigh the disadvantages.'

Less than two weeks later, on January 24, 1983, doctors from the UKHCDO met at a London airport with Austrian pharma company Immuno to discuss the issue of viruses in Factor VIII. Dr Kernoff was there on behalf of the Royal Free, along with Dr Aronstam from Treloar's, Dr Craske from the Public Health Laboratory Service and twenty-one others. The meeting began with a presentation from Immuno about the research it had been doing to kill hepatitis in Factor VIII. A representative said it had tried adding chemicals from the food industry, then stored it at different temperatures. Early trials in chimpanzees had been successful, with the animals who received the Factor VIII showing no signs of non-A, non-B hepatitis after six months. Dr Craske, who had been leading a national hepatitis study of nearly four hundred patients, said hepatitis was rife among people with hemophilia, even in those who had only been treated with Factor VIII on a few occasions.

The doctors wanted more information but were divided on how to study it further without a test for non-A, non-B hepatitis. It would be expensive to run animal trials of this new, chemically treated Factor VIII on chimps, so they opted to use patients who hadn't been exposed to hepatitis before. The most obvious 'virgin patients' were recently diagnosed children, but two doctors flagged the ethical problems of using children for trials, especially when they 'may be safer on cryoprecipitate because of the possible toxic side effects of the added chemicals.' Having discussed it among themselves, the doctors settled on starting their next trials on adults who required large and frequent doses of Factor VIII. 'One could then go to children,' noted the minutes.

After lunch, conversation between the Immuno reps and hematologists turned to AIDS. Dr Craske summarized what they knew so far: eight hundred people in the US had been diagnosed with the syndrome and more than three hundred had died, making the mortality rate around 45 percent. The incubation period was anywhere from six months to two years. The mood of the meeting was muted and unworried, with the discussion circling back to how speculative their knowledge of AIDS was. The doctors admitted no one knew exactly what was causing the syndrome. One early suggestion that it spread through poppers, the party drug made from alkyl nitrite that was popular among gay men, had been disproved. Another theory was that it could be the result of an immune system overload from the high numbers of sexually transmitted diseases present in America's gay communities, including gonorrhea, syphilis and hepatitis. One researcher had suggested sperm itself could be toxic if it entered the bloodstream and came into contact with the immune system.

There was mounting evidence that the syndrome could be caused by a blood-borne infection. In a watershed case, a baby in San Francisco had shown signs of AIDS after receiving a blood transfusion from a donor who later died from it. Dr Arthur Ammann, the baby's doctor, was convinced the case proved the link between AIDS and blood – and epidemiologists in America agreed. Dr Ammann suggested people who were at high risk of contracting the disease should be excluded from blood donation.

But there were still people in the medical world who refused to believe AIDS could affect children or pass through blood. One of the skeptics was Dr Peter Jones, director of the hemophilia center in Newcastle upon Tyne and renowned pediatrician who had written a successful book about living with the condition. As an executive member of the World Federation of Hemophilia, Dr Jones had the trust of his peers as he spoke with certainty about AIDS: there would surely be more cases in America if it was in fact spread through blood. It had been around since the late 1970s, after all. 'The recognition of disease in a few haemophiliacs does not necessarily reflect the tip of an iceberg,' Dr Jones later wrote in an unsigned editorial in *The Lancet*. 'The links suggested by the American workers must be regarded as not proven. Whilst careful surveillance must continue, the reported cases do not constitute a strong argument for a change in treatment policy.'

There were other doctors at the meeting who were starting to feel concerned. They had noticed T-cell ratio changes in their patients treated with Factor VIII, while those who were still being treated with cryo were less likely to have the same changes. The group contemplated Dr Desforges's suggestion of moving patients to the lower-risk cryo. But rather than jumping to any conclusions, they decided not to take any action just yet. After all, one of them said, the American companies who made Factor VIII were 'very aware of the problem' and were 'taking some unspecified measures' to screen out gay and bisexual men from donating blood and organs. And what's more, there were still many unknowns. The doctors closed the meeting by discussing the theory that AIDS might not be caused by one infectious agent, but rather a 'barrage of viruses' including hepatitis and cytomegalovirus (CMV).

Back at the Royal Free, Doctors Tuddenham and Kernoff mulled the threat to their patients. They were anxious and highly puzzled about what could be causing AIDS. But America was the epicenter of the new epidemic and Britain was yet to see many cases in the general population. Dr Tuddenham understood that if AIDS was caused by a virus, it was more likely that blood products from the US would contain it. The Royal Free was buying the same commercial Factor VIII that American doctors were using – and he was injecting it into his patients on a daily basis.

For Dr Tuddenham, medicine – and life – came down to risk: the calculation of whether the benefits of something outweighed the potential consequences. We accept a certain level of risk in everything we do. On average, five people die each day in road traffic accidents in the UK, but people still drive. Ten people with hemophilia had fallen ill with AIDS in the US; the number was tiny compared to some twenty thousand Americans with hemophilia. And the cases felt far removed from the reality of Dr Tuddenham's patients in north London. Every day, patients came to the Royal Free with bleeds in their knees, elbows or, very occasionally, brains. They would be in excruciating pain. In rare instances, they would be in serious danger. So Dr Tuddenham reached for whichever Factor VIII he had to hand in the hospital. The treatment posed a potential risk, but with little more than anecdotal research to go on and no test for AIDS, the chosen path was conservative: keep using Factor VIII and monitor patients for signs of AIDS. 'There was a trade-off: improving quality of life and range of activities for patients versus the risk of deadly infections,' says Professor Tuddenham, as he is now titled. 'The balance as we perceived it in the early 1980s was still in favor of using the treatment that would treat and prevent life-threatening bleeds.'

In fact, doctors were under pressure from all sides to make the most of the miracle treatment. Dr Liakat Parapia had become head of the hemophilia center in Bradford in 1982, aged thirty-one. He was a young consultant who wanted to make a name for himself – and the way to do that was to move all his patients from cryo to Factor VIII. He felt compelled to do so by his colleagues at the UKHCDO and those in the Haemophilia Society. Factor VIII was billed as being more efficient and convenient for both doctors and patients. 'If we didn't move to concentrates, we were not considered a modern center,' says Professor Parapia.

★

Professor Tuddenham believes one man set him on his life's path: his mentor, Professor Arthur Bloom, the director of the hemophilia center at University Hospital of Wales in Cardiff. Bloom had a professorial look, with thick square-framed glasses, a horseshoe hairline and a wiry grey moustache. A traditional man, he would habitually wear a shirt and suit jacket, sometimes tweed, and he moved with a quick intensity. To Dr Tuddenham, Bloom was an engaging and dedicated doctor. In Cardiff, he called his patients 'my boys,' to show how much he cared for them. Like so many who worked in hemophilia care, he had a relationship with them that was almost familial. Patients trusted him, and his peers in the hemophilia world revered him. It was on Bloom's shoulders that the decision rested about how to address the developing AIDS question, because he was Britain's leading hemophilia doctor and chair of the UKHCDO. He was a key adviser to the Haemophilia Society and the Department of Health. His response would affect doctors' behavior, government policy and, ultimately, patients' lives.

On March 4, 1983, the CDC released its first trends report on AIDS, naming people with hemophilia as one of the four most at-risk groups for the syndrome, along with homosexual men with multiple sexual partners, intravenous drug users and people from Haiti. 'Blood products or blood appear responsible for AIDS among haemophilia patients who require clotting factor,' said the report. It also mentioned the San Francisco baby who had developed AIDS after receiving a transfusion. Reading the report in Cardiff, Bloom wanted to find out more about the danger AIDS could pose in Britain, so he immediately wrote to Dr Bruce Evatt, director of the Division of Hematology at the CDC, to ask for a full picture of the situation in the US. The two knew each other well and were on first-name terms, having met multiple times at international conferences.

Dr Evatt responded three days later in alarming detail. 'As you can imagine, AIDS is having a major impact on the treatment of haemophiliacs here,' he said. 'The evolution of the epidemic is occurring with a frightening pace.' He ran through the number of cases in America: over 1,150 in total, 40 percent of which had appeared in the past three to four months. There had now been thirteen confirmed cases in people with hemophilia, up from ten at the beginning of the year, with another five 'highly suspected.' Uniquely, people with hemophilia had developed PCP but not Kaposi's sarcoma. The youngest was seven; the oldest sixty-two. In addition, twelve people had developed AIDS after having a blood transfusion, most of whom were based in New York, Los Angeles or San Francisco. 'Locations where we would expect the majority of donors with AIDS to be,' said Dr Evatt. By way of explanation, he added that blood for transfusions tended to be sourced locally.

Dr Evatt went on to explain that eight people with hemophilia had died from AIDS in 1982, making it the second most common cause of death behind the more expected hemorrhage. So far, he said, the rate of cases in people with hemophilia was mirroring the pattern of the overall epidemic, in which cases had doubled every six to nine months since 1979.

Although he didn't put this in his letter, Dr Evatt had personally believed the scientific theory that AIDS was transmitted through an infectious agent that traveled in blood ever since he heard about the first three cases of PCP in people with hemophilia in 1982. He had found it hard to convince American pharmaceutical companies, blood bankers and the US National Hemophilia Foundation to accept his theory based on such a small number of patients. These groups all had vested interests in the problem lying elsewhere: blood bankers didn't want to spend huge amounts of money changing their collections, and companies wanted patients to keep using their Factor VIII. They all wanted more evidence – and they were happy to wait for it.

In talking to Bloom, Dr Evatt had a chance to convey his suspicions – and to warn Britain to take action. He closed with a portentous warning: 'I suspect it is a matter of time before you begin to see cases in the United Kingdom.'

But Bloom didn't want to jump to conclusions, nor cause panic among British doctors and patients. Like those in America, he wanted more proof. He made more inquiries, writing to the pharma companies who made Factor VIII to ask for details about AIDS. One company, Alpha Therapeutics, assured him it was taking precautions to exclude people who could have the syndrome from donating plasma. Speaking about the cases in people with hemophilia, Alpha admitted that 'the evidence suggests – although it does not absolutely prove – that a virus or other disease agent was transmitted to them in Factor VIII.' But it stressed that patients still relied on the treatment both to keep them alive and to sustain 'a relatively normal lifestyle.'

While Bloom was grappling with this information, Kevin Slater came to the hemophilia center with his bewildering array of symptoms: anorexia, weight loss and oral thrush. Kevin had been assessed by one of Bloom's colleagues, who had diagnosed a potential immunological problem. When the results of Kevin's urine, blood and throat swab tests came back from the laboratory on March 17, they contained a worrying possibility: '? AIDS.' But Kevin was none the wiser; Bloom chose not to tell him. He suspected Kevin could be Britain's first hemophilia patient with the disease, but he couldn't be certain.

Bloom contacted Dr Craske and Dr Charles Rizza, director of the Oxford Hemophilia Centre, to ask what they thought the next course of action should be. Together, the three leading hematologists decided to write to their colleagues at the UKHCDO urging them to report any suspected cases of AIDS in their patients to Dr Craske at the Public Health Laboratory Service. 'It is most important that the extent of the problem is quickly identified so that preventative measures can be instituted as soon as possible to minimize numbers of cases occurring in the UK,' they wrote. They outlined the symptoms of AIDS, including a fever lasting for more than a week, swollen lymph nodes, unexplained weight loss, diarrhea, difficulty swallowing and thrush. Abnormal laboratory results, including an altered T-cell ratio, could also be a sign. They attached a form for doctors to complete and return to Dr Craske if they noticed any of these changes in their patients.

Kevin had some of these symptoms, but Bloom was wary of causing unnecessary alarm. If word got out that patients could be at risk of AIDS, they might refuse imported Factor VIII. If that happened, hospitals could face a crisis. Half of the UK's Factor VIII supply came from the US; there simply wasn't enough British Factor VIII. That could lead to a run on the older treatment, cryo. Not wanting to stoke fear, Bloom decided to keep his theory about what was ailing Kevin to himself – until he could be certain. He didn't fill out the form as per his own instructions, or send any information about Kevin's case to Dr Craske.

Towards the end of April 1983, just over a month after Kevin's test results were recorded with '? AIDS,' Bloom traveled to London to address the annual general meeting of the Haemophilia Society. Wanting to allay fears and ensure no one made any rash decisions about Factor VIII, he said he was 'unaware of any definite cases in British haemophiliacs.'

After delivering his mollifying speech, he took questions from the society's members. In this more relaxed conversational setting, Bloom couldn't help but veer off-script.

'We must not overlook the AIDS problems,' he said in response to a question. 'One of my patients may have a mild form of it.' And some other British patients had shown similar changes in test results. But he quickly brought himself back into line. 'Laboratory changes do not mean it is a serious disease. I do not know of any hemophiliac with AIDS in the UK, France or Germany. I do not think we need to get over-concerned about this. At the present time it would be absolutely wrong to curtail treatment.'

After the meeting, the Haemophilia Society sent a copy of Bloom's speech to its members, without his off-script remarks.

With this, Bloom had taken the stance he would maintain over successive months. He wanted patients to believe they didn't need to be scared, and for doctors to continue treating them with imported Factor VIII. They wouldn't have enough treatment to go round if everyone suddenly started demanding NHS-made Factor VIII. The gap could be filled with cryo, but it was less convenient. As chair of the UKHCDO and a senior member of the Haemophilia Society's medical advisory panel, Professor Bloom's word was to be trusted – and he delivered it with conviction.

Back in his office Bloom knew Kevin's symptoms were a sign that AIDS might become a problem in the UK, but he didn't want to let those concerns run away from him. He could very well be correct in his assertion that people with hemophilia would only develop a 'mild' form of the disease that was killing gay men. That was the line he would stick to.

Richard Warwick had been out of Treloar's for nearly a year by late April 1983, having left at sixteen to move back in with his family in Scarborough. Interested in early computers, he taught himself to code and used his spare time to design computer games that he sold on cassette tapes in local shops. One evening, he was in the living room with his parents, watching BBC Two on their rented color television, which was showing a new episode of the science documentary series *Horizon* called 'Killer in the Village.'

The documentary zoomed in on Greenwich Village, New York, where people were coming down with AIDS. American interviewees wore denim jackets, corduroy shirts and moustaches; some of them were painfully thin and spoke from hospital beds; others were still at home, working as artists and musicians. The interviewees described a worrying array of symptoms that were indicative of AIDS: dark spots on their skin, severe diarrhea, a form of tuberculosis that was common in birds but rare in humans, and a type of herpes called CMV. Health professionals had been told to look out for other symptoms, including a persistent fever, night sweats, a dry cough, weight loss of more than 10lb or 4.5kg in under two months, oral thrush and swollen lymph nodes. Across America, said the narrator, researchers were still trying to answer the most basic questions: How is AIDS transmitted? Is there an underlying infection that causes it? Why are gay men disproportionately affected? And, most importantly: Can anything be done to stop its spread?

The outbreak had first been identified in a small office in Georgia that was crowded with piles of paper and boxes of files by Sandy Ford, who worked for the CDC. With a reassuring voice, she told the documentary makers that she was in charge of distributing the best drug to combat a rare type of pneumonia, known as PCP. The drug, pentamidine, was restricted and Sandy had control of the world's supply. In 1981 her phone had started ringing far more than normal. Doctors wanted access to the restricted drug for their patients.

The sharp spike posed a conundrum – the patients had no underlying diagnosis that might have caused this pneumonia, such as leukemia. Sandy and the doctors she spoke to, most of whom were in New York and Los Angeles, started to piece together a pattern: these rare infections were all affecting gay men.

Seventeen-year-old Richard watched as researchers described their efforts to find out what could be causing this new syndrome. In research laboratories and doctors' surgeries, those on the front line had numerous theories that had slowly been ruled out. One prevailed: Could there be an infectious agent passed from person to person in blood and bodily fluids, like the virus that causes hepatitis B? Richard was all too familiar with that virus.

By the time 'Killer in the Village' aired there were three new AIDS cases in America every day, and it was estimated a million people there could have the syndrome by 1989 unless something was done (by the end of the decade the number of reported AIDS cases was approaching 118,000, while the estimated number of HIV infections was well over 700,000). Most cases occurred in high-risk groups: gay men, intravenous drug users and those who worked in the sex trade.

Forty minutes into the documentary, a moment came that made Richard's skin crawl.

'It's gay men and heroin addicts who may unwittingly have created the link to the next group,' the narrator said. 'In 1982 several hemophiliacs died. And others, as yet unaffected, are worried.' They described how some batches of American Factor VIII had been contaminated with AIDS, and how people with hemophilia there were having to decide whether they should give up their revolutionary treatment.

Dr Shelby Dietrich came on-screen with Steve, a patient with hemophilia, who was administering himself with Factor VIII. 'I would expect you've got some questions or feelings about this whole problem?' she said.

'Yeah, it's a little anxiety creating,' said Steve, smiling as he pressed his thumb down on a syringe to infuse. 'So they think it's in the Factor?'

'Well, yes,' said Dr Dietrich, looking down. 'The point is, hemophiliacs absolutely have to be treated for their bleeding problems – and you know that. And I'm sure it raises all kinds of questions, about what do I do now?'

'Whenever any of us hemophiliacs get together it's a topic of conversation that always comes up,' said Steve. 'I think everybody's a little scared – is *this* the infusion that's going to give it to me?' But he hadn't let these concerns dictate his own treatment. 'I'm not ready to give up the benefits of concentrates yet.'

Steve peeled off the tape that was holding the infusion tube to his wrist and pressed down with a cotton pad.

Richard knew those movements like muscle memory – mixing Factor VIII, pulling it into a syringe and injecting it into his veins. In Britain, this was the first he had heard about the risk of AIDS; his hematologist, Dr Swinburne, hadn't mentioned anything of the sort to him. And he hadn't been having the conversations with his peers that Steve described.

The successive details hit Richard one by one. Each batch of Factor VIII made in America contained the plasma of thousands of donors. Donations could be tested for signs of AIDS by checking the donor's ratio of helper and suppressor T-cells, but it would be expensive and time consuming. Gay men could be banned from giving blood.

The final scene showed people in a club, dancing in and out of pools of colored light. 'The British gay community is no longer just watching on the sidelines,' said the narrator. 'AIDS has already arrived in Britain. Do we already have the hidden seeds of an epidemic here?'

The Warwick family turned off the television. Distressed, Richard resolved to ask Dr Swinburne if he could move from one brand of Factor VIII to another: he wanted to stop taking Hemofil, by Baxter, and instead have Factorate, by Armour. Both were made in the US, but the documentary had indicated Armour was taking measures to screen donors. After he made the request, Dr Swinburne wrote to his local doctor in Scarborough.

'This young man, like many other haemophiliacs, was severely upset by the recent [TV] programme on AIDS,' she said. 'After discussions with myself and his parents, he would like to treat himself with Armour Factor VIII instead of Hemofil.' She added that all companies were 'busily engaged in screening out homosexuals, etcetera. In addition, Armour has a policy of collecting only from low hepatitis risk areas, which would correspond to low AIDS areas. I have not made any recommendations to the Warwicks and, in fact, said that I was not aware of any significant differences between the products. No UK cases in haemophiliacs have been reported in spite of millions of units of Factor VIII imported. Nevertheless, in view of their concern, I feel it would be wise to accede to their request.'

Across Britain, the people with hemophilia who had seen 'Killer in the Village' started to have difficult conversations with their doctors. Some asked to return to cryo. Others wanted to stick to Factor VIII manufactured in the UK and Europe. But the majority hadn't seen the documentary. To doctors, AIDS still felt like an American problem; there were just a handful of cases in the UK and neither they nor the Haemophilia Society wanted to spread concern, so they chose not to discuss it in any detail with patients. With little access to more information, patients trusted the experts – and the advice was to continue using Factor VIII.

In Cardiff, Kevin Slater noticed a new health problem. One of his testicles felt tender. Over the course of the afternoon it started to swell and became increasingly sore. As the pain developed, he became hot and flushed. He got antibiotics from the GP and went to bed in the hope he could sleep it off, but it persisted, spreading into his back. After two days, unable to endure it any longer, he got dressed and went to Cardiff hospital, where he was admitted as an emergency patient under Professor Bloom.

On assessment, Bloom found Kevin had epididymo-orchitis, a painful testicular swelling caused by an infection. His other symptoms now included oral thrush, repeat tonsillitis, a low white blood-cell count and a T-cell deficiency. In his notes, Bloom recorded a diagnosis: 'Acquired Immunodeficiency Syndrome new.'

Bloom couldn't keep his suspicions to himself any longer. On April 26, he filled out a form as per his own instructions. It had been three days since he had told the Haemophilia Society there were no

AIDS cases in patients in the UK, and over a month since Kevin had first presented with symptoms. Bloom ticked three of the suspected symptoms for AIDS: malaise, unexplained weight loss and enlarged lymph nodes lasting more than a month. He detailed Kevin's condition over five pages: recurring tonsillitis since 1977; candida in his mouth and throat; a swollen testicle; difficulties in swallowing; evidence of adenovirus, which causes a mild flu-like illness; and a reduced ratio of helper T-cells. Bloom noted that Kevin hadn't visited the US, he was neither gay nor a drug user and he had never had contact with an AIDS patient. But Kevin *had* received various brands of Factor VIII, from both America and Britain. At the bottom of the last page, Bloom added, 'Final clinical diagnosis: Probable acquired immune deficiency syndrome.' This time, he didn't use a question mark. He wrote that he had first suspected the disease in Kevin on March 17, when '? AIDS' was written in his medical notes.

But still Kevin was in the dark about the cause of his health problems. Because even as Bloom's thinking became more concrete, he chose not to inform his patient. He wanted to keep fear under wraps until he could be certain there was a connection between Factor VIII and AIDS.

Sue Douglas landed her job as medical correspondent at the *Mail on Sunday* in a roundabout way. She had studied physiology and biochemistry at university in the 1970s, testing scientific hypotheses on animals in the laboratory. She learned how to catch a rat with one hand, scooping under its front paws and clasping two fingers around its head. After university, she had moved to America to work as a management consultant at Andersen Consulting, the precursor to Accenture. Within a year, Sue realized she had chosen the wrong career and, in a move that took her friends and family by surprise, she pivoted into journalism. She returned to Britain to work at a medical magazine, before moving to South Africa to report on the repressive apartheid regime there.

In Soweto, she was at a riot when she saw a police officer beat up two children.

'We've got to stop this,' she said to her photographer, panic in her voice. 'We should intervene. That guy's going to kill them.'

'No,' replied the photographer. 'We just have to take the pictures and tell the story, so the world knows.'

That difficult moment taught Sue she could change things through her stories, not with her bare hands, by persistently capturing brutal truths in print and on camera. It cemented what she was beginning to understand: this was the career for her.

At twenty-six, Sue had that trait so often celebrated in journalists – she was fearless. With some important stories under her belt as a rookie reporter in South Africa, she returned to London to try to make her mark on the fourth estate. She got her first big break within a year at the *Mail on Sunday*, a new Fleet Street behemoth that had launched in May 1982. The tabloid stood apart from its sister publication, the *Daily Mail*, with its focus on investigative journalism and more centrist politics than the right-wing daily paper. Sue was a natural hire for the role of medical correspondent.

The *Mail on Sunday*'s newsroom was small in those early days, but it was full of invigorating noise and bustle. Reporters would spend their time picking up the phone and calling around sources. News editors would bellow across a dozen heads to an unsuspecting reporter. Frenetic fingers pecked away at typewriters. At the same time every afternoon, the whole building would vibrate as the printing presses started to roll for the daily edition. In the basement, men in shirt-sleeves assembled type onto hot metal machines. Sheets of paper were then squeezed through massive rollers at great speed. Soon after came another rumble as lorries arrived to collect the first edition of tomorrow's paper.

The headlines were a mixture of 1980s innovation – the one pound coin and the first CDs – accounts of turbulent social issues and Thatcher's standing ahead of the 1983 general election; the Iron Lady was hoping to tighten her grip on the nation even as unemployment spiraled out of control. There was one story Sue had been following in the medical press that would soon come to dominate the papers. In early 1983 most British newspaper editors – straight men who thought themselves the guardians of moral standards and family values – had been as yet reluctant to give too much space to AIDS. 'They were against anybody who wasn't like them,' says Sue. But editors would soon realize, with some cynicism, that they could sell papers by whipping up fear over the 'gay plague.'

The tip-off for Sue's first front-page story came in a casual, almost offhand way. It was spring 1983, and she was having a drink with Lorraine Fraser, an old friend and colleague from her days in medical magazines.

'I've got this interesting story, but I can't do anything with it,' said Lorraine, who worked for *General Practitioner* magazine, which was the wrong place to get the attention this story deserved.

Lorraine explained that she had recently been at a drugs conference where a doctor had raised concerns about something happening within his ranks. He was a hematologist in Cardiff, working under Bloom, and was worried about the safety of the blood products they were using.

'Will you take it on?' asked Lorraine.

'Of course,' said Sue.

Lorraine gave Sue the name of the doctor in the hope that she could get the full story out of him. When Sue contacted him, it wasn't clear if he would want to become a whistleblower; all he had done so far was talk to fellow hematologists in private. So Sue told him she was doing some medical research.

'I've got a background in physiology and biochemistry, and I'm really interested in the problems you're potentially facing with contaminated sources of blood,' she said.

The hematologist agreed to speak to her and she traveled to Cardiff, where he had a small office in one of the laboratories in the hospital's hemophilia center. The room was lined with books and had a window looking out over the main building. The doctor gave Sue the impression of being a learned man who was thoughtful and honest – everything she could have asked for both in a medical professional and in a source. He told her he was concerned for patients, but there would be consequences if he were to come forward. Sue earned his trust, speaking as an equal rather than a journalist seeking splashy quotes.

The hematologist told her that viruses had got into the British blood supply and patients had been coming down with hepatitis. Then he shared what he was most worried about: he had heard about two patients in Cardiff and London who had contracted AIDS after being given contaminated blood. At the time, there were only fourteen official cases of AIDS in Britain, but the true number was thought to be closer to a hundred, and there had already been five deaths. Thousands of people with hemophilia in the UK could now be at risk from their treatment.

The doctor put Sue in touch with colleagues at other hospitals who he knew would be willing to corroborate his theory. She spoke to more than half a dozen doctors off the record, and it became clear to her that some people within the medical community had serious misgivings. Yet those at the top had no formal plan to address the situation. Sue believed public attention – albeit a scary prospect for the doctors – was necessary. She spent a fortnight verifying what the first hematologist had told her.

With the story almost ready, she needed to be honest with her original source. She had obtained his trust through false means, by not telling him she was a tabloid journalist. At the end of the line in Cardiff, the doctor was worried. He could lose the confidence of his colleagues and possibly his job.

'It's a really important story,' said Sue. 'I've checked, and everything you said is true.'

He asked Sue not to use his name in the paper and she assured him she would be careful to protect his anonymity. With his consent, she contacted the University Hospital of Wales to ask for a comment on her finding that it was treating a hemophilia patient with AIDS. Bloom refused to confirm or deny the allegation.

Confident that she had nailed down the facts, Sue was ready to go to her editor-in-chief, Stewart Steven. He had resigned from the *Daily Express* after publishing a 'world exclusive' about Adolf Hitler's deputy, Martin Bormann, that turned out to be a hoax. And he had taken responsibility for a false story regarding a fictitious British Leyland slush fund. But he wasn't scared of backing his reporters – and he was 100 percent behind Sue. The story went through the newspaper's machine: it was combed through by subeditors, read by lawyers, placed on the 'splash' at the top of the front page, and given an attention-grabbing headline, 'Hospitals Using Killer Blood.' The piece was ready to go to press.

Sue watched the papers fly out of a chute in the bowels of the building. A man caught them and flung them into a waiting lorry. As the bundles piled up with 'Susan Douglas, medical correspondent' printed on the front, she had one of those rare flashes of clarity: this was a big moment in her career. Almost a year to the day after the *Mail on Sunday* launched, her name was on the front page.

Back in Treloar's at break time the next day, Ade was in the television room in his boardinghouse with his friend Juliet. They poured themselves a glass of squash and picked up a snack. Looking at the room, Ade noticed something out of place. On a small round table there was a discarded newspaper. He was used to seeing coloring books or the fortnightly *Smash Hits* magazine in the boardinghouse, but never newspapers – they were the reserve of the staff room. Children would have to sneak to the local newsagent to access them. At the age of twelve, Ade wasn't interested in newspapers; he wanted to be in a pop band, so he would go straight to *Smash Hits* when he saw it. But this newspaper was in a place that it shouldn't be. Usually so careful to ensure that nothing was left lying around, the staff had clearly missed this one.

Ade picked it up. It was a copy of the *Mail on Sunday* from that weekend, May 1, 1983. Along the top was a banner that said: 'EXCLUSIVE: Virus imported from US.' The headline, written in black, seemed to shout at Ade: 'Hospitals Using Killer Blood.'

'Killer blood,' he repeated. 'Juliet, is that us?'

'Oh no, it can't be you,' said Juliet. 'They wouldn't do that to you.' Then they read the article together:

BLOOD imported by the NHS from America could be threatening the lives of thousands of British people.

A sexually transmitted killer disease, which has struck more than 1,300 Americans, is present in contaminated blood used in transfusions and operations.

Experts revealed exclusively to The Mail on Sunday that two
men in hospital in London and Cardiff are suspected to be suffering
from the disease after routine transfusions for haemophilia.

The alarm rang, marking the end of break time. Ade dropped the
newspaper and went to his next lesson. He later heard that it was a
woman who worked in the cleaning staff who had left the newspaper
on the coffee table. She was never seen again at the school.

At 4 p.m., Ade was with another friend by the kitchen. Dave was
a tall boy from Sheffield and a few years older than Ade. They each
got a slice of fruitcake.

'Have you seen that thing in the newspaper?' said Dave. 'What's it
about? Are we going to get this fucking gay thing?'

In the final weeks of the summer term, the corridors were abuzz
with rumors about the new disease. Between lessons, the pupils with
hemophilia would compare notes on the latest things they had heard.
When they went to see Dr Aronstam they would ask him what was
going on. But they were too young to fully comprehend the dangers.
AIDS was in many ways a distant story for Ade and his classmates, not
a pressing everyday fear. One break time, the threatening epidemic
might be all they could talk about – were they in trouble? – but by
the time lessons came around and they had taken their places in the
art room or science lab, they had moved on. In the next break, they
might be discussing their nascent love lives or plans for the weekend.
They were more preoccupied with the messy and all-consuming
business of growing up. For Ade, that meant making sure he got his
hands on the latest pop releases, as he planned his exit from Treloar's
straight to an arena stage.

The differences between British and American Factor VIII
weren't completely new to the pupils of Treloar's. In the large
industrial fridges in the hemophilia center, Factor VIII bottles were
stored in sections according to their origin. Scottish products were
on the top shelf of one fridge, with those made by the NHS at
Blood Products Laboratory below. Another fridge contained the
imported American Factor VIII.

'This is Scottish, this is best,' Dr Wassef once said to Ade. 'If we can
get some more of this . . .'

Amid the growing disquiet, Ade started to get a sense that the American brands of Factor VIII – the ones named on his chronograph watch and other paraphernalia – might be more of a problem. That was seemingly confirmed one day in 1983 when he was waiting with his friend Simon outside Dr Aronstam's office. The door opened and the doctor came out with two people. Ade noticed their smart suits and cuff links and realized that it must have been their convertible BMW he had seen parked outside. Dr Aronstam was escorting them out of the building, a hand on one of their shoulders. Ade heard their American accents. Then Dr Aronstam said something unexpected: 'Don't come back here selling your shit to me again.' Ade could hear a rare charge of anger in his doctor's voice.

The two men left the hemophilia center and Dr Aronstam turned to Ade and Simon with a sharp look.

'Right, boys, who's next?'

On Tuesday, May 3, Sue Douglas was back in the office and ready to start working on a follow-up story when the editor called her into his office.

Oh shit! she thought.

Steven told her that a doctor had made a formal complaint about her to the Press Council.

Dr Jones, the Newcastle hematologist who had questioned how the San Francisco baby contracted AIDS, had criticized Sue for scaremongering. Her piece was 'neither objective nor accurate,' said Dr Jones:

> As an experienced doctor deeply concerned with the care of patients requiring blood transfusion, and in particular families with haemophilia, I take the gravest possible exception to this approach to reporting about illness. This sensational and highly exaggerated article has, not unnaturally, started a chain reaction involving other newspapers and radio and television, not only in this country, but abroad. As a result, this Haemophilia Centre and others throughout the country have been inundated with calls from worried families.

If Dr Jones was correct, Steven said to Sue, the paper had been grossly irresponsible.

Sue was confident she had done her homework, but she found it difficult to stop doubt from sneaking in. Over the next hour, she answered all the editor's questions about her reporting and how water-tight she believed it to be. All the while, her mind was spinning: Could this spell the end of her career in journalism just as it was getting off the ground?

The stakes were high. Sue's article was starting to generate horror among the public, with concerned readers bombarding the paper with phone calls and letters to ask for more information. Other newspapers and TV channels had picked up the story. If Sue was correct, people could already be infected. If she was wrong, patients could be mistakenly deterred from accessing vital treatments. But amid the backlash, Sue found support in the newsroom. The lawyers were all on her side and Steven said he would back her. She was buoyed by the paper's spirit of togetherness.

In journalism, there is always another enterprising reporter waiting in the wings. Andrew Veitch was Sue's rival at the *Guardian*, and also earning his keep writing about AIDS. Andrew was in his late thirties and had swung into the position of medical correspondent with a front-page story about genital herpes. Where other papers had neglected to cover the developing AIDS crisis in much detail before May 1983 – because of their prejudices around its associations with promiscuity and the gay community – Andrew had convinced editors at the *Guardian* that they should care about what was happening. Back in November 1982 he had written a largely ignored article about the risk to people with hemophilia, saying there was 'major speculation' that it could be 'carried in the blood.' In January 1983 he had said imported Factor VIII could pose a grave threat in the UK. But interest had been slim before Sue's front-page article. While Sue had to wait for the next Sunday to publish another story, Andrew followed up on May 2 with a report that the government was considering a ban on blood products imported from America.

Thousands of people, including babies and haemophiliacs, could be at risk from transfusions contaminated by what is thought to be an

AIDS virus. Some transfusion experts are believed to be recommending that present stocks of American blood products should be scrapped, and replaced by supplies from the Continent. Britain imports most of its Factor VIII, a blood–clotting agent needed by the country's 4,500 haemophiliacs, from the United States.

The next day, Andrew had a front-page story stating how health ministers had been told about the potential dangers of American blood products two years earlier, after a hepatitis outbreak at Treloar's in 1981.

Dr Aronstam was on the front line of the fallout from the media coverage. Some of the younger boys at Treloar's who had seen Sue's article had come to the hemophilia center in tears. Dr Aronstam couldn't sit back and watch the furor play out in the press; he wanted to calm the boys down. So he contacted Andrew at the *Guardian*. The outbreak of illness in 1981 wasn't hepatitis, he said, bending the truth. The Department of Health had made a mistake when it warned about the dangers of imported Factor VIII after those ten boys became ill, and it was more likely that the outbreak of sickness had been caused by a problem with the amount of protein in that batch. As well as falsely denying his patients had been infected with hepatitis, Dr Aronstam made an emotional appeal to Andrew. The stream of news was causing young children at Treloar's distress and the facts needed to be completely clear before half-baked rumors terrified his boys. 'Our patients are hysterical,' said Dr Aronstam. 'Every report brings hemophiliacs crying to us.'

Andrew also spoke to the virologist Dr Craske, who had brusque words of comfort. 'There is no cause for panic,' he said. The next day, the two doctors' words ran in the paper under the headline: 'Warning Against AIDS Panic.' Amid the state of confusion around the growing crisis, each party played for time, wanting more information before they took drastic action.

In the hemophilia center at Treloar's, Dr Aronstam hoped he had dampened the public fire for the time being. But in private, he knew a different story was playing out in the grounds of the school. Earlier that year he had started conducting a new set of tests on the pupils at Treloar's. From January 1983 following the airport meeting with his fellow doctors and Immuno reps, Dr Aronstam had begun monitoring his patients for signs of AIDS. He checked their T-cell counts, assessed their lymph nodes and looked out for weight loss, difficulty swallowing and rashes. By June, fifteen of forty-three patients had a reversed T-cell ratio.

The new word 'AIDS' meant more to some boys at Treloar's than others. Gary Webster wasn't able to push it to the back of his mind in the way Ade could, because he had already had to confront it. Gary was in his final months at Treloar's before leaving school for good in the summer of 1983. He had packed the near future with plans: he would turn eighteen, move in with his friend Stephen and start working as a tailor. One day, in the weeks before Ade found the *Mail on Sunday* with the 'Killer Blood' front page, Gary was called out of his tailoring class to go to the hemophilia center. On the way he met Stephen and they both remarked on how strange it was to be called to the doctor in the middle of the day.

When Gary and Stephen arrived at the hemophilia center, Dr Aronstam was waiting for them along with Dr Wassef and a nurse. The boys sat down and Dr Wassef began.

'I've got something to tell you,' he said, bypassing any small talk. 'There's something in your blood. We're not sure what it is, but it isn't good.'

There was a terrifying pause.

Then Gary and Stephen listened as the doctor told them they had the new deadly disease AIDS. He said they didn't know a lot about the condition and its implications, but he would do everything he could for them.

'What we can say is that it is incurable and we cannot guarantee you will be alive in two to three years,' he said, giving them a minute for the news to sink in. 'Have you got any questions?'

Gary looked at Stephen with disbelief; Stephen gave an incredulous laugh in return. In shock and not knowing how else to react, it was all they could muster. Gary was yet to have his eighteenth birthday. His head was filled with ambitions for his adult life: the gigs he could go to and the clothes he could make. He wanted to seize those opportunities, but they were being snatched away just as they were within reach. He didn't know what he could possibly ask.

Dr Wassef told the boys not to share the information with other students. And with that, he let them go back to class. Gary to tailoring; Stephen to computer studies.

Abdicating responsibility to tell Gary's and Stephen's parents what had occurred under their watch, Doctors Aronstam and Wassef left it to the boys to break the news to them. Gary waited a few weeks until he was at home one weekend on leave. Sitting in the living room with his parents, he steeled himself.

'I've got an infection . . .' he began.

As he spoke, Gary's mum became upset and he paused as she cried through the shock. When she recovered herself, she scolded her eldest son for the delay.

'Why didn't you tell us before?' she said.

His dad stepped in. 'He was waiting for the right time to tell us.'

But the right time for breaking news such as this simply did not exist.

Two days after Sue's article, Professor Bloom answered the phone to a journalist from the *South Wales Argus* who wanted to know about his AIDS patient. Bloom had managed to keep Kevin Slater's name out of the press and he batted this journalist away with a line about confidentiality. Then he sat down to write a letter to the Haemophilia Society. He was determined to nip concerns in the bud:

> Reports from America of AIDS in persons with haemophilia are causing anxiety to members of this Society and to their relatives. . . .
> It is important to consider the facts concerning AIDS and haemophilia. The cause of AIDS is quite unknown and it has not been proven to result from transmission of a specific infective agent in blood products. The number of cases reported in American haemophiliacs is small, and in spite of inaccurate statements in the press, we are unaware of any proven case in our own haemophiliac population. . . . Whilst it would be wrong to be complacent, it would be equally counter-productive to alter our treatment programmes

radically. We should avoid precipitate action and give those experts who are responsible a chance to continually assess the situation.

His advice remained the same: watch and wait.

The society shared Bloom's words in full in a letter to its members three days after Sue's article had been published. Its chairman, Reverend Alan Tanner, said the reports in the press had been 'unduly alarmist' and he wanted to 'reassure members.' They should keep following their doctors' advice and take their treatment.

Throughout that first week of May, Bloom was absorbed by conversations about AIDS. He attended a meeting with the Welsh Office along with people from the Health Authority, the National Blood Transfusion Service and the Communicable Disease Surveillance Centre. To these public health and Welsh government figures, Bloom outlined his patient Kevin's symptoms before addressing misrepresentation in newspapers. Bloom was clear on his position: the press was being sensationalist; the level of risk was low; and 'no established link' between AIDS and blood had been proven.

Bloom and the others at the meeting attempted to answer the looming question: If Factor VIII did give patients AIDS, what could they do about it? The obvious first step was to ban imported Factor VIII from America, the epicenter of the AIDS crisis. But half of Britain's Factor VIII was imported from there. At its full capacity, Britain's Blood Products Laboratory could service only half of their needs. In order to stop using imported Factor VIII, the doctors would have to reduce the number of patients they prescribed it to and halt prophylaxis altogether. Those would be 'far-reaching' consequences. The Haemophilia Society was keen for doctors to expand home treatment, which meant even more Factor VIII would be required, not less. After discussing the pros and cons, they decided it was best to stay the course. There was 'no justification on the basis of facts so far established to ban the importation of Factor VIII,' said the minutes to the meeting.

On 6 May – five days after Sue Douglas's 'Killer Blood' article was published and two days after Bloom told the Haemophilia Society there had been no proven cases in the UK – the weekly roundup from the Communicable Disease Surveillance Centre included a new case: 'Acquired immune deficiency syndrome has been reported in a twenty-year-old man with hemophilia in Cardiff. . . . This is the first report of AIDS in a patient with haemophilia in the UK known to CDSC.'

There was one doctor who pieced all of this together and came to the conclusion that Britain urgently needed to stop using American Factor VIII. Dr Spence Galbraith was the UK's leading epidemiologist, and from the start of his career he had been combative. In the late 1960s, he argued that the NHS needed a national epidemiological center to monitor disease patterns and prevent outbreaks. He lobbied for a decade before the government relented and agreed to open the Communicable Disease Surveillance Centre in north London, with him at the helm as founding director. Dr Galbraith was a modest man, who enjoyed tending to his garden on his days off, but he couldn't sit back and watch this impending crisis unfold without saying something.

When he heard the first case of AIDS in a person with hemophilia had been confirmed in Cardiff, he saw disaster coming. Added to the cases in America and the UK, he knew of three in Spain. The link between them? Factor VIII manufactured in the US. On May 9, Dr Galbraith sent a letter to the Department of Health with a firm recommendation: 'I have reviewed the literature and come to the conclusion that all blood products made from blood donated in the USA after 1978 should be withdrawn from use until the risk of AIDS transmission by these products has been clarified.'

Dr Galbraith didn't make the suggestion lightly; he knew how dependent Britain was on American Factor VIII. Attached to the letter, he included a report summarizing the six reasons why imported US blood products should no longer be used by the NHS. The first was that AIDS was 'probably' caused by a 'transmissible agent' in blood. Dr Galbraith cited Bloom's patient in Cardiff and Sue's 'Killer Blood' article. He acknowledged that, although the number of cases was currently small compared to the thousands of people who had been treated with Factor VIII, that could be because the incubation period for the disease was anything from several months to four years. Many more cases could yet appear. In the US, he added, gay men and intravenous drug users who donated plasma frequently could be incubating the disease without any outward signs.

'The mortality rate of AIDS exceeds 60 per cent one year after diagnosis and is expected to reach 70 per cent,' said Dr Galbraith. 'In conclusion may I say that I am most surprised that the USA manufacturers of the implicated blood products have not informed their customers of this new hazard. I assume no official warning has been received in the United Kingdom?'

Sue wasn't going to let Dr Jones's complaint to the Press Council blunt her pencil. Going silent would have indicated contrition – and other papers were busily writing follow-up pieces. So while the complaint worked its way through the regulator's system, Sue kept reporting. Amid the furor, her first article had opened doors to new sources. She tracked down the family of the hemophilia patient who was suffering from AIDS in London. Gradually, she regained her confidence – she had got it right.

In the week after her first piece, Stewart Steven arranged for her to have an off-the-record dinner with Norman Fowler, the secretary of state for health and social services. They met at Langan's Brasserie in Mayfair, a melting pot for establishment media types. Sue got the impression that Fowler understood the problem, but thought there was little he could do about it. She also spoke to the garrulous health minister, Ken Clarke, who was adamant that there was nothing to worry about. The more people she spoke to, the more she felt like a nuisance – so many powerful people wanted to sweep this under the carpet. It would be vastly expensive to overhaul hemophilia treatment and they didn't believe there was sufficient evidence to take such a drastic step.

In Newcastle, Dr Jones continued his campaign to assuage the fears of the public, going on television in mid-May to deny that there were concerns within the medical profession. Wearing a grey suit and blue tie, he spoke with steadfast assurance:

We have absolutely no doubt at all that the benefits are far greater than the risk, if the risk is actually there. . . . Despite what the newspapers say, there has only been one suspected, not confirmed, case of AIDS in a person with haemophilia in the United Kingdom. This is a very minor infection, if it is an infection. We don't have any proof that it's coming through blood. It's been blown up out of all proportion by the press. [I and my colleagues are] in no doubt whatsoever that everything continues for the moment as at present.

As the pressure from the Press Council increased, Sue worried that her reporting could spell the end for the *Mail on Sunday*. The Haemophilia Society had threatened to sue and a loss could bankrupt them. Eventually, the chairman of the Daily Mail and General Trust, Vere Harmsworth, the third Viscount Rothermere, summoned Sue to his office and spoke in that careful, terribly polite way associated with the British upper classes.

'I hope you've got this story right, young lady,' he said.

She assured him she had.

After a couple of weeks, the *Mail on Sunday* sent a detailed response to Dr Jones's complaint, explaining how researchers believed there was a 'very real threat' from American blood products. Norman Fowler and Ken Clarke 'have both been warned some time ago of this risk,' wrote George Woodhouse, managing editor of the *Mail on Sunday*. 'There is no dispute that it exists,' he added, even though many doctors and politicians were still trying to deny the connection.

The Press Council upheld Dr Jones's complaint, concluding Sue had manufactured an atmosphere of panic and fear, which had put people's lives at risk. The watchdog advised the *Mail on Sunday* to sanction Sue: she should be sacked for incompetence. Steven assured her he would do no such thing and, in a vote of confidence, promoted her to features editor. 'It was about shooting the messenger,' says Sue. A couple of years later Sue was vindicated when the Press Council overturned its decision against her.

In 2023 a man contacted Sue to say he believed her reporting had saved his life. After reading her 'Killer Blood' article, his parents had fought his doctor to stop treating him with Factor VIII.

On May 17, 1983, researchers at the Pasteur Institute in Paris discovered a novel virus in a patient with AIDS. The team, led by professors Luc Montagnier and Françoise Barré-Sinoussi, had found the lymphadenopathy associated virus (LAV) in a sample of a lymph node from a thirty-three-year-old man with symptoms of AIDS. The discovery was momentous, but not conclusive. When they published their results in full on May 20 in the journal *Science*, Professor Montagnier said more research was needed to find out if LAV actually caused AIDS. Until they had that proof, the uncertainty about how AIDS was spreading would continue.

With every passing day, the British newspapers bearing Sue's words of warning became chip paper. But the developing epidemic was finally cutting through. On May 25, 1983, after more than 558 deaths in the US, the *New York Times* ran its first front-page story about AIDS. 'Our findings indicate that AIDS is spread almost entirely through sexual contact, through the sharing of needles by drug abusers and, less commonly, through blood or blood products,' said Dr Edward Brandt, assistant secretary of health and human services in the US government. The battle against AIDS was a 'number one priority.'

4. Missed Warnings

In the weeks before Clair's twenty-first birthday, Bryan asked her to marry him.

'Yes,' she said.

They started making plans for a wedding in the countryside.

Having scrimped for a couple of years, they managed to save £2,000 to cover a deposit for their first home. Setting down roots, they bought a semi-detached house in Leamington Spa for £23,000, with three bedrooms and a garden that stretched for a hundred and twenty feet. They were proud of their first home: it marked the beginning of their lives together. They talked about the children they would fill it with and the memories they would create.

There was no reason for them not to have children. Hemophilia might be a hereditary condition, but it passed from mothers to sons, so there would be no risk of their children being born with the bleeding disorder. True, if they had a daughter, she could be a carrier of the gene and might in turn pass it down to any sons she had. But the days when someone with the condition would not live into adulthood were long gone by the early 1980s. They were still young, brimming with aspiration. Before they had a family, Clair and Bryan wanted to establish their careers. Time was on their side.

On May 21, 1983, Clair and Bryan got married. Clair was slight, with loose wavy hair and a wide smile. Bryan had shoulder-length shaggy hair and a light brown beard. In front of a fast-moving river, fields stretching into the distance behind them, Bryan held Clair by the waist and they both smiled for the camera. They could now seize the future and whatever it might bring together, as a married couple.

The weather grew warmer as the summer holidays approached Treloar's in 1983. Before sending pupils home for the break, Doctors Aronstam and Wassef wrote to their patients' GPs with an update about AIDS at the school. Dr Wassef gave each doctor the results of their patients' 'AIDS related tests' and an assessment of whether they were showing signs of the disease. Dr Aronstam was both frustrated and worried by the 'current hysteria around AIDS,' which he expressed to one doctor whose patient's shoulders and elbows had seized up after they refused treatment. Dr Aronstam said he had tried to reassure the patient there was a 'very small risk numerically' of him contracting the disease. What he hadn't told them, which he shared with the GP, was that the patient had lost weight and had an inverted T-cell ratio that was similar to that seen in people with AIDS.

As Dr Aronstam monitored his patients for AIDS in secret, he became increasingly anxious about what could be coming for them. But when anyone asked him about the threat, he would consistently tell them there were thousands of people with hemophilia in the UK, and only two had the syndrome. He followed the advice of Professor Bloom and chose to keep pupils and their parents in the dark.

A week before Ade was due to go home for the holidays, he went to the hemophilia center for a final injection of Factor VIII: either Hemofil from Baxter or Koate from Bayer, the two main products he was being given at Treloar's around that time. Every year, Ade's family would go on holiday to Worcester, where he would ride his skateboard, hang out with relatives and escape for a couple of weeks. But as the others packed their suitcases and talked excitedly about the fortnight away, Ade couldn't get out of bed. Everything was too loud; their voices rang through the house and around his head. He had a painful ear infection, but the symptoms didn't stop there. He also had a temperature and night sweats, vomiting and diarrhea. His glands swelled up behind his ear and under his armpits. One side hurt so much he couldn't close his arm. Food lost its appeal. Ade's mum took him to the GP, who prescribed antibiotics. But they didn't seem to have any effect. His ear continued to ache, an acute pain that travelled into his jaw. They went back to the GP.

'It's probably glandular fever,' said the doctor.

It was the first time Ade had really heard of that illness. His mum considered canceling the trip to Worcester, but he insisted he could manage the journey. For three hours in the car, he bore the pain.

Once there, he spent two weeks on the sofa. In the final days of the holiday, Ade finally felt well enough to go for a cycle. But he had only just started to enjoy himself when he cut his elbow. It wouldn't stop bleeding. Scared to inject himself with Factor VIII, he went to the garage to look for some superglue. His uncle found him before he did more damage to himself and encouraged him to have his treatment.

All summer Ade was overcome by a malaise that refused to dissipate. He was thirteen and his mum put the symptoms down to growing pains. Ade disagreed; he was properly ill.

When Dr Galbraith's warning letter had arrived on the desk of Dr Ian Field in the Department of Health in May 1983, the government was on an election footing. There was a month to go before Britain went to the polls and the atmosphere in the cabinet was tense. Thatcher was determined to maintain power even though her cutthroat economic program had made her widely unpopular. Unemployment had doubled in the four years since she first took power, with more than three million people out of work by 1983. She had increased taxes to curb inflation, which contributed to the public's overall dissatisfaction. Despite her low approval ratings, there was still hope. She had recently overseen a decisive victory in the Falkland Islands, and the left was divided between Labour and an alliance between the Liberal and Social Democrat parties. But the Conservative Party had to work hard if Thatcher were to be reelected.

Thatcher's focus on the election left her silent on one developing crisis: AIDS. She was reluctant to intervene in what she saw as a problem associated exclusively with the gay community. Having been raised a Christian, she believed in 'family values' and prided herself on having a 'firm moral code.' She wanted no connection with this new illness and the liberal lifestyle that came with it. Later, Norman Fowler, her health secretary, went so far as to say she was 'neurotic about getting too associated' with AIDS. Following Thatcher's lead, AIDS was low on the government's priority list, her cabinet also reluctant to comment on what they thought was a problem connected to sexual mores. To them, it was not the business of government. And so they presided over a string of fatal delays. Scientific experts in the Department of Health discussed forming a working party on AIDS in 1983, but abandoned the idea in favor of ad hoc conversations. The Expert Advisory Group on AIDS was eventually established two years later. And the government didn't launch its AIDS educational campaign until 1986, by which point there had been 370 recorded AIDS deaths in the UK.

Into this hesitant and distracted government came Dr Galbraith's letter. Following Sue's 'Killer Blood' article, the Department of Health had sought advice from Professor Bloom and the Haemophilia Society, both of whom cautioned it not to jump to conclusions about AIDS being transmitted through blood, nor to introduce a ban on US blood products. Such hasty action could leave doctors and patients in the lurch, they said, creating a dangerous situation where bleeds couldn't be treated. Preparing Thatcher for a potential grilling at Prime Minister's Questions on May 4, the Department of Health had decided the 'line to take' was: 'There is as yet no con- clusive proof that AIDS has been transmitted from American blood products. The risk that these products may transmit the disease must be balanced against the obvious risks to hemophiliacs of withdraw- ing a major source of supplies.' The greatest risk was still from bleeds, according to the ministry, and imports of Factor VIII should continue.

On reading Dr Galbraith's letter, civil servants thought he was making a big leap, given the available evidence. Dr Diana Walford was senior principal medical officer and a key government adviser on AIDS, having treated hemophilia patients as a doctor before joining the Department of Health. She could see from the early cases that there was an epidemiological link between AIDS and hemophilia, but she didn't believe there was enough evidence for a draconian ban on American Factor VIII. On her assessment, following Dr Galbraith's advice would have cut the amount of treatment available to patients in half, leading to severe rationing – and they didn't even know if AIDS was caused by a blood-borne agent. But her calculations failed to take into account a reintroduction of cryo and a pause in prophy- lactic treatment. Despite the severity of language used by Dr Galbraith, who was the only epidemiologist to advise the government on AIDS, the letter he sent to Dr Field wasn't shared with any government ministers. Years later, Norman Fowler, Ken Clarke and their junior ministers claimed they had never seen it.

Meanwhile, the American pharmaceutical companies who made Factor VIII lobbied the Department of Health to keep importing their products. Cutter, which was part of Bayer, used the same rhetoric as the doctors, saying sensationalist reporting had led to 'false conclusions' and that it was only 'an assumption that AIDS can be transmitted by certain blood products.' Cutter said, 'It is unclear whether the syndrome contracted by haemophiliacs really is the same as the AIDS syndrome contracted by other high-risk groups.' Armour wrote to hemophilia center directors to say there was 'little evidence' of a link between AIDS and its products. They wanted to make sure the UK continued to buy as much of its Factor VIII as it had in the past.

Word was spreading about the danger as cases of AIDS sprang up in new places. On June 23, 1983, the Council of Europe sent a list of recommendations to member states saying doctors and patients should be warned about the 'health hazards' of Factor VIII. It said countries should avoid using Factor VIII made from pools containing a large number of plasma donations, which is how US companies manufactured it. British civil servants believed there had already been plenty of information about AIDS published in medical journals and reports from the Communicable Disease Surveillance Centre, and they therefore didn't need to tell doctors or patients about the potential dangers of Factor VIII. But patients weren't aware, and as the UK continued to import Factor VIII from America, they were given no choice over which treatment they received.

A few weeks later, on July 13, the Committee on the Safety of Medicines, which had been set up after the thalidomide scandal to advise the UK Licensing Authority on new drugs, decided that Factor VIII did carry a risk of AIDS. However, it also said the chance of people contracting it was small and that it wouldn't be feasible to withdraw American Factor VIII from the NHS. Balancing the risk, it advised staying the course. Joseph Smith, director of the National

Institute for Biological Standards and Control, wrote to Bloom and asked him to keep the recommendations 'confidential, largely because of the commercial implications.' That line would later cause real controversy: Had financial concerns driven the Department of Health in this life-or-death matter?

Concern was growing in pockets of Westminster. Gwyneth Dunwoody, Labour MP for Crewe and Nantwich, asked about AIDS and hemophilia in Parliament for the first time. She wanted to know how many people with hemophilia had died from the disease and what the shortfall would be if the NHS just used British Factor VIII.

As health minister, Clarke was in charge of disseminating the Department of Health's message on AIDS and throughout the summer he repeated a canned response: there was little to be concerned about and treatment should continue.

On June 9, Thatcher won the general election in a landslide victory that gave her a 144-seat majority, an increase of fifty-eight MPs. With her government safely reinstalled, Clarke turned to a task that had been awaiting his reelection: putting his name to a leaflet about AIDS and blood donation. Civil servants had spent weeks going back and forth on the language they should use. In keeping with Thatcher's and Clarke's unwillingness to break the taboo and talk about promiscuous sex, it was decided they would not explicitly mention gay men as being at greater risk. Thatcher later asked Fowler if they really needed to include a line about 'risky sex' in another educational campaign, which she feared could make people 'experiment.' He replied that that part was essential if they were going to warn people about how the virus was spreading. Rather than taking forthright action, the government decided to provide some information in the hope that those who were most at risk would choose not to donate. As a show of goodwill, they offered donors counseling on the question of AIDS, but people who would be receiving blood and blood products weren't offered equivalent support.

There was one passage in the leaflet about how AIDS spread that caused civil servants a great deal of consternation. Dr Walford's initial draft said: 'There is no conclusive proof that AIDS can be transmitted by blood, cryoprecipitate or Factor VIII concentrates. But the assumption is that such transmission may be possible.' The government was unwilling to step away from the narrative given to them by Bloom and big pharma that the risk was yet to be confirmed, which conveniently required less action on their part. So civil servants watered Dr Walford's language down. By the time Clarke signed the leaflet and it went out to the public, the 'assumption is that such transmission may be possible' had been removed.

At the beginning of September, the leaflet was posted to the British public, accompanied by a quote from Clarke in which he repeated the comforting words he and his colleagues had used throughout the summer: 'It has been suggested that AIDS may be transmitted in blood or blood products. There is no conclusive proof that this is so.'

In the middle of June 1983 Kevin's condition worsened. Two illnesses combined to leave him in a terrible state. He had a chest infection as well as a vomiting bug. Once more he got in the car and went to Cardiff. Kevin was still unaware about what was causing his bout of poor health. All he knew was that he felt dreadful. With 'AIDS' written in his medical notes by Bloom, the doctor who assessed him when he got to the hospital knew to test him for PCP, one of the infections associated with the syndrome.

Kevin was now fighting off potential pneumonia, but Bloom decided it was best to downgrade his diagnosis of AIDS from certain to probable. There was no test for AIDS, which meant he could blur the lines depending on who he was talking to. He and Dr Rizza wrote a letter to hemophilia center directors saying, 'So far one possible case has been reported to our organization. This patient [Kevin] conforms to the definition published by the CDC in Atlanta, Georgia, but cannot be described as a definite case. We are not aware of any other definable patients amongst the UK haemophiliac population.'

Bloom and Dr Rizza recommended a new policy that might protect some patients if the fears were true: children and patients with mild hemophilia should be restricted to cryo and NHS Factor VIII. 'Because of the increased risk of transmitting hepatitis by large-pool concentrates, this is in any case the usual practice of many,' the doctors wrote. Another option was Desmopressin (DDAVP), which could increase the concentration of factor VIII in a person's blood. Adult patients and those with severe hemophilia could continue to be treated with imported Factor VIII. But the advice wasn't mandatory: doctors should treat patients in the way that made the most sense for their center.

'We have not laid down hard and fast regulations, since the details of treatment will depend on local circumstances,' said Bloom to a doctor in Scotland. 'I do not think that anyone is complacent about the situation but I think that we all agree that it would be counter-productive to ban the importation of blood products.'

In his hospital, Bloom started using cryo and NHS Factor VIII for minor problems and people with mild hemophilia, as well as children. All other patients were treated with imported Factor VIII, but restricted to one brand 'to reduce donor exposure.'

At Treloar's, Dr Aronstam tried to increase the amount of NHS Factor VIII he used, but he didn't overhaul the pupils' treatment altogether, continuing to give them a mix of imported and home-made alike, regardless of their age. With thousands of bleeds to deal with each year, his priority was well-stocked fridges and ease of treatment. Really, he preferred Baxter and Armour's Factor VIII because they could be administered in a few minutes rather than the twenty it took to prepare the NHS version. The American manufacturers had also been generous in helping the school and funding its research. When Cutter failed to give him a research grant, he prioritized products from other companies; Cutter then sought to redress the shift. In 1983 NHS Factor VIII was the most used product at Treloar's, but Baxter's Hemofil followed closely behind. By 1984, Dr Aronstam was trying to remove the school's dependency on the commercial brands, but still more than half of the Factor VIII prescribed there was imported.

Doctors Tuddenham and Kernoff at the Royal Free received Bloom's message clearly and altered their treatment accordingly. From now on, British Factor VIII would be reserved for younger patients in the hope they wouldn't become infected. Most of the adult patients had been injecting themselves with Factor VIII for a decade, so had potentially already been exposed. Children and those who had received fewer doses, by comparison, were less likely to have contracted viruses. Earlier in the year, after the CDC reported that AIDS spread through blood, Dr Kernoff had written to Armour to say 'profound changes' to imports of Factor VIII may soon be required because of the risk. But rather than refuse Armour's Factor VIII, he teamed up with the company to study 'the relative morbidity associated with exposure to different blood products.' Armour would provide £12,396 for the salary of a laboratory technician who would spend a year helping Dr Kernoff look for immune abnormalities in their patients.

Since each hemophilia center was responsible for buying its own Factor VIII and setting treatment policies, some hospitals continued to use more imported products than others. Suppliers were sometimes able to exert influence through a cozy relationship, funding doctors' research and investing in their centers. In 1981 distributor Inter-Pharma offered St Thomas' Hospital in London kickbacks for buying Bayer and Baxter's Factor VIII. For every 250,000 units the hospital purchased it would get £400. If it ordered four million units, the kickback would be £8,500. (It's not clear how widespread this practice was, or how great was its influence.)

In July 1983 the Haemophilia Society asked Bloom if he would like to update its members on the situation regarding AIDS. Since his last update two months earlier, when he had said he was 'unaware of any proven case in our own haemophiliac population,' he had confirmed Kevin's diagnosis and French researchers had isolated the LAV virus. But Bloom didn't believe the situation had materially changed. He said it wasn't worth sending another message until they knew more.

Around the same time as Bloom doubled down, Kevin's diagnosis was recorded in the Department of Health's epidemiological table, along with thirteen cases of AIDS in England and Wales unrelated to hemophilia.

Bloom's ambivalence persisted over the following months. He continued to use careful, noncommittal language when discussing Kevin's diagnosis and the potential contamination of Factor VIII. Sometimes, he would say Kevin had 'suspected' or 'not confirmed'

AIDS. At other times, it was 'probable.' Privately among his colleagues in Cardiff and in Kevin's medical notes, the diagnosis was definitive. But in public, when Bloom was making statements that would dictate policy in hospitals and government, he was less sure. One thing was clear from Bloom's pronouncements: *if* Kevin did have AIDS, he had only a 'mild' case.

Professor Bloom was at the sharp end of the developing crisis in hemophilia care. He had to look after his patients in Cardiff, keep up to date with the latest news from the US, counsel hemophilia doctors, liaise with the Haemophilia Society and advise the Department of Health. But as he spread the message that there wasn't enough proof to conclude AIDS was transmitted through Factor VIII, he privately believed there could be more cases. From April to June 1983 Bloom knew of at least seven other patients who could develop the syndrome, including Kevin's brother, Paul, who also had hemophilia. He had a suspicion about which batch of Factor VIII Kevin may have contracted AIDS from, and he wrote to other doctors whose patients had been treated with the same batch. In a letter to Dr Aronstam, Bloom warned: 'Although our patient may not be suffering from AIDS, I nevertheless thought you should know.' Dr Aronstam replied to say that his pupil 'exhibits none of the stigmata of AIDS.'

Bloom could still have believed the numbers were small and a ban of imported American Factor VIII wasn't feasible, but there is also a chance that he sensed the rising danger and was trying to hide a much bigger problem he feared was coming down the track. Whatever Bloom's motivation, his equivocations would prove to have fatal consequences.

Dr Tuddenham traveled to Stockholm in the summer of 1983 for the World Federation of Hemophilia's annual conference. These meetings were well attended by doctors from around the world, as well as representatives from pharmaceutical companies. Doctors could learn from one another about the latest research in hemophilia care, and the companies could showcase their new products. International conferences were such a good networking opportunity that the companies would often pay for leading doctors to attend, providing them with lavish hospitality: first-class flights, five-star hotels and expensive meals. On one trip, a company took Dr Tuddenham and his wife to Istanbul. They were treated to a pleasure cruise down the Bosporus and a dinner with fine wine.

But Stockholm would be different for Dr Tuddenham. He was regarded internationally as one of the researchers who had isolated the factor VIII protein back in 1979. His opinion carried real weight, a gravitas he wanted to use to jolt the companies who made Factor VIII into taking notice of the AIDS problem. And he wasn't the only one.

Dr Evatt from the CDC faced a full audience as he told the attendees about the AIDS situation in the US: they now had sixteen cases among people with hemophilia, eight of whom had died. He knew of five confirmed cases abroad. Dr Evatt said there was strong epidemiological evidence that AIDS was passed through an infectious agent in blood, given the groups who had so far been affected and the pattern of transmission between close contacts. His assessment met with a mixed reaction. Some listeners thought he was overplaying the risk; others were already nervous.

For Dr Peter Foster, head of research and development at Scotland's Protein Fractionation Centre, panic set in. That night, he wrote a letter to his colleagues back in Edinburgh to convey his fear: 'The US manufacturers and clinicians are doing their utmost to play down the situation,' he said. 'We may only be seeing the first puffs of smoke from the volcano.'

Dr Tuddenham took a different tack. Rather than cause alarm, he wanted to encourage his colleagues and the pharma companies who made Factor VIII to think about safer treatments. 'We need an alternative to these products that are so dangerous,' he said. He suggested they could revert to cryo. But there were many doctors and hemophilia organizations who believed the 'miracle' benefits of Factor VIII still outweighed its risks. He also mentioned a version of Factor VIII made from pig plasma, which his colleague Dr Kernoff had been researching at the Royal Free alongside Speywood. Perhaps they could use that instead.

'Who is to blame for this deplorable situation, the results of which are being discussed in the seminars on hepatitis and AIDS?' he continued, urging everyone to apply their scientific brains to the problem. 'Frankly, we're all in this together: doctors, patients, national blood centers, commercial fractionators. We must recognize the deficiency and take drastic steps to bring coagulation factor purification into the 1980s.'

He urged pharma companies to step up their research into killing viruses in Factor VIII (a couple of them had developed products that had been heated or chemically cleaned, but they were yet to become widely available). He didn't see this as a long-term solution. 'I do not consider that heating and irradiating blood products to remove things that shouldn't be there in the first place is anything other than a temporary measure of desperation,' he said. Ultimately, he wanted to accelerate the creation of a synthetic treatment that didn't require human plasma at all, a process that was in the works with his isolated sample of the factor VIII protein.

The pharma representatives went very quiet. Most of them were sales staff, as opposed to scientific researchers, and when Dr Tuddenham tried to talk to them after his presentation they didn't give much away. From their offices in America, the companies were earnestly pushing back against the CDC's conclusion that AIDS could be transmitted through their products. They knew there were billions of dollars to be made each year in selling Factor VIII, even if it could be infected with hepatitis and the potential cause of AIDS. But some within their ranks had started to sweat about the idea that they could be infecting customers.

Back at the Royal Free, more of Dr Tuddenham's patients developed troubling symptoms. His colleague Dr Christine Lee documented an array of problems connected to the immune system, including weight loss, septicemia, herpes zoster, rare pneumonia and swelling of the lymph nodes. They suspected – while praying they were wrong – these could all be related to AIDS.

When Ade returned to school for the autumn term in 1983, he didn't experience the usual flutterings of excitement. Instead, he had a cast around his elbow and a persistent earache. He wasn't the only child who had been suffering through the summer holidays. A boy who had joined the school a year earlier had lost a lot of weight. Richard Campbell was a geeky teenager who lived in Burnham House with Ade. He loved making model airplanes and was often seen in his dorm room attentively gluing new parts to the three or four planes he had on the go. Richard had wanted to join the RAF, but realized that with the limitations of hemophilia, he would never be able to see the dream through. Regardless, he had his models. Richard was funny and well liked, but he could also cut a lonesome figure.

Ade thought Richard looked different after the summer. He was pale and gaunt, almost skeletal. Having once had a healthy appetite, he had been turned off his food. Like many children with hemophilia, Richard had suffered from a few sore throats and temperatures in recent months, but nothing out of the ordinary. Now he was withdrawn and unlike himself. A greyish color, with dark circles around his eyes. Noticing Richard looked almost translucent, Ade thought he would mention it.

'Richard, have a look at your eyes,' said Ade, trying to get his friend to talk to him. 'They're a bit dark.'

'Oh, I'm in some trouble,' said Richard, his head lowered. 'I'm not very well.'

'You'll be fine,' said Ade. But he wasn't so sure.

October half-term came and went. When Ade returned to school for the second half of the term, Richard was nowhere to be seen. He never came back to Treloar's. In the run-up to Christmas, there was an announcement in assembly: Richard had passed away.

Ade thought, with the shock of a discovery, *I'll never see him again.* The boy who had come to Treloar's as a hysterical lad had left as a shadow; his model airplanes left behind. But as was the harsh reality at a school for children with life-limiting conditions, the day continued. Teachers taught lessons; children were mischievous.

When the boys went to the hemophilia center, the fear resurfaced. They asked the doctors and nurses probing questions: What happened to Richard? Could it be coming for them, too? The doctors replied that a virus or something similar had got into Richard's Factor VIII. They didn't know much more than that. But the doctors were clear that the boys shouldn't be worried.

Years later, Ade would meet a relative of Richard and have his suspicions confirmed: Richard had been the first pupil at Treloar's to die from AIDS.

On September 6, 1983, as Ade and Richard had returned to school for the new term, a fifty-eight-year-old patient at Bristol Royal Infirmary joined Kevin Slater as the second reported case of AIDS in a British person with hemophilia. Before the month was out, the man had died, becoming the country's first official AIDS death outside of the gay community.

In the *Mail on Sunday*, Sue Douglas reported his death as a 'scandal.' She said his death certificate would list 'renal failure' as the cause, meaning the hospital would avoid an inquest into how he had died. 'Everyone who knows about [him], his doctors as well as the Government's watchdog committee, the Communicable Disease Surveillance Centre, knows that the real cause of his death was that he was given blood infected with AIDS,' wrote Sue. In an editorial that ran alongside her piece, the newspaper said, 'The suppression of the facts of [his] tragic death and the lack of an inquest point towards a conspiracy of silence.' Sue and her editors believed the cover-up went all the way to the top of government.

The article brought another complaint flying down Fleet Street. Dr Jones said the paper had once again reported misconceptions that were 'causing a great deal of suffering' to people with hemophilia. 'Susan Douglas uses her lack of knowledge in an attempt to mount a campaign against the importation of blood,' said Dr Jones, who preferred American commercial Factor VIII to the NHS version because of how easy it was to use. 'Once again there is a misleading headline: "Victim of AIDS because a blood donor was infected." At this time, there is no proof that this particular death was connected with the importation of blood from America.'

A few weeks later, Andrew Veitch reported in the *Guardian* that doctors had confirmed the man had 'almost certainly caught the disease from contaminated supplies of the blood-clotting agent Factor VIII, imported from the US.'

In the Department of Health, Andrew's article was photocopied and shared among politicians and civil servants. One of those who read it scribbled a note next to it asking senior medical officer Dr Walford, 'Is it OK for me to continue to say "there is no conclusive proof that the disease has been transmitted by American blood products"?' On the same piece of paper, Dr Walford replied, 'Yes it is OK.' Dr Walford didn't believe the man's death changed anything. The department had already known about the cases in Bristol and Cardiff. And there was still no scientifically proven connection between AIDS and blood. Dr Walford could see no justification for amending their language. Again, the government decided to carry on waiting for more evidence.

At the end of October, Simon Glenarthur, the junior health minister whose remit covered blood products, received a scathing letter from Clive Jenkins, who headed up the trade union that represented NHS laboratory and technical workers:

> I would like to put on record my disagreement. . . . You say that there is no conclusive evidence that AIDS is transmitted through blood products. I would argue that the evidence is very strong. There are now about twenty American haemophiliacs with AIDS and this figure is likely to underestimate the risk because of the apparently long incubation period. Haemophiliacs in Europe (using US derived products) are contracting AIDS in locations where the disease has not previously existed.

Jenkins then cited a paper the Department of Health itself had written which said there was 'strong circumstantial evidence' that AIDS could be transmitted through blood.

Glenarthur replied, 'It remains the case that there is no underlying conclusive evidence.'

The department wanted to make sure people with haemophilia continued to accept their treatment. It had bought Bloom and the pharmaceutical companies' argument that patients would face a 'greater risk' if they refused Factor VIII.

On November 14, following months of rising fear, Ken Clarke made a statement in Parliament about the risk of contamination in blood products. In a debate in the House of Commons, Edwina Currie, Conservative MP for South Derbyshire, asked him what advice his department had given to hospitals about imported Factor VIII carrying AIDS. Clarke reached for the response prepared earlier: 'There is no conclusive evidence that acquired immune deficiency syndrome is transmitted by blood products,' he said. 'Professional advice has been made available to [hemophilia] centers in relation to the possible risk of AIDS from this material.' Ministers and officials repeated the phrase 'no conclusive proof' for months to come.

In December 1983 the Haemophilia Society accepted Kevin's case of AIDS was 'confirmed' and, in a move that conveyed Professor Bloom's true thinking about the dangers of blood, he told his Cardiff hospital colleagues that 'of course his blood should be treated as infective.' All the while, the majority of patients were oblivious of the risk they faced every time they injected themselves with commercial Factor VIII.

On April 23, 1984, a team of researchers in the US announced a breakthrough. Dr Robert Gallo headed up a research group at the National Institutes of Health in Maryland, where he had discovered the first human retrovirus known as the human T-lymphotropic virus type I, or HTLV-I. Nearly a year had passed since Montagnier and Barré-Sinoussi at the Pasteur Institute had discovered the novel virus LAV, but they had struggled to prove it caused people to develop AIDS. Dr Gallo and his team had now succeeded in identifying an HTLV variant, HTLV-III, as the cause of AIDS. (HTLV-III was renamed the Human Immunodeficiency Virus, or HIV, in 1986.) They had found evidence that a majority of patients with AIDS had antibodies for this retrovirus. HIV gets inside helper T-cells and destroys them while replicating itself, then spreads through the body. Their findings ran in *Science* on May 4 with the conclusion that 'HTLV-III may be the primary cause of AIDS' marking a turning point in the world's understanding of this new killer illness.

With that finding, the British government officially dropped its stance that AIDS couldn't definitively be connected to blood products.

But it didn't alert the public to the change for another eight months. Wrongly believing that 'public interest had waned,' the Department of Health waited until December 1984 to acknowledge publicly that AIDS could definitely be transmitted through blood. In the meantime, doctors continued to treat patients as they had before. 'At what point did we firmly decide as a group that it was time to stop importing?' says Professor Tuddenham. 'We never did take that decision.'

Meanwhile, the number of patients requiring treatment kept growing. One day in 1984, Dr Tuddenham received a telephone call from a woman in Iran whose young son had recently been diagnosed with severe hemophilia. The family had enough money to be able to travel for treatment and she was thinking about moving to London.

'No,' said Dr Tuddenham, almost as a reflex. 'Don't come here. Stay where you are and avoid the treatment we're giving.'

Dr Tuddenham's advice might just have saved the boy's life – he avoided being infected – but there was an uncomfortable cognitive dissonance to Dr Tuddenham's actions, and those of his colleagues across Britain, as they continued to inject patients with imported Factor VIII. 'We had to treat hemophilia and control the immediate life-threatening situation of uncontrolled bleeds,' says Professor Tuddenham. 'We bought Factor VIII from America because that's where they were making it. And we continued slowly infecting more patients.'

Dr Aronstam lived in the countryside near Treloar's with his wife, Gill, their three children and two spaniels. They had a detached family cottage with a large garden and swimming pool. On occasion, he liked to invite some of his hemophilia patients over for an afternoon, to enjoy the sanctuary away from the bustle of the school. In the summer of 1984, Ade had been having a difficult time recovering from the illness of the previous year and several recent debilitating bleeds. His joints were aching and he had to miss a school trip to the New Forest. His school work had suffered and his home life was tense. Three years had elapsed since his dad passed away and his relationship with his adoptive mum had started to deteriorate. Added to that, he was becoming a teenager: hormones were swirling through his veins, along with the regular doses of Factor VIII. His friend Sean was struggling, too, with the recent death of his mum. One weekend, Ade and Sean were staying behind as the other children went home on leave, so Dr Aronstam invited them over to his house for the afternoon. They could drink lemonade and swim in the pool.

That afternoon, Ade met Dr Aronstam's son and swam with his wife; it was good, wholesome fun. As the sun was going down, Ade offered to help clear up, carrying the tray with the empty glasses back to the small kitchen in the summer house. But he stopped before he got that far. Dr Aronstam was standing over the sink, his head bowed, leaning heavily on his hands. He rocked gently back and forth. Ade noticed that his eyes, usually bright and kind, were filled with tears. Underneath were grey circles. Dr Aronstam was clearly in pain; Ade didn't know what to do with their roles reversed.

Sean broke the silence from behind him.

'Doctor A, are you OK?' he said. 'Why are you upset?'

Dr Aronstam sighed, a deep guttural sigh. Then told the boys slightly too much. 'We've fucked up,' he said. 'We've messed up, boys. *I've* messed up. It's all gone wrong.'

Ade and Sean couldn't make out what the doctor meant. Ade stayed quiet.

'Are we going to be OK, Dr A?' asked Sean. 'Are we all right?'

'We'll do our best,' said Dr Aronstam. 'We're going to do our absolute best for you.'

Sean persisted. 'Are we sick?'

Dr Aronstam said something vaguely cryptic about stormy weather and the road ahead. With tears in his eyes, he had one last promise for Ade and Sean. 'I'll be there for you; we'll be there for you.'

But that flash of emotion by the pool was a rare lapse for Dr Aronstam. Back in the hemophilia center, he took the view that although the T-cell changes in some patients were 'a very worrying problem for all of us in haemophilia care, at present the general view is that while the disease is horrific, the numerical risk of it is nevertheless small and should not deflect us from the appropriate treatment.' As such, he continued to prescribe courses of prophylactic treatment and used whichever US-imported brands he had to hand.

In fact, 1984 saw the highest usage of Factor VIII to date at Treloar's because of an increase in prophylaxis, more than half of which was imported.

The memory of that afternoon stayed lodged in Ade's mind. Fear grew from a kernel of doubt about Factor VIII to a hideous worry that something bad could happen to him and his friends. He was just fourteen. Ade tried to get answers from his mum when he went home to Portsmouth: How serious was AIDS? Could he be at risk? Eventually, after becoming unsettled by Ade's questioning, his mum decided to ask the doctors herself. She was at Treloar's to watch Ade sing in the school choir and they stopped by the hemophilia center together.

'I need to stop Adrian worrying,' Margaret said to Dr Wassef.

'There is nothing wrong with Adrian's treatment, Mrs Goodyear,' he said with utter certainty. 'There's nothing you need to be concerned about. I've told Ade but he doesn't listen.'

As his doctor and mum reaffirmed one another, Ade couldn't help but think his doctor was lying. He had an unshakeable feeling that something terrible was on the horizon and he was no longer certain he could trust Dr Wassef. Ade had no idea the doctors had been assessing them for signs of AIDS for nearly two years, nor that Gary and Stephen had already been diagnosed with it, nor that Richard Campbell had died from AIDS-related illness.

A sample of the retrovirus discovered in France, LAV, was making its way from Paris to London. First, it took a train from the Pasteur Institute. Then it boarded a ferry across the English Channel. But a series of delays meant the courier carrying it ran out of time and had to leave it in a locker in Waterloo Station. There, it died.

Professor Montagnier in Paris had been trying to send the sample of the virus to Professor Richard Tedder, head of virology at University College London's Medical School. Tedder had spent the last few years creating an antibody test to detect HTLV-I. When AIDS emerged, he had quickly suspected it was caused by a virus, because of the similarities with hepatitis B. In response, he had made a concerted effort to treat his patients with cryo rather than Factor VIII.

He had also tried to convince the Department of Health of his suspicion at the start of 1983, and asked for its help in researching the cause of AIDS. But the ministry rejected his request and discouraged him from researching the theory that it was spread by a 'transmissible agent.' Tedder had continued his research regardless.

After the virus died in the locker in autumn 1983, Tedder had to wait until February 1984 before he could secure another sample. Once he had it in his laboratory, he managed to create an early antibody test for HTLV-III within seven months. If he had received the first package, Britain 'would have been six months ahead of where we were in September 1984,' Tedder later said. 'It grieves me that we lost six to nine months . . . I still weep about it.' It was just one of many delays, exasperating and mundane, in the fight against AIDS. But with his test now developed, Tedder could transform the UK's understanding of AIDS because doctors could now find out how many of their patients had antibodies for the virus.

Tedder invited hemophilia doctors to submit blood samples from their patients for testing. They dutifully complied without informing their patients, not wanting to alarm them prematurely. Tedder tested two thousand samples from gay men, intravenous drug users and those with hemophilia. His results revealed the true scale of the disaster that was about to hit the British hemophilia community. A third of those who had been treated with Factor VIII tested positive for HTLV-III antibodies. Kevin had, in fact, represented the tip of the iceberg. And Dr Aronstam's tears on that summer afternoon began to feel all the more prescient.

With these concerning results in hand, Professor Bloom brought the hemophilia center directors together on December 10, 1984. By then, there were over six thousand reported cases of AIDS in the US, including fifty-two among people with hemophilia. The UK had 102 cases, with three confirmed in people with hemophilia. Before they had the HTLV-III test, doctors had been able to hedge AIDS diagnoses and downplay the risk of Factor VIII, as Bloom had done with Kevin and Dr Aronstam had done with Gary and Stephen. But now Tedder said it was 'likely' all those people who had tested positive for HTLV-III antibodies were infected and would go on to develop AIDS. There was still debate among the doctors in the room, and researchers internationally, about what a positive test actually meant for patients. Some believed having antibodies for HTLV-III was a good sign, indicating a patient had recovered from the virus. Others thought just a small portion of those who tested positive would go on to develop AIDS. But Professor Tedder and Dr Evatt at the CDC believed HTLV-III was the infectious agent that caused AIDS and all those who had tested positive would go on to develop serious illnesses.

'Haemophiliacs who are positive should be considered a high risk until the situation becomes clearer,' said Bloom.

The doctors discussed what they should tell patients about the early HTLV-III tests. Dr Kernoff suggested that, given the high percentage of people with hemophilia who had been exposed to it, they could give everyone some information without telling them their actual test results. But Bloom wasn't convinced of the benefits of sharing anything until they knew more; it could cause too much distress. He concluded that every hemophilia patient should be tested as soon as possible, but – staggeringly – doctors shouldn't tell them their test results unless they asked.

In that meeting, Bloom finally conceded that 'one has to accept, for the present, that it is difficult to avoid the argument that [Factor VIII] constitutes a risk.' Together with a few colleagues, he created a set of recommendations for hemophilia centers, which listed the available treatments in descending order of safety. Imported American Factor VIII was the most dangerous: 'almost certain to be contaminated.' But even after the test for HTLV-III had become available and over a thousand people with hemophilia tested positive, doctors continued to prescribe imported Factor VIII. They told themselves their patients needed this wonder drug and that severe bleeds were still the most common cause of death. Although Bloom recommended other treatments should take precedence, he said doctors and patients could make up their own minds. The patients themselves, though, were rarely given a choice.

★

In March 1983 the American Food and Drug Administration (FDA) granted a licence to Baxter's Travenol Laboratories for a new version of Factor VIII that had been heated to kill the viruses in it. Throughout that year, the other three companies who made Factor VIII in the US – Alpha, Armour and Bayer – quickly followed suit. By February 1984 they all had licences for a heat-treated version of Factor VIII that was pitched as safer, because the temperature should inactivate viruses.

But the British government was skeptical, about both whether this heat-treated Factor VIII was actually safe against AIDS and how much more expensive it was. In June 1983 the National Blood Transfusion Service wrote to the Department of Health to say there was no evidence the potential agent behind AIDS could be killed with heat, and that this new treatment would cost twice as much as their old one. The Transfusion Service was concerned that if patients and doctors heard about this product and started demanding it, the spiraling price would 'play havoc' with their finances. They paid little attention to the reduced hepatitis risk.

The Department of Health replied that costs would not affect its decision, but the 'potentially major financial consequences' could be used to argue that doctors should wait for clinical trials before adopting it. Again, safety was not discussed.

Dr Mark Winter was director of the hemophilia center at Thanet General Hospital and, like others in his position, he was in charge of buying Factor VIII for his patients. In spring 1984 he decided to take matters into his own hands. Alpha, which had a licence to produce heat-treated Factor VIII in America, had a manufacturing plant in Norfolk. Dr Winter approached Alpha with a few other doctors from hospitals in Sheffield and London.

'We're aware of this licence in the US,' he said. 'Do you think you would be able to get supplies for us?' He knew he could prescribe named patients medicine that was yet to be licensed in the UK.

Alpha said yes, but it would be 50 percent more expensive.

At this point, heat-treated Factor VIII wasn't proven to be safe against AIDS, but Dr Winter was deeply concerned for his patients and wanted to do something to decrease the risk. It was a difficult decision, but he decided it was worth it: heat-treated Factor VIII was unlikely to be *more* dangerous than the version they were currently using. So, in May 1984, Dr Winter became one of the first doctors in the UK to start treating all his patients with heat-treated Factor VIII.

Professor Bloom castigated him, calling the decision 'mad.' Other doctors in the UKHCDO agreed. Without Bloom's support and a national recommendation to use heat-treated Factor VIII, it was difficult to persuade hospitals to spend 50 percent more on it.

Confirmation that Dr Winter had been right came in September, when *The Lancet* published research showing heating Factor VIII to 68°C for several hours substantially reduced the risk of HTLV-III. The virus had a fatty casing around it, which dissolved with heat, thereby deactivating it. Before the end of the year, *The Lancet* published an editorial saying it was 'indefensible' to not switch patients to this new treatment. The advice was followed in the US and Scotland, where doctors were told to stop using unheated Factor VIII.

But in England and Wales, the transition was slower. Health minister Ken Clarke still wasn't satisfied with the evidence. He wanted more expert advice on whether heat treatment was 'a proper protection against AIDS' or if something else would be more effective. Cost was still a consideration. Bloom was equally reticent, taking three months before he came around to the idea that heat-treated Factor VIII was safer. In November 1984 he wrote to the Department of Health to say change might soon be needed: 'It looks very much that we are going to be driven into using heat-treated concentrates. It could give unfavourable publicity if these concentrates are freely available in the USA and, say, Germany, but are not licensed in this country.' In December he said he would move all of his patients to heat-treated Factor VIII, but only when his stocks of the older treatment ran out.

Dr Aronstam switched the Treloar's boys to heat-treated Factor VIII as 1984 drew to a close, eating up the budget of the hemophilia center. But for many boys it was too late. As years passed, Dr Aronstam blamed the government for not giving hemophilia center directors a clear enough lead when it came to heat-treated Factor VIII, which he wished had been introduced months earlier.

At the beginning of 1985 the Department of Health finally recommended all doctors should use heat-treated Factor VIII. But six months later, many hemophilia centers were still prescribing the original, unheated version. The delay was in part caused by confusion. Some doctors questioned whether it was safer to use heat-treated Factor VIII made with dangerous blood from America, or the NHS Factor VIII, which was unheated. Britain's Blood Products Laboratory didn't introduce its own heat-treated Factor VIII until March 1985 and didn't start testing blood donors for HTLV-III until October of that year.

Having himself prevaricated for months, Bloom hypocritically criticized such sluggishness in June 1985, saying it was unjustified and had 'disturbing implications.' But still there were some hospitals in England and Wales that used imported, unheated Factor VIII until late 1985. There was never a mandatory recall of the unheated version from British hospitals.

Potentially lethal Factor VIII was injected into the arms of people with hemophilia for more than two and a half years after the first case of AIDS in a British hemophiliac appeared; eighteen months after HTLV-III was discovered as the cause of the syndrome; and more than a year after heat was found to kill the virus.

In Cwmbran, Kevin's health was deteriorating. He had acute pneumonia and a severe case of herpes. He was plagued by a persistent cough and headaches. There were times when he would vomit and others when he felt shivery. He had been living at home with his mum, who cared for him as his health got worse and worse. It had been a while since he had been able to go out with his friends, because he was so fragile, and he had stopped working long ago. He continued to lose weight, disappearing in front of his family's eyes, while also developing sores on his body and occasionally coughing up blood. Having been back and forth to the hospital many times, he was admitted for the last time in June 1985 with pneumonia. In his medical notes, a doctor wrote that he was as 'weak as a kitten.'

Kevin was put into an isolation ward completely alone. Staff were reluctant to enter his room, so his family had to bring him food.

They were used to him being treated with disdain and a lack of compassion – when people in their small village discovered Kevin had AIDS, they began crossing the street to avoid him. The postman left letters at the end of the drive. In his final days, Kevin had lost so much strength he couldn't even hold a glass of milk. It was down to his family not just to bring him supplies, but also to feed him.

On June 23, 1985, aged twenty-two, Kevin died. The funeral director was scared to enter his room to collect his body because of the risk of contracting AIDS.

When his brother, Paul, heard Kevin had passed away, he wanted to run out of the room; but he was so fragile himself that he could barely walk. By then, Paul had also been diagnosed with HTLV-III and was starting to become ill. He was so frightened about what was going to happen to his body that he cut himself off from those closest to him, splitting up with his partner, the mother of his child. He wanted her to be able to live, even as he died. Paul remained a good father and would see his daughter on weekends. The hardest part was to think of leaving his child behind.

Over the next five years, Paul's weight dropped to four and a half stone. In an attempt to mask his condition, he would wrap bandages around his legs before putting on his trousers and layer himself with multiple jumpers to try to bulk himself out.

On August 4, 1991, Paul passed away, aged thirty-one. His daughter was eleven.

'Paul, Kevin and their parents trusted the medical staff to give them safe medication,' said Lynda Maule, the mother of Paul's daughter. 'Sadly that did not happen.'

5. Lethal Injections

Bryan arrived at Wonford Hospital in Exeter for a routine hemophilia appointment in early March 1985. The morning had been cool and overcast, with the clouds clearing after lunch to reveal an early spring blue sky. He and Clair had moved to Devon after Clair was offered a job as a senior archive conservator there. Seizing the chance for a new beginning, they had sold their first house in Leamington Spa and set themselves up afresh in a Devonshire village. It was an idyllic life, remote compared to the Coventry corridor of their upbringings, with easy access to ruddy countryside.

At the hospital, the doctor asked Bryan if he wouldn't mind doing a blood test. It would only take a couple of minutes. Bryan was used to having needles pierce his skin, but the doctor explained this was a new test that had only been available in British hospitals for a few months, which could identify if someone had the virus that caused AIDS, known as HTLV-III.

Unlike many former Treloar's boys, Bryan hadn't sought to surround himself with other hemophiliacs. He had left the school long before the rumors about Factor VIII and its dangers began. Living in the countryside, neither he nor Clair followed the news closely; the television was one of those trappings of modern life that was superfluous in their new rural setting. As such, Bryan knew little about HTLV-III and didn't have an easy way to get more information beyond asking his doctor. Details were still trickling over from America in early 1985. In the face of scant helpful detail in the press, the British gay community had begun relying on people who traveled to the US to bring back the latest reports about AIDS in medical journals and magazines. The London Gay Switchboard had started operating an AIDS helpline to disseminate information, but in the days before the internet it was much more difficult for the general public to research new diseases and epidemics. What's more, Bryan had been lucky to have avoided sickness from blood-borne viruses to date. He had proudly recounted to Clair how his doctor told him he had been exposed to hepatitis so many times through Factor VIII that he had developed antibodies to the virus. Not knowing much about AIDS, Bryan agreed to do the test. It would be good to be sure he didn't have HTLV-III.

Later that week, when he had a moment to himself, Bryan wrote a note in his diary: 'I had a blood test on the 4th March to see if I am carrying the disease AIDS. I won't know the result till six or eight weeks . . . I hope it's negative. For Clair's sake, if nothing else.'

Six weeks later, Bryan went back to the hospital for the results of the test. This time Clair went with him. Bryan's doctor and a nurse joined them in a consulting room. Not delaying with any pleasant-ries, the consultant began in a neutral tone.

'You've tested positive for HTLV-III,' they said. 'You will go on to develop AIDS.'

There was no cushioning the news or couching it in uncertainty. The consultant told Bryan he most likely had two or three years left to live.

Clair and Bryan sat there as the consultant told them they should use condoms when they had sex. The nurse handed Clair a box of rubber gloves and told her to 'protect herself' by avoiding contact with his blood. How odd, she thought, to have to protect herself from her own husband. Beyond that, there was little further informa-tion they could offer right now. Research was still underway, and there weren't currently any treatments. Having delivered the news, the doctor stood up and said they would leave the young couple alone for a minute. 'There was no counseling, no discussion, no empathy,' says Clair. 'It was, here's a diagnosis, here's the prognosis, bye.' Their future together had suddenly been cut short. And yet the devastating news had been delivered with an air of strange inconse-quentiality. Could it really be true? In shock, they were left to come to terms with Bryan's diagnosis on their own.

As Clair and Bryan left the hospital to return home, they were both quiet. Clair didn't know what to say; Bryan had no words to express what he was feeling. What they didn't know – and wouldn't until decades later – was that Bryan had been tested for HTLV-III without his knowledge nearly a year earlier, in June 1984. The positive result had been written into Bryan's medical records, but no one had told him. Throughout that time, as doctors withheld the truth, Clair had been at risk.

The scale of the AIDS crisis was only just emerging in 1985, but it was clear that it was a deadly disease. Even the word was something to be feared. After the first generation of tests were licensed for use, over four thousand people in Britain tested positive for HTLV-III. At that point, around three hundred and fifty people had died from AIDS-related illness in the UK. With little detailed information to hand, the British public was beginning to panic. And with panic came prejudice. Rumors circulated that the syndrome could be caught from teacups and toilet seats. Before long, people would stop shaking hands. The headlines from both the UK and US were terrifying. Tabloids had branded the growing epidemic the 'gay plague' and were soon running daily stories with sensationalist headlines that encouraged hatred towards anyone with the syndrome. In July, the actor Rock Hudson became one of the first celebrities to announce publicly that he had tested positive. Word spread that the Hollywood heartthrob of the 1950s had been secretly gay. Newspapers obsessed over the story and, as public fear morphed into stigma, Rock Hudson became the subject of a raft of homophobic jokes. After he died, on October 2, 1985, the cruel comments continued.

At their new home in Devon, Clair and Bryan were still receiving the previous owners' newspapers, which included *The Sun*. After Hudson's death, *The Sun* ran a piece with the headline: 'I'd shoot My Son If He Had AIDS, Says Vicar!' A full-width photo underneath the headline showed Reverend Robert Simpson aiming a shotgun at the face of his eighteen-year-old son, Chris. Reverend Simpson was concerned that AIDS would 'be like the Black Plague. It could wipe out Britain.' In the years to come, he said, the country would be divided, with family pitched against family. To help prevent the apocalyptic vision from coming true, Reverend Simpson outlined his desire to ban gay men from taking Communion so the illness couldn't spread via the chalice. And he would take a strong line at home, too.

'Chris would not get closer to me than six yards,' said Reverend Simpson in the newspaper. 'He would be a dead man.' He added, 'And that would go for the rest of my family, as well as strangers.'

Clair and Bryan came to dread the next day's headlines. They felt like they were being attacked in their own home. But they couldn't escape the news: there were reports of people saying those with AIDS should be branded with tattoos or sent to an island, like people with leprosy had been until just a few decades earlier. Clair and Bryan heard stories about people losing their jobs and children with hemophilia being kicked out of school. People would physically move away if they knew someone had come into contact with the virus. Families found slurs painted onto their houses. Anyone who was positive for HTLV-III was seen as a pariah. Bryan and Clair decided to keep the news of Bryan's diagnosis to themselves for fear of rejection or physical attack. Eventually, they chose to tell their parents and close family.

The reality took a while to sink in. Bryan tried to act as though nothing had changed, while Clair was paralyzed by the thought of what was to come. Then, one day, Bryan told Clair he had made a decision for both of them.

'If I'm going to die, I want to be back with my family,' he said.

They started making arrangements to go back to the Midlands. Less than a year after they had moved into their Devonshire home, they sold it. Bryan reapplied for his old job running petrol stations in Leamington Spa and Clair found a new role at Coventry City Records Office. As they packed away their things, they couldn't escape the thought that they were boxing up their dreams before they'd had a chance to realize any of them. With all their possessions, the couple climbed into Bryan's classic car and drove a hundred and sixty miles north. Clair was twenty-four and Bryan was twenty-seven. They had been married for two and a half years. And they were returning to the Midlands for the final years of Bryan's life.

★

Late one morning in May 1985, fifteen-year-old Ade was called to see Dr Aronstam at the Treloar's hemophilia center. He wasn't the only one – four other boys were told to go with him. Ray, the friend he shared a dorm with, was one of those in the group, along with Dave from Sheffield. It was strange, Ade thought, to have an appointment with so many fellow pupils. They would often go to the center in pairs when one of them had a bleed, and they sometimes had treatment sessions together. But this felt different.

Dr Aronstam was waiting for them in an examination room, along with Dr Wassef, two nurses and a physio. Ade got onto the bed and three boys sat alongside him. The fifth boy took a chair next to them. They were packed tight, with ten people in the stuffy little medical room. Dr Aronstam looked at the boys, who fell quiet.

'You may have heard that Factor VIII isn't as clean as it should be,' said Dr Aronstam.

He described the range of viruses the children had caught from their treatment, including multiple strains of hepatitis – A, B and a new type they were calling non-A, non-B – as well as CMV, Epstein-Barr virus and parvovirus. Dr Aronstam said parvovirus usually affected only dogs, but some of them had received a human version. One of the other boys barked, trying to lighten the mood. Ray elbowed him in the ribs. Dr Aronstam's tone was reassuring; this wasn't anything unexpected. Ade sensed he was trying to keep the atmosphere forcibly relaxed, but his smile was tense. The boys tried to follow as Dr Aronstam started to use technical language, such as 'helper T-cells' and 'CD4 lymphocytes.' The minutes dragged on, Dr Aronstam talking about the different effects Factor VIII was having inside their bodies. Eventually, he arrived at the reason he had brought them all to the hemophilia center.

'You may have heard of the virus HTLV-III,' said Dr Aronstam. 'Some of you have it.'

Dr Aronstam's eyes looked glassy as he lifted his arm to do something unheard of. He went around the room from left to right and pointed at the boys in turn.

'You have; you haven't; you have; you haven't; you have got HTLV-III,' said Dr Aronstam.

Ade was one of the 'you haves.' He had HTLV-III, the virus that caused AIDS.

There was a moment of silence. The sun cut a sharp beam through the blind and Ade focused on its glare. Around him, as he tuned out what was happening in the room, one of the nurses started to cry.

'So how long have we fucking got, then?' snapped Dave, who was also positive.

'We don't know,' said Dr Aronstam. He told the boys there was a lot they didn't know. The virus was the same as that which was causing boys in America to get sick, but that didn't mean they would get ill in the same way.

Ade had seen enough to know the 'boys in America' meant the adult men shrinking in their hospital beds. Gaunt faces and hollowed-out eyes.

'At the moment it's two to three years, but we believe it's going to be longer,' said Dr Aronstam. 'You could be gone by eighteen or twenty. But we will do all we can for you. We'll do our very best.'

All Ade heard was *two to three years*.

Dr Aronstam stressed once more that he would go to the ends of the earth to protect them, but the words felt meaningless, inconsequential.

Before Dr Aronstam let them go, he had a piece of advice for the boys. The school had already appeared in media stories about AIDS, and he didn't want the pupils to come under any more fire, so he told them not to share their viral statuses with anyone, including their peers. They had just been given the worst news in front of their classmates, without the support of their parents. Dr Aronstam finished talking and signaled they could leave the room.

Ade climbed off the examination bed and filed out with Ray and Dave. Waiting in the corridor outside was another group of five boys, who were about to receive their verdicts. Ade saw his own terror reflected in their faces. He left the hemophilia center as those next five went into the examination room, thinking about how Dr Wassef had lied to him.

Outside, Ade squinted into the bright spring sun. He felt hollow, as though he had been robbed of something elemental – of the right to enjoy the day's beauty and warmth. His time was now limited. Dave stormed past him, furious and swearing profusely. Ade and Ray went after him, in the direction of the horticulture department. Dave picked up a pot and threw it against the wall of the hemophilia center.

'We're dead; we're all fucking dead,' he shouted, as the pot smashed. 'You've fucking killed us.'

With shards of pottery scattered at their feet, Dave stormed off, leaving Ade and Ray behind. Ade looked at Ray, his dorm mate who he had once battled with for a BAXTER chronograph watch. His friend who had also been diagnosed as HTLV-III positive. Not knowing what else to do, the two boys hugged. In a quiet space hidden from the rest of Treloar's, they tried to offer one another as much comfort as they could, their arms wrapped tightly around each other. They were both fifteen. The stages of grief would come for Ade, starting with denial and anger, before reaching depression. But for now, he stood there in the quiet and hugged Ray.

Ade didn't have time to process the bombshell that he had been infected with a fatal illness, because he was told to return to class. By 2 p.m. he was in a science lesson. He had just been told he was going to die and yet there he was looking at a blackboard and listening to a teacher drone on. How could he be sitting here in damn Biology – it didn't make sense.

Ade went into that examination room with four other boys; he is now the only survivor. Ray and Dave died from AIDS-related illness within a year of each other in the early 1990s. The other two have since passed away from complications of hepatitis. Of the five boys who were waiting in the corridor to go into the examination room after Ade, there are just two survivors. From the early 1970s to the late 1980s, over 122 children with hemophilia went to Treloar's school. Around half of them were infected with HIV. All contracted hepatitis C. At least seventy-two have died from their infections; just thirty-two are still alive. 'Everything they could have been,' says Ade. 'It chokes me.'

Dr Tuddenham knew tragedy was approaching the Royal Free's hemophilia center, but he didn't anticipate how far-reaching it would be. The hospital tested every patient in the center for HTLV-III. Unlike at Treloar's and some other hospitals, the Royal Free obtained consent before conducting the tests. The results soon built up, with a sheet of paper for each patient. As Dr Tuddenham and his colleagues sifted through the pile, they came to realize that a tragedy of enormous scale had befallen the hospital. He found the results horrifying. Around half of their two hundred and fifty patients had tested positive for HTLV-III. Nearly all of their adult patients with severe hemophilia A who required Factor VIII had been infected.

For every diagnosis, there was the most difficult conversation to be had. Patients and their families were invited to the Royal Free to meet with a nurse and psychosocial worker. The whole family was taken into a private room to hear their loved ones be given a death sentence. "This is the diagnosis," one of the clinicians would say. "We don't have a treatment for it yet. It will get worse and we don't know how long you've got to live."

While his colleagues broke the news, Dr Tuddenham retreated to his laboratory.

'We had no idea it was going to be as bad as it was,' says Professor Tuddenham. 'That was the beginning of the tide that washed over us and took half our patients from us.'

Those were nightmarish weeks in the corner of the Royal Free that housed one of Britain's largest hemophilia centers. Patients were receiving awful news whenever they visited the center. As the dire disclosures filtered through the unit, staff tried desperately to keep morale up.

Across the country, the number of positive test results climbed. Between 1970 and 1991 around 1,250 people with hemophilia in Britain tested positive for HTLV-III – all infected by contaminated blood products.

Dr Tuddenham had given his patients a treatment that was going to kill them. It was the worst experience a doctor could have. By 1986 he decided the situation in the hemophilia center was just too harrowing. Having watched two patients die from AIDS-related illness, he knew he wouldn't be able to cope with the coming disaster – the shattering experience of caring for patients who were dying. And so when an opportunity came up, he left the Royal Free, escaping into full-time research.

'This looks like HTLV-III developing into full-blown AIDS,' said the junior doctor who had been called to help Joe, the aspirational mod who was married to Frankie.

Joe was lying on a trolley bed in the Queen Elizabeth Hospital in Birmingham. Frankie was by his side and his dad was outside, parking the car. It was early in 1985 and the three of them had rushed to hospital together after Joe collapsed at the cabinetmakers where he worked. He had been suffering from a urinary infection and was in the workshop's toilets when he passed out and fell to the floor. Frankie didn't have a driving license – they couldn't afford a car – so she had phoned Joe's dad. They picked Joe up together and raced twenty-five miles to the hospital in Birmingham. Now, Joe was with Frankie in a side room at the hospital, surrounded by beaten-up trolleys and oxygen bottles, awaiting assessment.

When the doctor said those words – 'full-blown AIDS' – Joe and Frankie looked blank. They hadn't heard about HTLV-III and had little awareness of AIDS. Joe was only twenty-one; Frankie was nineteen. Like Clair and Bryan, they didn't follow the news. If they had seen anything about AIDS, it was the pictures of emaciated gay men in American cities. But they had never been to the US. They were a young married couple in rural England, who enjoyed zooming around on their scooter with their dog in the sidecar. At home, they didn't watch television or read the news. Joe was cut off from the hemophilia community so the rumors hadn't reached him. The doctor gave them scant information.

Nearly six months passed and Joe and Frankie were left wondering if Joe actually had HTLV-III and, if he did, what the implications were. But throughout those months of not knowing, there was a more pressing issue at the front of Frankie's mind: she was pregnant. She was still a teenager; young to become a mother, let alone in these circumstances.

Frankie and Joe quickly got the impression theirs was a unique situation. Doctors seemed to know little about AIDS and whether it could be passed from a mother or father to a child. While they waited for confirmation that Joe had HTLV-III, Frankie had a momentous decision to make. Should she have the baby or terminate the pregnancy? The doctors had implied there was a risk to Joe and the baby, but told her little else. She felt like she was being swept along by a current. Because of the stigma surrounding AIDS, she couldn't seek advice from her family, and even talking to Joe was difficult. No one had the language to really discuss what was happening. Not only was there an unspecified risk to the baby, but if Joe did have AIDS, that meant he was dying. The prospect was too terrifying to tackle head-on. Both of them found it difficult to voice any thoughts about what they should do. Time dragged on. They buried their heads in indecision.

With the arrival of summer, Frankie went with Joe to his hemophilia doctor to ask for advice. Frankie was petrified. While there, both of them agreed to do a blood test for HTLV-III. Following the appointment, Joe's hematologist wrote to Frankie's GP about their predicament.

> The current concern amongst the haemophiliacs regarding the acquired immune deficiency syndrome (AIDS) has been causing us to modify our advice to haemophiliac patients who wish to undertake a family at the moment. Our present advice to these couples is that they should not have children until the infectivity of the AIDS virus has been clarified. . . .
>
> I would consider that, in view of the current nationally agreed advice given to haemophiliac patients, together with the likelihood of Joe being positive for HTLV-III antibody (70 per cent of our severe haemophiliacs are positive) that the possible risks of transmission of the HTLV-III virus from Joe to his wife and hence to a foetus is sufficiently likely to represent grounds for termination under the Abortion Act.

Frankie's GP replied that the situation was 'rather frightening.'

The couple were told that if Joe tested positive, the risk that the baby could have HTLV-III was sufficient for Frankie to terminate the pregnancy. But they couldn't wait for Joe's test results, because Frankie was already in her third trimester. When she tried to ask for more advice, she was met with a lack of support and vague information. No one seemed to know anything about AIDS. Ultimately, she was left feeling like she had little choice. She agreed to have a termination under what she felt was pressure from their doctors. By the time she reached the decision, she was seven months pregnant – but that didn't matter in what doctors believed was an unprecedented situation.

On a Friday in August 1985, Frankie and Joe arrived at the maternity unit at the hospital. The staff were immediately cold towards them. Joe was told to go to the waiting area, while Frankie was taken to a room on her own, which had been plastered with biohazard stickers ahead of her arrival. From that moment, the doctor and nurse who saw her were dressed from head to toe in protective gear: she couldn't see their faces. Because of the late stage of her pregnancy, Frankie had to be induced into labor. She was alone for hours, not allowed to leave the room nor have Joe accompany her for support. When she was screaming out in pain during contractions, she had no one's hand to hold. She felt like she was on death row.

After the ordeal was over, a doctor came to check on her. He examined her and made sure she had recovered enough to be discharged. But before leaving the room, he said something to Frankie. It was something she feared had been on everyone's minds as they shut her away to give birth and attended to her in full protective gear.

'Women like you should be sterilized,' said the doctor.

Returning home, Frankie and Joe tried to bury the nightmare, never speaking about it again. Three days later, on Monday morning, Frankie was back at work. She needed to keep earning money for their mortgage, and she couldn't risk anyone finding out what she had been through. Still recovering from the trauma of labor, her breasts started to leak.

Joe and Frankie's HTLV-III results came back after her termination. Having waited weeks for the answers, they went to the hospital together to hear the verdict. The atmosphere in the room was matter-of-fact as the doctor told Joe he had HTLV-III, and approximately three years to live. Joe struggled to absorb the news. Inside, he felt like a healthy twenty-one-year-old – not someone who supposedly had a deadly disease.

Frankie's test results were negative, but it was hard for her to feel relieved. She hadn't been infected with HTLV-III when she had the termination and now her husband was dying.

In the years that followed, Frankie never told her parents about Joe's diagnosis; or that she had been pregnant; or that she had had a termination. She felt too guilty about the situation and that she would be unable to give her parents the joy of grandchildren, especially her father, who adored kids. Slowly, she closed herself off from the people she loved.

To this day, she cannot console herself over the decision to terminate her pregnancy seven months in – nor understand how she came to make it. She is tearful as she tells me, 'I have felt for many years that I was a murderer.' She still wakes up and thinks of herself in this way.

Bryan became obsessed with living for the moment. With a death sentence hanging over him, he wanted to enjoy what time he had left; to make the most of his life with Clair. But he became understandably irascible. Sometimes he was angry about what was happening to him. At other times, he wanted to forget it all. But his main goal was to live, to urgently tick off the hopes on his bucket list as a means of fighting the terror of a premature death. Back in the Midlands, close to his family, he and Clair bought a new house – their third in less than three years – and threw themselves into renovating it. By day, they would go to work; at the weekends, they would fix up their new home.

Those months weren't easy. In search of answers and support, Bryan tried to reconnect with old friends from the hemophilia world of his childhood. Those who had contracted the virus had found themselves ostracized from society. Most were sinking under the mental toll like Bryan, who became increasingly resentful of having been infected with this illness. He stopped taking care of himself and started drinking heavily. Clair knew he was traumatized, but couldn't see a way to help him. He pushed her further and further away until they ended up separating. She was heartbroken.

After just a few months, they met to discuss getting back together – the time apart had been difficult for both of them. They talked and talked like they used to during those long summer evenings at the petrol station, going over their hopes for the near future and what they wanted their lives to look like. On deciding to move back in with each other, they determined that they would pursue their dreams regardless of Bryan's condition. Above all else, they wanted to start a family. They wanted a reset. They were stubbornly clinging on to hope.

Bryan had been HIV positive for over a year. In that time, Clair hadn't contracted the virus. Maybe it wasn't as infectious as people thought. They decided to speak to Bryan's hemophilia consultant to assess their options. At the hospital in Coventry, Clair took the lead.

'We would quite like to have a baby,' she said.

The response wasn't encouraging. 'It's not a very good idea,' the doctor replied. 'But if you want to go ahead, we'll monitor you.' The consultant didn't tell Bryan if he could actually father a child, given his HIV status, nor what the risks to Clair and their potential baby would be. But the doctor was the expert and didn't seem too concerned, so Clair thought it would be all right. She agreed to go back to the hospital once a month to do a blood test to see if she was pregnant – and if she had contracted HIV. Leaving the room, Clair and Bryan believed they had the green light to start trying for a baby.

Every month from September 1986 Clair went to the hospital for her regular checkup. With each visit the HIV tests came back negative, as did her pregnancy tests.

One day in early summer 1987, Clair was riding her motorbike when she started to feel unwell. She pulled over and rested before returning home. Over the coming days, her flu-like symptoms developed and she became more unwell than she had ever been before. There was an intense fever and deep aches. When her temperature subsided and she started to feel better, Clair went for her monthly checkup at the hospital. She wasn't pregnant; but this time her HIV test was inconclusive. The doctor asked her to do another one.

Clair and Bryan refused to entertain the idea that she could have contracted HIV. Neither of them could take any more bad news. Walking through the streets of Leamington Spa and trying to suppress their anxiety, they saw pictures of California in the windows of a travel agent. Clair was reminded of a holiday they had taken to Santa Barbara a few years earlier to visit some friends. In a moment of rare impulsiveness, they decided there and then to book flights. They would go to America! See their friends, and forget about the hospital, hemophilia, HIV and pregnancy.

When they were sitting on the plane, in the air over the Atlantic, Clair suddenly remembered something. She had been feeling so numb, trying so hard not to think about the next potential blow that was about to befall them. She turned to Bryan.

'I forgot to ask for the results of my test,' she said.

Bryan hesitated. He had already spoken to the nurse. 'It came back positive,' he said, not knowing how to cushion the news. 'They told me.'

Clair felt like she was living someone else's life. Looking out of the window at the ocean below she thought of all she had experienced in the last two years: getting married, moving to Devon, being told her husband would die of AIDS, trying for a baby, then finding out she was HIV positive. In that moment, she felt wholly dissociated from the reality of their lives. As if other people were experiencing these problems, not them. As the news sunk in, she realized she would have to find yet another way to survive.

Landing in America, amid the Hollywood hills and dramatic Pacific coastline, the pain melted away. For a brief time, they could each be someone else. Forgetting their reality was easier than confronting it.

Treloar's was reeling after dozens of pupils discovered they had HIV. In an attempt to contain the virus, staff introduced a 'six-inch rule': pupils weren't allowed to sit within six inches of the person next to them. To enforce the policy, some teachers carried measuring tapes around their necks or in their pockets. Initially, when little was known about how the virus was transmitted, staff thought pupils' saliva and tears could be dangerous. Children with hemophilia were treated as hazardous. For a term in 1985 they were given disposable bed linen to protect the cleaning staff. It made Ade feel isolated and diseased. When his bed was ready to be changed, he would put the used sheets in a yellow biohazard bag that was kept in the corner of his dorm room. He learned to wash his own clothes, too.

Amanda Beesley was a member of the care staff in Burnham House, where Ade lived. She had to get used to a new set of protocols. If blood spilled on the floor, they had to clean it up carefully to prevent further infections. Staff had ready access to disposable gloves and sterilizing fluid. But the hardest thing was comforting the children who had HIV. Amanda knew how to steer children through conversations about death, because there were other pupils at Treloar's who had life-shortening conditions, such as muscular dystrophy or cystic fibrosis, who might not live into adulthood. But AIDS was different. So little was known and so much was rumored. Staff felt ill-equipped to offer the necessary psychological support.

The children with HIV were distracted by the painful deaths they might face in the coming years. Those who had avoided infection were fearful of contracting it from Factor VIII or their peers. Tension built within the school. Boys got into fights in the playground; friendship groups splintered.

Every time Ade went to sick bay he was reminded that he was riddled with infection. He learned how to calculate his T-cell ratio and put condoms on a banana. He knew in great detail what was happening inside his body, in terms of not just hemophilia but HIV as well. Although there was comfort from Dr Aronstam and his medical colleagues, Ade reached a point where he didn't want to visit the hemophilia center anymore.

The majority of staff were supportive, but there were a few who were obsessed with AIDS, harboring prejudices seen in the tabloids. One even said the children with the virus would have to move to a remote island. Dr Aronstam wanted the identities of pupils with HIV kept secret from those outside the hemophilia center, so everyone would be treated equally, but some members of staff were persistent in their attempts to find out their names. Dr Aronstam said that if anyone asked the boys for their test results, they should report it straight to him, which Ade did when a careers adviser tried to coax his diagnosis out of him.

In the world outside the school, the language around AIDS had become apocalyptic. While Ade and his friends were too young to pay much attention to the newspapers, the media scaremongering about AIDS had been ramped up to new heights. Downing Street was conspicuously silent on the matter until 1986, when Thatcher's government finally intervened in the crisis with a £5 million public information campaign that only added to the fear. The infamous 'Monolith' advert caught the attention of Ade and his friends. It opened with an explosion in a dark quarry that shot fragments of rock and a propulsion of water into the air. 'There is now a danger that has become a threat to us all. It is a deadly disease and there is no known cure,' said actor John Hurt in a grave voice-over. Threatening music clanged in the background. A close-up showed workers' hands chiseling black rock. 'The virus can be passed during sexual intercourse with an infected person. Anyone can get it, man or woman. So far it has been confined to small groups – but it's spreading.' The word *AIDS* appeared out of the darkness, etched in white on a black tombstone.

'Protect yourself,' said Hurt, as the tombstone fell to the ground. 'If you ignore AIDS it could be the death of you. So don't die of ignorance.'

A bunch of white lilies was flung on the tombstone, as smoke hovered eerily in the middle distance. Beneath was the statement: 'Issued by the Health Departments of the United Kingdom.'

In April 1987 Princess Diana eased some of the public anxiety when she opened the UK's first AIDS ward at Middlesex Hospital in London. On camera, she shook the hand of someone with the syndrome without wearing gloves or protective clothing. 'HIV does not make people dangerous to know,' she said. 'You can shake their hands and give them a hug. Heaven knows they need it. What's more, you can share their homes, their workplaces, their playgrounds and toys.'

In the quiet of their dorm rooms, Ade and his friends who had been diagnosed with HIV – Ray, Dave and Simon – had to contend with the inconceivable idea that they were going to die as boys. 'The worst thing they did was put two to three years on it,' says Ade. When they were first given their diagnoses, many of them had normal T-cell counts and weren't showing any symptoms of AIDS. But after receiving their death sentences, at least nine of Ade's friends had started to drink heavily.

Ade's relationship with his mum was already difficult and he had been warned over and over about the hatred faced by people with AIDS, so he chose not to tell her about his diagnosis. Eighteen months later, in 1986, Dr Aronstam finally wrote to Ade's doctor in Portsmouth to inform them he had HIV and to ask them to let his mother know. Having administered the treatment that had given him the virus, Dr Aronstam didn't know how to tell her himself.

Not long after Ade turned sixteen, his family life broke down. His mum was convinced doctors didn't harm people; she had told Ade he was lying about the dangers of Factor VIII. Both Dr Wassef and the Haemophilia Society had told her Factor VIII was safe. But now she was scared of her own son. She told Ade he had brought shame on her and was violent towards him. The abuse came to a head when she said she didn't want him around anymore. Aged seventeen, Ade moved into Kerr House children's home in Portsmouth for the school holidays.

Hemophilia had become a dirty word, associated as it was with AIDS. In the streets of Portsmouth, children would shout insults at Ade. 'Don't come to Ade's aid, he's got AIDS!' Whenever he was at the children's home for the weekend or during school holidays, he willed time to pass more quickly so he could get back to Treloar's. Even though it was the place where he had been infected with HIV, it still felt like a safe haven. He had friends there who knew exactly how he felt, because they also had hemophilia and HIV. After ten months of Ade going to the children's home during the holidays, two members of Treloar's staff invited him to stay with them. Despite everything, they and Dr Aronstam were his surrogate guardians.

One afternoon at Treloar's, the pressure became too much for Ade. He was in his dorm room alone, supposed to be doing his homework. His friends were all at homework club, but he had been given permission to work from his room. That sometimes happened when pupils were recovering from a bleed. Ade looked at the objects scattered across the small area he called his own: a single bed next to a desk that doubled as a chest of drawers. There were three furry animal toys looking up at him with googly eyes. The words ARMOUR and ALPHA were on ribbons attached to them. Next to them he had stationery, an organizer and a calculator, all branded with the names of pharma companies. Names that reminded him of the fear, of his fractured home life, of the newspaper headlines scaremongering about AIDS. Names that seemed to be screaming at him, 'You're going to die.'

Rage rose up his throat. How could he focus on something as banal as homework when he had been told he was going to die?

Seeking an outlet for his anger, Ade picked up one of the furry toys and tried to rip it apart. He tugged as hard as he could, but it wouldn't give. Instead he tore its eyes off, one by one. For a second, sorrow for the toy overtook his anger. Then he noticed the chronograph watch, with its blue sheen, brown leather strap and BAXTER branding. He grabbed the watch and banged it on the edge of his desk. Striking it against the wood, he felt the glass crack beneath his hand. Silence vibrated around him after each shattering blow.

Concerned that a member of staff might hear the noise, Ade changed tack. They wouldn't react kindly to him smashing up his possessions when he was meant to be doing homework. He couldn't face a confrontation in this state. With his thumb, he managed to pry the back off the watch. He twisted out the first springs with a pen. Then piece by piece, he took the chronograph watch apart from the inside out. He worked methodically, destroying the prize he had been so eager to attain.

Half an hour later, Ade's desk was covered with watch innards. He was calm again, though breathing heavily. As he looked at the pieces, Ade felt an overwhelming sense of guilt about what he had done. To bury the feeling, he swept the parts into the watch's soft leather carrying case and shoved it into his drawer.

For years that case remained hidden at the back of Ade's wardrobe, taunting him. When he opened the doors and saw it there, he told himself he would get someone to put it back together. But he never got around to it. Decades later, the broken watch has long disappeared, and Ade regrets the loss: it would have been a prime piece of evidence.

The year Dr Aronstam gave Ade and his classmates their HIV diagnoses, he released a book titled *Haemophilic Bleeding: Early Management at Home*. Drawing on the years he had spent treating and studying pupils at the school, he outlined the best ways for doctors and parents to look after children with the condition – and how to make the most of the Factor VIII revolution. In the opening pages, Dr Aronstam thanked his colleagues at Treloar's, as well as head teacher Macpherson and his own family who had 'uncomplainingly given up their rights' to his time. At the end of the preface, he also thanked an American pharma company.

'Armour Pharmaceutical Co. Ltd have generously contributed to the production costs of this book,' wrote Dr Aronstam. 'It is through them that it will be available to the public at a subsidized price. This help is gratefully received.'

The sole reference Dr Aronstam made to infectious diseases in his Armour-subsidized book was buried late in chapter twelve, in a section about prophylactic treatment: 'The risk of complications such as hepatitis and AIDS makes prophylaxis unacceptable to some doctors and some haemophiliacs,' he wrote. 'I feel very strongly that this is a matter you should consider after discussion with your own doctors.' And yet he had never had those conversations with his own young patients – or their parents.

Inside the hemophilia center, Dr Aronstam was trying to get a handle on the wreckage caused by Factor VIII. By 1986 he had forty-three patients who were HIV positive, many of whom were starting to show signs of AIDS. They were experiencing greater problems with their health as well as socially. 'There are gloomier predictions about, which suggest that up to 100 per cent of the infected haemophiliac population will eventually succumb to the virus,' wrote Dr Aronstam in a report. 'The bare facts do not reveal the cataclysmic impact of the HIV/AIDS problem on our haemophilia centre. The patients, their families, the haemophilia centre staff and the community all around us are all profoundly affected and will continue to be so for many years to come.'

His patients were plagued by prejudice inside and outside the school. Counseling had become a significant part of his job, and he couldn't escape the guilt of having given his patients a death sentence as he tried to hand them healthier, freer lives. Many had begun to 'live a life haunted by fear,' he said.

The ripples of the HIV disaster spread throughout Britain's hemophilia population, with tragedies mirroring one another in Devon and Newcastle, Cardiff and Belfast. People lost their jobs, were told they couldn't get life or travel insurance, had mortgage applications refused and were strongly advised not to start families. Colin Smith was two years old when Professor Bloom told his parents in a hospital corridor that their son had HTLV-III. In their Welsh community, people nicknamed them the 'AIDS family' and sent them into isolation. Their home had 'AIDS DEAD' spray-painted across it and crosses scratched into the front door. Their car was vandalized. At school, Colin's brother endured children taunting him, shouting, 'Your brother's got AIDS!' His father lost his job. Colin died aged seven.

There were families in which multiple members were infected with HIV: two brothers in the Farrugia family from north London; Jason and Leigh Peach at Treloar's; Gareth and Haydn Lewis in Cardiff; Suresh and Praful Vaghela in Coventry. Of these, only Suresh survives. People developed alcoholism and depression; they were made homeless, separated from their partners, lost contact with close family members. The pattern was repeated wherever contaminated Factor VIII was in use: the US, Canada, the UK, Ireland, France, Germany, Portugal, Italy, Greece, Austria, Sweden, Japan, Taiwan, Hong Kong, Israel, Iran, Iraq, India, Pakistan, Australia, Argentina, Colombia, Mexico, South Africa, and many more. In the prime of their lives, boys and men with hemophilia whose dreams had only recently been made possible by Factor VIII were obliterated in just over a decade.

Richard Warwick had left Treloar's in 1982, missing the rising panic and wave of infections that would soon hit the school. Six years later, in 1988, he was twenty-three and had been dating his girlfriend Tina for nearly a year. Richard thought she was his soulmate, and quickly asked her to marry him. He was still suffering from health problems. His epilepsy had developed from nighttime seizures to attacks in the middle of the day. There had been times when he had ended up in hospital after having a fit while walking down the street.

When Richard went to his GP to discuss the severe epileptic attacks he had been having, he was offhandedly given a new diagnosis: 'You do know, Richard, that you're HIV positive, don't you?' asked his doctor.

Richard's heart started pounding. He certainly hadn't known. Without his knowledge, doctors had tested him for HIV numerous times since December 27, 1984. The very first test had come back positive.

'Why has nobody told me about it in four years?' he demanded.

The GP had no answer. Some doctors believed they were helping patients by withholding their HIV statuses in the early years of AIDS. Given there was no treatment, and how upsetting a diagnosis was, there were those like Richard's doctor who chose to keep it to themselves. That way, their patients could continue to live normal lives. The mere fact of having taken an HIV test could be enough to prevent people from getting a mortgage. But Richard was furious. He was engaged to Tina and had been putting her in danger.

With his HIV diagnosis, answers about his health problems started to fall into place. By 1988 it had become apparent that patients newly infected with HIV could develop an illness that looked very similar to glandular fever. On other occasions, the illness associated with seroconversion, the body's initial response to an HIV infection, looked more like flu. Now, Richard's unconfirmed bout of glandular fever in 1981 made sense: it had in fact been his seroconversion with

HIV following infection from a contaminated batch of Factor VIII three years earlier. The same was true of Ade's sickness in 1983 and Joe's in 1984. That made Gary, who had glandular fever at Treloar's back in 1978, one of the earliest British patients to seroconvert with HIV from Factor VIII.

It would take longer for researchers to connect HIV to Richard's other health problems, but it eventually became clear that the virus could also cause patients to develop epilepsy. The seizures that had started during the night when he was a schoolboy, and which had developed into an unpredictable burden, were in fact a sign that the virus was attacking his brain.

When Richard left the doctor's office, it was dark and raining. As soon as he got through the door back home, he asked Tina to come upstairs with him. Slowly, he shared the horrific news with her. Through tears, she told him it didn't matter; she loved him and still wanted to be with him.

A year later, Tina found out she was pregnant. It had been an accident. They were married, but knew the dangers involved. Their doctor told them in no uncertain terms that Tina should have an abortion. The risk of the baby having HIV was too high. Added to that, Richard believed he was living on borrowed time. He was still having epileptic fits and was halfway into the two years the GP had said he would live. The couple were devastated. It was their first and only chance to have a child, but Tina had a termination.

As the 1990s dawned, Bryan was planning a once-in-a-lifetime road trip. He was going to drive to the very north of Scotland and travel by ferry to the Orkney, Shetland and Faroe Islands, before landing in Iceland. The whole trip would take around five weeks, with Clair flying to meet him in Reykjavík for a fortnight. Bryan had spent time carefully converting his new Land Rover into a camper van; he had come to believe money was there to be spent, even if it was in short supply. He had been forced to quit work because of his health and missed the late nights on the forecourt watching the tankers roll in, but planning this road trip had provided a welcome distraction.

Clair, who was also HIV positive, was working twice as hard at her dream job in conservation at the Shakespeare Birthplace Trust in Stratford-upon-Avon. While she was still healthy, she needed to support their lifestyles, and wanted to banish any existential dread through the academic pursuit of making sure the past survived into the future. For Bryan, enjoying life had become a necessity. He was agitated about making the most of the time he had left and wanted to seize the day, packing in all the things on his bucket list. And he had always wanted to visit Iceland. Clair helped him get the Land Rover ready, sewing a set of curtains for the back windows and making cushions for the living area. As a leaving present, she bought him a portable voice recorder so he could document the trip.

By the time he was putting the final decorative touches on the Land Rover and planning his route, Bryan was feeling the time pressure. He had been told he had just a year and a half to live, a prognosis that felt worryingly more exact than the one he had received back in 1985, given how his health was declining.

Bryan was being treated with azidothymidine (AZT), a revolutionary treatment for HIV widely touted as the drug that could cure AIDS. But he wasn't convinced by it. Originally developed in the 1960s as a cancer treatment, AZT had been shelved after it was found to be unsuccessful. In 1987 it was fast-tracked for approval by the FDA for use in AIDS cases following a trial with fewer than three hundred patients, which was cut short after sixteen weeks and declared a success. Proponents said AZT would delay the onset of AIDS, but critics believed it caused more problems than the infection itself. In the early days of the epidemic, AZT was prescribed in doses so high they could be toxic. Bryan started to worry about what AZT was doing to his body, but was told it was the best treatment available. Accurate information was difficult to come by so he had no choice but to trust his doctor. Clair later discovered he was on a megadose of the drug, and despite sticking to a strict regimen, he became more ill.

In 1989 a lump appeared on Bryan's neck. He watched it grow, concerned about what it signified. His doctor said he should have a biopsy. While at the hospital for the procedure, he needed a dose of Factor VIII. The nurse treating him did something Bryan had never experienced before: she made him collect the Factor VIII from the fridge himself. He did as he was told and went through the familiar motions of mixing the powder with distilled water, drawing it into a syringe and injecting it into his arm. It was obvious that the nurse had not wanted to touch him. When Clair arrived at the hospital to collect Bryan, she found him visibly upset about the way he had been treated.

The results of the biopsy added to the couple's litany of bad news. The lump on Bryan's neck was cancerous: he had non-Hodgkin's lymphoma. At the time it was incurable and a sign Bryan had 'full-blown AIDS.' That was when he learned he had eighteen months to live.

Bryan then had a course of radiotherapy, which destroyed the hair follicles on one side of his face and neck. Having worn a beard, he resorted to shaving. The radiotherapy reduced the lump for a limited time, but the signs of his future were everywhere. When he was in hospital for treatment, staff would bring a recliner chair to his bedside so Clair could sit with him. Before he became too unwell, Bryan had tried to track down an old friend from Treloar's to see if he had been infected – and, if so, how he was coping. By the time Bryan found the friend's contact details and called him, it was too late. His family gave Bryan the news that his friend had very recently died from AIDS-related illness. Feeling shaken, Bryan went to pay his respects at the funeral. The death hit him hard. Now, as he lay in hospital receiving cancer treatment, a plaque on the recliner that Clair sat in by his bed-side remembered that friend who had been killed by contaminated Factor VIII. Bryan couldn't help but think of it as an omen.

Bryan desperately wanted to maintain his adventurous life. Clair could see he was losing a lot of weight and declining physically, as much as he tried to hide it. Determined not to be beaten down, Bryan set off on the thousand-mile journey to Iceland in 1991. He made his way through the swollen hills in the north of England and across the mountains of Scotland, driving towards the ferry terminal at the uppermost edge of the UK. As he waited for the first boat to the Orkneys, he was feeling animated.

Eventually landing in Iceland, he was awed by the vast, imposing landscape, at once beautiful and desolate. There was certainly a sense of it being a country in the making. Bryan drove through streams and up mountain roads, playing the radio loud as a backdrop and documenting everything from the spectacular to the mundane. There were days when the clouds hung so low they obscured the visibility. But before long they would break to reveal blue skies and glistening sunshine. He saw lakes filled with icebergs the size of his Land Rover and as clear as glass.

When Clair joined him, Bryan felt at ease driving through the deserted landscape. They saw wild Icelandic horses and geysers spitting mud. They bathed in the Blue Lagoon, Clair's long hair flowing behind her in the milky water. For breakfast, Bryan would cook bacon, eggs and baked beans on a camp stove in the shadow of mountains.

'I've just taken photographs of some of the flora,' said Clair into the voice recorder as wind hurtled past the Land Rover's windows. 'It's beautiful, warm and sunny. But in the distance there's a black cloud hanging over.'

They continued driving towards a mountain obscured by the cloud.

They ate dinner at the summit and ventured out into the volcanic sand desert, where the quiet was deafening.

After their fortnight together drew to a close and Clair flew back to England, Bryan started to feel lonely. The weather had turned, and with Clair suddenly absent the Land Rover felt too big for one person. Feeling down, he would call home as often as he could in an attempt to lift his mood. But Clair couldn't always answer. Once, after he had tried calling her without success, he decided that an extended holiday on his own wasn't a good idea. Better to have Clair with him to keep his spirits up when they started to flag, he thought.

As his car turned south towards home, their reunification in sight, Bryan's mood improved. 'The old adage about making hay while the sun shines certainly applies to this part of the world,' he said. 'Everybody's making hay.'

He determined that when he reached Tórshavn in the Faroe Islands he would start writing a full diary: an autobiography. While he still had time.

When Bryan got home, however, Clair noticed a dramatic change in him: he was completely emaciated. Bryan had coped with hemophilia throughout his life, with the pain and inconvenience it brought. He had to, because he had been born with it. But not AIDS. He had been infected with this deadly virus, and he was becoming ever more resentful about the fate that had been wrongfully assigned to him by his medical treatment.

Over the next two years, Bryan's health grew progressively worse. Chemotherapy for his non-Hodgkin's lymphoma failed to have the intended effect. He developed severe pain in his jaw, which he tried to remain stoic about, but Clair could see it was bothering him. On assessment, it was discovered that the previous radiotherapy had destroyed part of his jawbone. In January 1993 he had excruciating surgery to reconstruct it. It was successful, but it was merely cosmetic; it didn't change the fact that he was dying.

By this point, Bryan was in and out of hospital in Oxford. Not wanting to lose his independence, he insisted on being an outpatient. Time at home with Clair was more valuable than that spent with hospital staff whose caution around him was a constant reminder that he had AIDS. Clair stayed at his side through it all. When he was in hospital, she was there to make sure they gave him medicine on time, to bring him food at regular intervals and to support him emotionally.

One day in early March 1993 Clair and Bryan were in the kitchen at home. The rain had been beating down for weeks and Bryan seemed somehow different to her; his spirit was receding. Standing there in their third home, in the house where they had planned to have children, where they lived when Clair herself had been diagnosed with HIV and where Bryan was now fading away, the young couple hugged. It was an intense and prolonged embrace, both of them clinging to one another.

'I don't want to die, I'm too young,' said Bryan. He was frightened for himself and for Clair. 'I've got so much I want to do. I don't want to die. What's going to happen to you?'

'It's OK,' said Clair, trying to comfort him as much as she could. 'I'll be all right.'

Clair didn't know whether she was telling the truth, or if those were just words Bryan needed to hear. Later, when she thought back to that moment, she believed she had given him permission to die. He was thirty-four; she was thirty-one.

Relentless bad weather accompanied them as Bryan was hospitalized in the final stages of AIDS. On March 13, 1993, Clair was visiting him in hospital one morning when he asked her to help him sit up in bed so he could look out the window. He wanted to see the hospital grounds in the rain. Clair held his foot so he could lift himself up.

Outside, there was a solitary magpie.

'One for sorrow,' said Bryan.

Even though he was now in hospital permanently, Clair kept the inevitable reality at bay in her mind. She was busy distracting herself, taking a mathematics course at the Open University alongside her job at the Shakespeare Birthplace Trust. As Bryan slept, she would sit on the end of his hospital bed or in an armchair next to him and take out her books to study calculus. That afternoon Bryan was dozing, so Clair went to ask the nurse if she could borrow a video player. She had a recording to watch for her course. The nurse looked at her, not answering. Instead, a consultant came over and pulled her to one side.

'You do know he's going to die?' said the doctor.

'Yes, of course I do,' said Clair quietly.

'No, I mean now. In the next few hours.'

Caught off guard by the directness, Clair cried for the first time. After years of buildup, the inevitable was about to happen.

Having calmed down, Clair called Bryan's parents and brother, who drove to Oxford from the Midlands as quickly as possible. She sat next to Bryan, holding his hand while they waited for his family, and thought: *Who is going to be there for me when it's my turn?* It was easy to forget, given Bryan's condition, that she also had HIV. She was terrified at the prospect of dying alone in a hospital where she would be treated like a pariah.

By the time Bryan's family arrived, his breathing was labored. He had slowly lost consciousness while Clair waited. Surrounded by his family, Bryan took his last breath around 10 p.m.

Just shy of ten years after their wedding day, Bryan passed away, leaving Clair a widow. A part of her shut down. Now, she was left alone in a hostile world with her own terminal diagnosis.

In the days after Bryan's death, the clouds cleared for the first time in weeks. Remembering the searching look he had passed across the hospital's garden when he saw the solitary magpie, Clair felt desolate. The quiet crashed in.

She was afraid to tell anybody outside her close family what had happened to Bryan for fear of how they might react. Instead of telling people he had AIDS, she told them he had died of cancer.

Years after his death, Bryan's oral diary remained on the recorder he had taken to Iceland, his voice preserved while the world turned. Buried among his memories of the wilderness and the excitement of his holiday with Clair, Bryan had recorded his theory of life. In a wan tone, his voice faltering, he said: 'All the things that happen to you are sent as a trial. And when your number is called up, your number's called up. There's nothing you can do about it. The things that are sent to try you are to somehow test your strength, I guess. Just goes to show how quickly life can be snatched away from you. Enjoy everything while you can, especially each other and your loved ones.'

6. Evasion

One former doctor and politician felt a tragic sense of irony as he watched the story of AIDS and hemophilia unfold. David Owen had been dreading a crisis spawned by Britain's reliance on American blood products ever since he had been minister for health and social security from 1974 to 1976. Owen came from a family of doctors, and from the early years of Factor VIII had been aware that it was potentially dangerous because it was made from human plasma. In fact, the danger of blood products imported from the US had been a subject of debate between doctors and politicians ever since Factor VIII was licensed in 1973.

There was a prevailing philosophy in global medicine that blood and organs should be donated, rather than sold. According to this lore, giving blood and signing up for organ donation – either before or after death – should be acts of altruism. If donors were compensated financially, the dynamic would change because of the monetary reward. In Britain, along with most Western countries, blood and plasma donation had always functioned on what is called the 'gift relationship': people give blood to help others, knowing they won't receive any benefit themselves. The term had been coined by pioneering social policy researcher Richard Titmuss in 1970. Factor VIII produced in Britain at Blood Products Laboratory and the Protein Fractionation Centre was therefore made from donated plasma.

But the US, with its free-market ethos of untrammeled capitalism, had different rules. There, it was legal to pay people for plasma donations. Private companies set up shop and paid for plasma, which they then sold to pharmaceutical companies, who in turn used it to make Factor VIII. Owen had been paid to donate blood himself when he was a student traveling in Greece, and he understood how money changed the motivation.

On December 1, 1975, an investigative documentary broadcast in the UK revealed the dangers of American plasma. The episode of ITV's *World in Action*, a weekly current affairs series that uncovered corruption and underhanded behavior, was called 'Blood Money' and it showed a queue of people outside the Blood Donor Center in the impoverished downtown Skid Row district of Los Angeles, where shop fronts were boarded up and homeless people congregated. People went in, gave plasma and left with cash in their hands. That plasma was then used to make hemophilia medication. Because of the source, Factor VIII produced in the US had a higher chance of being contaminated with viruses, the narrator said. In the manufacturing process, the blood of thousands of donors was pooled together, multiplying the risk. In comparison, Factor VIII produced in Britain was made by pooling just a couple of hundred voluntary donations. The reporter showed how the consequences were already playing out: people with hemophilia were contracting hepatitis. Excluding paid-for donors had been proven to lower the transmission of hepatitis B.

Owen believed Britain should expect more from its blood products – and other leading doctors agreed. Dr Judith Graham Pool, who discovered cryo at Stanford University, wrote to federal officials in 1974 about President Richard Nixon's plans for a national blood policy and advised against the use of paid donors. His policy 'in no way requires or even encourages the use of volunteer blood for Factor VIII but assumes a continuation of the dangerous, expensive, wasteful, and unethical purchase of plasma by pharmaceutical houses,' she said. Her teacher at Stanford, Dr Joseph Garrott Allen, wrote to Britain's Blood Products Laboratory warning about how 'extraordinarily hazardous' American Factor VIII, was owing to the high hepatitis rates among donors. He said screening and testing for hepatitis was ineffective and that Britain should avoid importing Factor VIII until America moved to a voluntary system of donating.

That advice was echoed in sage medical circles in 1975. The World Health Organization advised countries to use voluntarily donated blood collected in their own countries. And a number of British doctors, including Dr Mark Winter from Thanet General Hospital, who would become one of the first to introduce heat-treated Factor VIII, wrote to the Department of Health to say it should reconsider importing commercial blood products from America because of the hepatitis risk.

Owen had tried to address the danger by laying out a plan to make Britain self-sufficient in blood products. British people would be encouraged to donate blood and plasma, while the laboratories that made Factor VIII in the UK would be given proper investment. Within two years, by 1977, the country would be self-sufficient, said Owen. At the time, Britain produced just 30 percent of the blood products it used. Owen invested £500,000 in speeding up plasma collection and the plan to gear up the work of Blood Products Laboratory began.

But a year into his plan, Owen was promoted to minister of state for foreign and commonwealth affairs and his vision for a country that could sustain its blood-product needs was cast aside by the Department of Health. Inadequate funding meant the expansion of buildings and equipment faltered, while the public didn't rise to the challenge of donating enough plasma.

In the meantime, doctors in Britain's hemophilia centers started exploring ways to make the most of the new miracle treatment and ramping up its use through prophylaxis. Arguments about self-sufficiency were shelved by the government due to the expense, and it instead approved the importation of increasing amounts of Factor VIII from America to meet the growing demand. By 1983, with the AIDS threat becoming very real, Britain was importing half of its supply – and the warnings about the risks of pooled plasma were ignored and unheeded.

Solicitor Graham Ross was working in his Southport office in 1986 when a married couple came to him for help. He liked to think of himself as 'the resolver,' someone who could find a way through tricky legal scenarios with his amiable manner and smiling eyes. The husband in this couple had HIV, which his doctor said he had contracted from his hemophilia treatment, and he wanted to know if there was any legal recourse. Graham had recently been working on a vast medical case involving some twelve thousand people who became addicted to benzodiazepines because of doctors overprescribing. From what the couple said, Graham thought they could have a similar case.

Graham set about gathering evidence, speaking to the doctors and researchers who had played major roles in hemophilia treatment and poring over sheaves of documents. He quickly learned that blood was a 'sewer of infection,' and that little had been done to protect people with hemophilia from viruses in their treatment. The first mistake he found was that politicians, manufacturers and doctors hadn't learned lessons from the spread of hepatitis in Factor VIII. Rather than think of hepatitis as a problem to be fixed, they had accepted it as an unavoidable side effect. That complacency had left patients entirely unprotected when a more deadly virus entered the blood pool, paving the way for HIV to spread. Dr David Dane, a leading virologist, told Graham, 'Whilst you can only ever identify so many viruses, you know there will be others.'

Given he was bringing the case in the UK, Graham decided to focus on how the government had failed to protect people from dangerous American Factor VIII, rather than going after the foreign companies. David Owen's ditched plan to make Britain self-sufficient in blood products had been followed by other failed attempts. Most came after a public outburst, such as an investment of £1 million in 1981 after the reports of multiple children at Treloar's contracting hepatitis. When AIDS emerged, health minister Ken Clarke had announced his own £20 million plan for self-sufficiency, which involved building a new Blood Products Laboratory plant at Elstree. Work began in May 1983, but the Association of Scientific, Technical and Managerial Staff said it would have required at least £30 million to make Britain self-sufficient. As the lab was slowly built, the government then denied the risk of AIDS being transmitted through blood.

Targets for self-sufficiency were repeatedly introduced, then pushed back: it would be achieved by 1985, then 1989. In the meantime, the Department of Health authorized increasing imports of Factor VIII. When the new Blood Products Laboratory opened in 1987 England and Wales were still using the same ratio of imported

Factor VIII as they had been a decade earlier. But self-sufficiency could have helped prevent the devastating crisis among people with hemophilia. Only a few batches of Factor VIII made from UK-sourced plasma were contaminated with HIV. In Scotland, which became self-sufficient in the early 1980s, the rate of AIDS in people with hemophilia was far lower. Had the relationship between Blood Products Laboratory and the Scottish Protein Fractionation Centre been better, it could have helped fill the gap in England and Wales.

Graham gathered enough evidence to show the government's consistent underinvestment in Blood Products Laboratory meant Britain had never produced anywhere near enough Factor VIII, leaving doctors with little choice but to rely on American imports when a deadly illness was spreading there. Whereas Scotland had withdrawn imported Factor VIII and replaced it with the heat-treated version at the end of 1984, England and Wales had taken an extra year to switch all patients to the safer version.

More people who had contracted HIV from Factor VIII came to Graham, and before long he was representing some eight hundred patients in the UK. He was one of around seventy lawyers who joined together to represent 926 people who had been infected with HIV. Together, they wanted to prove the Department of Health had been operationally negligent. From the outset Graham had thought it would be difficult to get the government to admit to mistakes and he wrote to the Haemophilia Society, saying that 'the final outcome would be some element of no fault compensation for all haemophiliacs.'

By June 1989 the lawyers had enough evidence to launch one of the UK's first group legal actions. The 926 victims sued the Department of Health, along with secondary organizations that had played a part in the tragedy: the blood transfusion service, the medical licensing authority and the Committee on the Safety of Medicines. Their main claim was that the government's failure to make Britain self-sufficient in blood products had put patients at risk from imported Factor VIII. In addition, Graham and the other lawyers alleged that the Department of Health had delayed the introduction of heat-treated Factor VIII, not responded adequately to the AIDS crisis and breached its duty of care under the National Health Service Act of 1977.

Professor Bloom and his colleagues at the UKHCDO rallied to support the Department of Health with its case. For the defense, Bloom wrote a two-hundred-page description of the events as they had unfolded.

In a volte-face that revealed how deep his guilt ran, Dr Aronstam decided in early 1990 to support the patients. Living with the shame of what had happened at Treloar's on his watch, he had slowly retreated from tending to patients personally since 1986, and now wanted to help them more widely in any way he could. Growing frustrated with his colleagues' apparent disregard for the tragedy that had befallen those in their care, he recused himself during a UKHCDO meeting where they were discussing the lawsuit, saying he was assisting the patients with their case. At the end of the session, he resigned from its AIDS group altogether.

Around that time, Ade had a bleed in his elbow. He was still living in Hampshire and his nearest treatment center was the old sick bay in the grounds of Treloar's. Ade walked through the familiar doors and found Dr Aronstam in his office, still working into the evening. The doctor was staring at his desk; he looked like a broken man.

'Don't worry, you did your best,' said Ade.

'No, we messed up,' replied Dr Aronstam. 'AIDS didn't need to happen. The Public Health Laboratory Service have let me down. They set me up.' He was referring to the place where Dr Craske had conducted research into hepatitis and then AIDS.

Ade tried to comfort his doctor. 'You've done your best; this is just an accident,' he said.

Deflated, Dr Aronstam poured them two brandies. The doctor and his infected patient sat in the hemophilia center where so many young children had contracted HIV and drank together.

When Ade later learned how much Dr Aronstam had known about the dangers of AIDS from 1982 onwards, and the extent to which he had failed him and his friends, he would think about this moment again and again. Part of him wanted to hate Dr Aronstam for having harmed them. But he still had a tenderness for his doctor, knowing how desperately he had tried to help save their lives once the full scale of AIDS became clear.

★

In 1988 former health minister David Owen became resolute: the government had put people in danger. Desirous of an investigation, he lodged a complaint that year with the Parliamentary and Health Service Ombudsman about what he believed was 'gross maladministration' by successive governments. In his complaint, Owen wrote, 'The crucial commitment to become self-sufficient in blood products was made when I was minister for health, a commitment made after careful consideration and quite a bureaucratic battle, in order to avoid the necessity for imported blood products. I am appalled that this commitment was never secured. As a result, infected blood has been introduced long after it need have been.' Owen waited months before a reply arrived from commissioner Sir Anthony Barrowclough.

More disconcerting was a discovery he made when he tried to access his private ministerial papers from his time in office. He asked a colleague to arrange an appointment with the Department of Health so he could examine his old documents from the mid-1970s to see if they could shed any more light on the failures. But the department said there were no papers for him to see – they had recently been pulped. Owen's colleague scribbled down a note: 'Papers have been destroyed. Normal procedure after ten years.'

Owen had heard about a thirty-year rule which prevented former ministers from sharing their private papers within three decades of leaving office without seeking permission. But after doing some digging, he discovered there was no such precedent for disposing of ministerial papers after just ten years. He still had access to all his papers from when he was minister for foreign and commonwealth affairs, some of which went to the National Archives and others to the University of Liverpool. He couldn't understand why his papers would have been destroyed without him being offered them for his records – especially as he was still a politician and actively involved in the controversy. He tried to raise the issue with the commissioner, but again Barrowclough was slow to reply.

When Barrowclough eventually responded to Owen, he said he had decided not to proceed with the investigation because he believed Owen's desire for self-sufficiency had been driven by financial reasons, not safety concerns. Only one memo about Owen's self-sufficiency drive had survived the cull, and it outlined how expensive it would be, given the financial pressures already placed on the NHS. 'Does it not follow – given the state of medical knowledge at the time – that the UK product would have been seen as carrying neither a lesser nor greater risk than that of imported Factor VIII?' wrote Barrowclough.

Owen was outraged. He protested that had he wanted self-sufficiency because of contamination fears, not financial prudence. But Barrowclough wouldn't budge.

In November 1989, Owen made an impassioned plea to his colleagues in Parliament to help people with hemophilia who had contracted HIV. Every MP, he felt, bore some responsibility for the UK's failure to achieve self-sufficiency in blood products, a government policy that had been announced in the House of Commons but was never realized. He told the House:

> I feel personally responsible . . . I have tried to persuade the parliamentary ombudsman to investigate this issue but failed. If ever there has been a clear and graphic case of maladministration, this must be it. We are all responsible. It is no use trying to buy off a court case with an inadequate payment given grudgingly. In Canada, sums as high as £150,000 are being paid out. In Germany, there have been supplements of more than £160,000.

But Owen was an opposition MP, leader of his own offshoot Social Democratic Party, and the government simply ignored him.

The UK government had given small payments to support people with hemophilia who were infected with HIV, but when measured against what they were experiencing, the amounts were derisory. In November 1987 the government announced it would make a £10 million payment to the Hemophilia Society to set up the Macfarlane Trust to help hemophiliacs who had been infected with HIV through contaminated NHS blood products. The payment was voluntary and didn't come with an admission of guilt: John Major, chief secretary to the treasury at the time, had warned his colleagues that giving victims a 'sympathetic response' might 'give rise to court action against the Government because of the implication of negligence.' Divided between the 1,250 or so people who had been infected with HIV and their families, the amount available per person was around £8,000. People could apply to the Trust for income top-ups, one-off grants and other support for items such as a washing machine or winter fuel. But the amounts were often pitifully small, and grant applications were regularly denied. Claimants felt like they were begging for mere scraps as they left their jobs and progressed to AIDS.

The case Graham Ross was building was set to be one of the biggest compensation claims ever made in Britain. On all sides the pressure was high: the government wanted to avoid an embarrassing and costly court case; people infected with HIV wanted justice before it was too late. By the beginning of 1990, 163 victims had developed AIDS and 110 had died. It was thought at least fifty more could die before the court date in a year's time.

Graham felt confident after Lord Justice Tom Bingham said he believed 'the tragedy was avoidable' and could 'have been prevented' if the Department of Health and others had acted differently in the 1970s and '80s. 'Grave errors of judgement were made by the government,' said Lord Bingham. But a win for the victims wasn't a certainty. Britain's courts recognize that government departments, particularly the NHS, have limited budgets, and that giving more money to one patient group would have meant taking it away from another. Rather than criticizing government policy, Graham and the seventy lawyers for the victims needed to prove negligence in how Blood Products Laboratory had been run, both in its failure to become self-sufficient and in its slow introduction of heat treatment.

Overseeing the case was Justice Harry Ognall, a former QC who was best known for prosecuting Peter Sutcliffe, the 'Yorkshire Ripper,' who murdered thirteen women. One morning at the end of June 1990, Justice Ognall made a rare move. The lawyers on both sides were in court for a regular update when he told them he had a note to give them.

'In order not to be misunderstood, I have written it out,' he said, before handing each of the lawyers a copy.

In it, Justice Ognall acknowledged how important this case was. The result would have significant consequences for the NHS, he said, as well as the people who were suffering as a result of their HIV infections. To his mind, there was only one way forward. The government had to be conciliatory: its lawyers shouldn't see this as a legal game to be played in court, but should try to find a settlement that worked for everyone involved. That way, the plaintiffs wouldn't be dragged into a lengthy court battle while their health rapidly deteriorated. And, perhaps crucially, the government would save face.

Graham was stunned. He had never seen a judge push for an agreement like this. *The Times* obtained a leaked copy of the letter and ran a piece about Justice Ognall under the headline 'A Wise Judge.' Seizing on the opportunity, Graham and his team asked the defense for £90 million in compensation for their victims, amounting to almost £100,000 per infected person.

But Justice Ognall's advice had caused a rift in the government. Thatcher thought the particulars of government decision making shouldn't be aired in public, but she also didn't want to compensate victims; she was certain her government hadn't done anything wrong. Her secretary of state for health, Ken Clarke, agreed. He insisted the tragedy was 'no one's fault.' The Department of Health hadn't known of the dangers at the time, he said, so he and his colleagues couldn't have behaved any differently. He fought back against the idea that a settlement was in the government's best interests: paying a vast sum of money when it had done nothing wrong would open the floodgates for no-fault compensation. 'It would have grave consequences for medicine in this country if compensation was paid whenever a patient who had been treated properly by his or her doctors later suffered awful side effects or died,' said Clarke, who feared Britain becoming 'like the American system, where every doctor has a lawyer, and everybody pays huge compensation every time a treatment fails.'

But chief medical officer Sir Donald Acheson urged the government to settle the case, wanting to avoid handing over sensitive and potentially incriminating documents from the 1980s that outlined decisions made by ministers and civil servants as contaminated Factor VIII was imported.

'Senior officials will face an embarrassing public cross-examination when the case reaches trial next March,' wrote Claire Dyer in the *British Medical Journal*. The evidence, she said, would include documents that showed how slow the government had been:

> In 1983 the department received advice from the United States that blood donors should be asked specific questions designed to screen out high-risk donors. Instead, it issued a leaflet asking those at risk not to give blood. Routine testing for HIV was not started until October 1985, although tests were available in late 1984. Heat treatment was not introduced until April 1985.

The *Sunday Times* started a campaign for 'The Forgotten Victims,' calling for an end to the Department of Health's secrecy and revealing that 'a growing number of politicians believe money should be paid without the need for legal action.' One piece told the story of Gerard Hillary, a sixteen-year-old with hemophilia who had passed away from AIDS-related illness in 1989, weighing just three stone. It was a stark reminder of the devastation yet to come for hundreds of people.

With the lawsuit still underway, MPs were applying further pressure on the government to compensate victims. To reduce the heat, Clarke announced the government would give each infected person £20,000, again as an ex-gratia payment, but he stressed that the government still planned to defend itself from the allegations in the lawsuit: 'I don't believe that the Health Service is legally liable for what occurred,' he said. 'It's an appalling tragedy and just a consequence of the spread of AIDS in America and the then-state of knowledge about blood products and the availability of the blood products some years ago.'

Graham Ross and his clients thought the sums of money were too small, given the damage people with hemophilia had been exposed to. He pushed on with the case, planning for an open hearing in court. At the same time, he knew there was a risk the victims could lose. If Justice Ognall ruled this was a policy case, not one of operational negligence, his clients would be left with nothing. It was a high-risk strategy. He knew fault was there, but that didn't necessarily mean he could prove it in law. And time was of the essence. By November 1990 over two hundred people with hemophilia had developed AIDS and one hundred and thirty had died. The number of claimants had risen by some three hundred people to more than twelve hundred.

As the end of 1990 approached, AIDS was still considered a death sentence. When the government rejected Graham's initial request for £90 million, lawyers and experts on both sides knew the claimants were likely to live for only another five or so years – a prognosis that was tragically accurate for the majority of them. On this basis, the lawyers eventually found a compromise. The Department of Health offered an ex-gratia payment of £42 million to victims to settle the case. Thatcher's government wouldn't accept liability and the money shouldn't be considered compensation.

On December 12, 1990, before claimants had even been informed about the offer, the new prime minister, John Major, announced in Parliament that the HIV litigation had been settled. Graham and the other lawyers quickly started calling their clients, some of whom felt coerced into accepting the offer: if they didn't all agree, no one would receive anything. A civil servant in the Treasury later criticized the Department of Health for these underhanded tactics, scrawling on an official document that, 'vexing' as the department's handling had been, 'it turned out as well as (or better than) we might have expected.' But, the anonymous Treasury mandarin added: 'I will however make clear again to the Department of Health that this was no way to do business.'

The British government had succeeded in shutting down further investigation just six years after more than twelve hundred people with hemophilia had tested positive for HIV. The ex-gratia money would be divided between those with HIV and their relatives. Infected children received £21,500, single adults £23,500, infected partners and children £23,500, adults who were married without children £32,000 and infected adults with children £60,500.

Pharmacist Brian Brierley had been loath to settle. He felt betrayed by the medics who had told him his treatment was safe, and he wanted justice. But he knew he was dying. Having once been a large, burly man, Brian had lost so much weight he was barely recognizable. When he went to the HIV litigation meetings with his wife, he could see that he was just one of many victims who were visibly unwell. For them, the three-month wait for a court date could well be too long. He ultimately agreed to put pen to paper and accept the deal. By then, he had pneumonia. Brian passed away at the beginning of 1991, aged forty-nine, still angry at those who had told him his treatment was safe. His share of the money arrived with his widow and two sons six months after his death.

Alcohol had become an anesthetic for Joe. Day after day, he would sit on the sofa, watching television and drinking. Frankie was out of the house most of the time, working four jobs and trying desperately to keep them afloat. While her husband became increasingly despondent, she had to pay the mortgage and look after the house. Joe was dying; she couldn't criticize how he chose to spend his final years, but she had to be responsible for the two of them.

After the HIV litigation was settled, Joe and Frankie went to see their lawyer in Coventry to discuss the final amount they would be due. They were married, but didn't have any children so Joe would get £32,000. With Joe's ill health, they had been falling slowly into debt, getting behind on mortgage payments and having to ask Frankie's parents for help. The settlement money gave Joe an opportunity to put things right and secure their future. In a rare flash of maturity, he wanted his lawyer's help to make a plan for when the money landed in his bank account.

'So what do you think I should do with it?' Joe asked the solicitor, thinking he might offer them some investment advice.

'Spend it,' the solicitor said. 'You're going to die. Has that not sunk in?'

Joe was in denial, living in a senseless limbo as he waited for the symptoms of AIDS to arrive, with no idea when they could hit. The doctor had given him three years, but no one knew exactly when the countdown had begun. He didn't feel unwell, aside from the occasional bleed from hemophilia, but he had lost the drive to live. Rather than investing the money, he and Frankie splurged on a trip to Disney World in America, a Jeep, a tanning sunbed and an early mobile phone that cost £900, even though Joe knew very few people he could call with it.

Joe had grown accustomed to receiving bad news in a blunt, insensitive way. In 1995 his doctor tested him for another chronic virus that he was suspected to have contracted from Factor VIII over a decade earlier: hepatitis C.

'By the way, I have the results – do you want to know?' inquired the doctor nonchalantly.

'Do I need to ask?' replied Joe, who could tell what was coming.

'It's positive,' the doctor replied, before running through some of the symptoms of hepatitis C: fatigue, jaundice, confusion, itchy skin and weight loss. Left untreated, it would slowly attack his liver and could lead to cirrhosis and cancer. But the doctor didn't want Joe to be too concerned. 'I wouldn't worry about it. You have to prioritize things. Your hemophilia is going to come above the hep C. HIV and AIDS is at the top of your list.' In the shadow of HIV, everything else paled.

Despite the doctor's insouciance, Joe had just discovered a second crisis in hemophilia care that doctors and politicians had seen coming. Since the 1970s, groups of specialist doctors had been conducting research into non-A, non-B hepatitis – a new strain of the blood-borne virus that appeared to be more potent and chronic – and had recognized that it was a major cause of liver problems in people with hemophilia. By the time hepatitis C was isolated in 1988, doctors had known for well over a decade that it was more serious than other forms of hepatitis. The first test for it was available within a year but was only licensed in the UK in 1991. Hepatitis C could lie dormant for twenty to thirty years, slowly attacking the liver and causing excruciating chronic pain, as well as itchy skin, digestive issues and mood swings. As the liver degraded, toxins could build up in the blood, affecting brain function and giving people brain fog. When symptoms appeared it was often too late. Long term, people with hepatitis C could develop both scarring on the liver (cirrhosis) and liver cancer.

For the 1,250 people who had HIV, this additional diagnosis was presented as nothing more than a subplot. But across Britain, a new cohort of hemophiliacs were about to discover that, although they had avoided HIV, they had still contracted a life-threatening virus. Nearly every person with hemophilia who had been treated with Factor VIII in the 1970s and '80s tested positive for hepatitis C, up to an estimated five thousand people in the UK, excluding those with HIV who were 'co-infected' with two chronic, potentially lethal viruses. As HIV attacked people's immune systems, hepatitis C was slowly destroying their livers.

The government had made sure this new virus wouldn't cause further legal problems. After Graham Ross and his clients agreed to the settlement, it added an extra clause: claimants had to waive the right to sue again for contracting hepatitis through blood products.

The idea had come from Dr Andrzej Rejman, senior medical officer in the Department of Health. On February 22, 1991, with the HIV settlement agreed but not yet signed, Dr Rejman had a new piece of advice for his colleagues: 'I believe that any that are HIV positive would have to agree not to raise hepatitis in any further litigation.' Dr Rejman knew there was long-standing evidence of the severity of hepatitis C and its prevalence in people with hemophilia. He also knew thousands were yet to discover they had the virus, since, for the past year hemophilia doctors had been testing their patients for hepatitis C without telling them. Almost everyone who had infused unheated Factor VIII, and a similar treatment for hemophilia B called Factor IX, was positive. The doctors chose to withhold this hepatitis data from the Haemophilia Society. Everyone who had signed the settlement in the HIV litigation had waived their rights to take further action over hepatitis C before they knew they had contracted the virus.

Dr Rejman later admitted he had shopped around for expert witnesses during the HIV litigation and asked doctors like Bloom to tone down their witness statements. Lawyers can ask witnesses to clarify details in their statements, but what Dr Rejman did as a member of government shouldn't happen. Senior civil servants in the Department of Health also confessed to one another that their legal case hadn't been watertight. Discussing a way to prevent another lawsuit over hepatitis C in 1995, civil servant J. C. Dobson said they had settled the HIV litigation not because of the 'special plight' of people with hemophilia, but 'on a straight calculation on the balance of risk that the court would in fact have found it negligent if the case had come to trial.'

People with hemophilia had been betrayed by the British government, forced to accept a bad deal on the assumption they wouldn't be around long enough to fight back.

7. Survival

Professor Jean-Pierre Allain considered fleeing the country. If he made it to somewhere on the African continent – to a country that didn't have an extradition treaty with France – then he might escape the inevitability of being sent to prison. His wife, Dr Helen Lee, had been supportive throughout the whole 'ghastly process' and was willing to entertain the possibilities: where he could go, how he would get there and when she could join him.

It was 1993 and Professor Allain was meant to be an internationally respected doctor. He was a professor at Cambridge University, having previously worked at a pharmaceutical company in America and, before that, the Centre National de Transfusion Sanguine, France's national blood transfusion center. He had conducted research alongside his fellow professors Montagnier and Barré-Sinoussi as they discovered LAV. But now he was contemplating the life of a fugitive – on the run from what he thought of as vengeful patients, an aggressive media and a government that would rather string up an innocent person than accept responsibility. There were people out there who wanted him to be locked away for life; who thought he was guilty of far worse than the charges of fraud he was on trial for. In some circles, the words 'poison' and 'manslaughter' were being uttered.

A similar tragedy to that in Britain had unfolded in France, with more than twelve hundred people with hemophilia out of four thousand contracting HIV. Unlike their British neighbors, who had tried to sweep the tragedy under the rug with a legal settlement, the French government had blamed its leading doctors in order to protect itself. Citizens wanted justice. Prison sentences were looking likely. Allain was one of four doctors who had been arraigned for 'deception over the quality of a product.'

Allain maintained that he was a reasonable person who had dedicated his life to his patients. He had treated them with more care than his own children – or so his sons would always say, in a rather back-handed compliment. As seriously as he entertained the idea of absconding – of getting on a plane to the African continent and finding somewhere new to live with Dr Lee – he knew ultimately that it wasn't the responsible thing to do. Allain had to face the French legal system. In his heart, he didn't feel like a guilty man, but he could see from the way the trial was going that the panel of three judges might swing against him. And he would end up in jail.

Allain had always been the kind of person who spoke in a level, considered way; the professorial type. He had a relaxed air, with a ready smile and a glass-half-full outlook. At twenty-six, he had become head of hemophilia at a French boarding school. Like Dr Aronstam, he had cared for a significant number of children, and had pioneered home treatment with Factor VIII in France. After six years at the school, Allain moved to the national blood transfusion center in Paris, where he became head of research and development for plasma products. It was here that the difficulties began.

In the summer of 1983, following reports of Americans with hemophilia coming down with AIDS and noticing signs in some of their own patients, Allain and Professor Jean-Pierre Soulier, the director of the transfusion service, had a suggestion. At the annual meeting of l'Association française des hémophiles, the French hemophilia association, they raised the idea of a temporary return to cryo. Until they understood more about AIDS and the risk of its transmission through Factor VIII, it would be wise to take precautions. But they were met with ardent resistance. The health ministry wanted to continue its Factor VIII drive and patients didn't want to regress to the days of cryo. The president of the hemophilia association encouraged patients to protest if their doctors tried to move them back to cryo.

Later that year, when the first French person with hemophilia developed AIDS, Allain and Soulier launched a major national research project: the AIDS-Hemophilia French Study Group. Around thirty experts joined them, including Montagnier and Barré-Sinoussi, who had recently discovered LAV. They collected samples from more than four hundred people with hemophilia to look for signs of AIDS. Allain wasn't too concerned about the syndrome at that point – none of his thirty patients was showing signs of it – but he was curious to know if something was in their blood. Montagnier and Barré-Sinoussi's discovery of LAV enabled the creation of a rudimentary antibody test and a pattern started to emerge: cryo resulted in lower incidence of antibodies than Factor VIII.

As the study ran into late 1984, Allain believed they had enough information to warn patients about the risk of AIDS and give them their own test results, but his suggestion sparked fierce debate among the researchers. One camp insisted they didn't have enough information – they still didn't know if being positive for antibodies meant a person had recovered from the virus or actually had AIDS. Allain didn't want to leave patients in the dark. When it became clear his side was going to lose, his best friend resigned from the study; if they weren't going to be open with patients, he didn't want to be part of it. Allain wrestled with the idea of resigning himself. He wanted patients to know what was happening, but there were still so many questions to answer and *he* was coordinating the research. After discussing it with his wife, he decided to stay the course. Six months passed before his colleagues finally agreed to inform patients about AIDS and their test results. Unlike doctors in the UK, he didn't give his patients a prognosis. 'Because we didn't know,' says Professor Allain. 'This idea you're going to die in two years is rubbish because it wasn't the case. It's difficult to know what's wrong or right when you don't know the answer. As usual, there are the pessimists and optimists. Typically, I was on the optimists' side.'

French people with hemophilia later criticized doctors for having underplayed their diagnoses, saying it meant they hadn't understood the severity until it was too late, and they had infected their partners or were dying themselves.

The tensions worsened in late 1984, when Soulier stepped down as director of the transfusion service and was replaced by the handlebar-moustached Dr Michel Garretta, a condescending figure whose attitude was contrary to everything Allain represented. Allain had watched with horror that August as Dr Garretta had blown an opportunity for France to introduce heat-treated Factor VIII after causing a row with Immuno. In his determination to get a good financial deal, Dr Garretta had let negotiations for France to access the company's heat treatment technology fall apart. In Allain's opinion, if Dr Garretta hadn't been so stubborn, France could have started using heat-treated Factor VIII by the end of 1984.

When Dr Garretta took up his new role, Allain was insistent: it was imperative they introduce heat treatment. In an urgent letter, Allain told Dr Garretta they had missed a vital opportunity and he needed to reconsider the deal with Immuno. If he didn't, he would be responsible for a swath of people with hemophilia being infected. Dr Garretta finally listened and by October 1985 France was heating its Factor VIII. 'Because of this stupidity we lost six months,' says Professor Allain. 'It shows how damaging emotions can be instead of rationality.' The fight ultimately backfired, though, and in December 1985, after months of hostility, Dr Garretta sacked Allain. Although he won compensation for unfair dismissal, Allain left the French transfusion service and moved to the US. His wife, Dr Lee, had a job at Abbott Laboratories, which had developed the ELISA test for HIV, and it agreed to give him a position, too.

In prioritizing homemade unheated Factor VIII, France's health ministry was responsible for putting people with hemophilia at risk. Although blood was donated in France, its Factor VIII ended up being just as contaminated with HIV as the American version, because blood had been collected in the center of Paris and in prisons throughout the AIDS crisis.

Allain's difficulties with the law had started when he was living in Chicago in 1990. Winter was closing in and he was at work when his phone rang. By now, he was medical director in the AIDS and hepatitis division of Abbott Laboratories and enjoying the relative quiet after his tumultuous final years in France. From his small office, he organized a conference that brought pioneering AIDS researchers Professor Montagnier and Dr Gallo together for the first time. As Allain picked up the phone, he had no idea that the conversation he was about to have would trigger legal proceedings against him.

The caller introduced herself as Anne-Marie Casteret, a French journalist who wrote for the weekly magazine *L'Événement du jeudi*. She told him the French government had in April 1989 agreed to compensate people with hemophilia, but only if they agreed not to sue the blood transfusion service, a sequence of events not dissimilar to those in Britain. Victims became suspicious the government was trying to cover up its mistakes.

'Can I come and talk to you?' asked Anne-Marie.

Allain certainly had material that would help her. When he left France, he had taken copies of internal memos from the transfusion service with him. In one document from April 1985 a colleague had said all of their Factor VIII was infected. Another from that June was from a worried doctor to Dr Jacques Roux, director general of health, which said, 'I am very concerned about the situation in which we find ourselves. We know that every day we are injecting blood products from LAV-positive donors which will cause seroconversion in the recipient, who may in turn infect his family. How many cases of AIDS will we be responsible for in this way?' A letter from July said that unheated Factor VIII 'must be used until stocks are depleted.'

Allain told Anne-Marie he would need to think before agreeing to help. That night, he stayed up until 2 a.m. with his wife discussing whether or not to give Anne-Marie his side of the story. Handing over the internal documents would make him a whistleblower and troublemaker. But his colleagues had shown him little respect throughout the AIDS crisis. Indeed, they had fired him for insisting on what he believed was the right course of action. Dr Lee was more skeptical about Anne-Marie's intentions as a journalist. Thirty years later, when I arrive at the couple's home in leafy Cambridgeshire, she expresses the same reservations: Can I be trusted to tell the truth, or will I misconstrue the events as a scandal? Intermittently throughout my interview with Professor Allain, she comes into the room and says to her husband, 'I don't think you should be doing this interview.' Back in 1990 she had been more certain:

'You need to be really careful,' she warned. 'Don't give Anne-Marie the documents until you know a lot more about what is really happening.'

But Allain was open to the idea of helping his former patients. He felt like he had done the best he could, and he still thought fondly of those he had left behind in France. In spite of his wife's concern, he agreed to help.

Back in France later that year, Anne-Marie wrote a blistering article based on the material Allain had given her, which contained such an explosive account of how slow doctors and politicians had been to react to AIDS that the government was left with little choice but to announce an inquiry. A couple of months later, at the beginning of 1991, a judge who was investigating the case arrived in Chicago to interview Allain and ask for documents he had shared with the journalist. Allain couldn't shake the feeling that the judge had a preconceived notion that doctors had deliberately allowed the infections to happen. He tried to explain that the crisis had been unavoidable, and that doctors had done the best they could with the information available.

Soon after that conversation with the judge, Allain moved to England to take up two new roles: professor of hematology at Cambridge University and head of the East Anglian Regional Blood Transfusion Service. Dr Lee stayed behind in the US and they shuttled back and forth. But his position was more precarious than he realized, because he was implicated in a civil case the judges were building.

At the end of 1991 the French government passed legislation to compensate people with hemophilia who had been infected with HIV with a grant of Fr100 million (£10 million). The maximum each person could receive was Fr2 million (£205,000), which was paid in four installments and treated like a lifetime pension.

Behind the scenes, French prosecutors had been investigating multiple doctors, including Professor Allain, Dr Garretta, Dr Roux, and Dr Robert Netter, head of the French health laboratory. They soon had enough evidence to charge the four doctors with distributing a product they knew to be defective. From March to October 1985, the judges alleged, the doctors had knowingly continued to manufacture and prescribe dangerous unheated Factor VIII. Allain was accused of colluding with Dr Garretta, the person he had fought for two long years, to continue treating patients until older stocks ran out. His efforts to explain to the judge that this was an unavoidable disaster had been fruitless. Although he believed he had done the best he could and was innocent, he now had to prove to his country that he wasn't guilty.

Former Treloar's pupil Stephen had a series of mounting health problems in the early 1990s. He lived with his parents on their pig farm in Norfolk where he had grown up, and where he had brought his best friend, Gary Webster, home in the summer holidays so they could work together for spending money. Stephen was engaged to be married and was busy planning his wedding with his fiancée. He didn't want to admit to himself what was happening inside his body, so he tried to hide it, continuing to make plans for the future behind a mask.

Gary was based in Southampton, where he worked as a tailor, putting to use the skills he had learned in his final years at Treloar's. He had a girlfriend and, like Stephen, was doing his best to forget about the fact that he had HIV. In their late twenties, he and Stephen would still get together with their school friends in the countryside near Treloar's. They would spend long weekends at a friend's house, bringing their partners along and watching motor racing like they had done back in their school days. Together, they could have unencumbered fun, thanks to the deep history they had shared at Treloar's, even making light of their traumatic experiences.

Over the course of those weekends, Gary started to notice that weight was falling off Stephen. His friend had always been bigger than he was, but as Stephen's health deteriorated he was slimming down so much they were nearly the same size. Stephen would tire more easily and found it difficult to join in activities that used to be a breeze for him. Having tried to suppress what was happening, Stephen finally opened up to Gary.

'I think I've got it,' said Stephen, meaning that his HIV had progressed to AIDS.

Not one for outward displays of emotion, Gary responded in the way that felt natural, with gallows humor. 'Join the club,' he said. He, too, was becoming unwell.

Still in their twenties, they were already well acquainted with the pain of going to the funerals of their peers. One of the first was for a boy Gary had started at Treloar's with. The school held an annual old boys' reunion, which Gary and Stephen had initially attended with enthusiasm after they left. But as time went by and their friends passed away in increasing numbers, the reunions became less and less well attended. Eventually, Gary and Stephen stopped going altogether. They found it too bleak.

Stephen's condition gradually worsened. He pulled out of the weekends in the Hampshire countryside with his friends and Gary missed the acceleration of his illness. When Gary received a phone call from Stephen's dad, it came as a shock.

'Steve's ill,' said his dad. 'He's in hospital. He's got pneumonia and he wants you to come up.'

Gary was recovering from an infection himself, so his parents drove him to Norfolk to visit Stephen in the small village hospital where he was being cared for. At his best friend's bedside, Gary tried to find the right words.

'Hey, mate, how are you doing?' he said.

Stephen didn't appear to notice he was there.

They had been through so much together – from staying up late at Treloar's, making calls on the Citizen's Band radio and sneaking to concerts in London, to the terror of receiving their HIV diagnoses. Stephen was the person Gary had spent his summer holidays with. The friend he had moved in with after leaving school. But now they were diverging for the first time in their lives; Stephen's deterioration with AIDS-related illness was moving at a much faster rate.

Gary said goodbye to his childhood best friend. All the while thinking: *That's coming for me.*

Two days later, Stephen's dad phoned Gary to say his son had passed away.

The trial of the French doctors opened on June 22, 1992. In a strange turn of events, Professor Allain was in the dock alongside his former colleague and adversary Dr Garretta, as well as Doctors Roux and Netter. The prosecutor accused them of knowingly infecting patients with AIDS, presenting internal documents from the transfusion service that Allain had handed to them, which showed they had discussed the risks of Factor VIII while continuing to treat patients with it.

Allain and his former colleagues argued they had been dealing with an unprecedented situation and that knowledge of AIDS had emerged slowly. But Professor Montagnier testified that Allain's national AIDS study hadn't followed ethical principles and that doctors had put patients at risk through repeat infections. 'Montagnier was part of the group, one of the leaders in the discussions and co-authors on the papers,' says Professor Allain. 'All of a sudden he decided it was unethical.' Another leading virologist who had lobbied not to tell patients about the risks of AIDS testified against them. Allain couldn't help but think his former colleagues were reframing history to protect themselves. Meanwhile, he also pointed the finger away from himself as the four doctors distanced themselves from one another.

Allain's wife, Dr Helen Lee, took the stand and said her husband had had 'many violent confrontations with management,' including Dr Garretta, as he tried to make the transfusion service change course by informing patients and bringing in heat treatment.

As the trial progressed through the summer of 1992, Allain started to lose faith. Patients he had treated since they were young children turned on him. He had been so close to one family that he and Dr Lee had visited them when they moved to Egypt back in 1984. Of their two sons, one was infected with HIV. The other had avoided infection after Allain managed to give him an early version of heat-treated Factor VIII. The professor found it unbearable to listen as their mother verbally eviscerated him on the stand. When four brothers from another family testified against him, he broke down in tears, feeling betrayed.

Patients condemned the doctors throughout the trial, sometimes shouting 'Assassins!' when the proceedings became too much. The press portrayed them as criminals. To overcome the contradiction between the ostensible care Allain had shown his patients and the seemingly calculated risks he had taken with HIV-infected Factor

VIII, the media decided he was like Dr Jekyll and Mr Hyde. Outwardly benevolent and caring, but behind closed doors a callous villain. The criticism didn't end there. In some circles, Allain was compared to Josef Mengele, the Nazi SS officer known as the Angel of Death for the deadly experiments he conducted on prisoners at Auschwitz. One furious group of activists blew up Dr Garretta's car.

Dr Lee was living in Chicago during the trial, but she flew across the Atlantic as often as she could to support her husband. One of Allain's sons from his first marriage came to the courthouse for just two days, before resolving that he wouldn't watch another minute of the proceedings.

'I don't have to come anymore,' he said. 'I know you're innocent and you're going to be convicted anyway. So why should I waste my time?'

In the face of the vitriol, Allain's nerves frayed. After a particularly forceful session from the prosecutor, he went to a side room and sobbed uncontrollably. He knew the prevailing winds were against him.

'There is nobody as deaf as the one who doesn't want to hear,' said his lawyer, by way of explanation.

Four months after the trial began, France's largest court, the Tribunal de grande instance de Paris, had reached a decision: the four doctors had failed to protect their patients from HIV infection by distributing Factor VIII that was potentially contaminated. Three were found guilty.

'The deliberate nature of the actions of Dr Garretta and Dr Allain and their intent to deceive the victims is amply demonstrated by the investigation,' said the court. 'As physicians, they had greater power to deceive and they disregarded a basic rule of ethics.'

The court held Dr Garretta, Allain's former colleague and adversary, primarily responsible for the HIV infections of people with hemophilia and sentenced him to four years in prison. 'He ignored, thrust aside or short-circuited opponents to his policy,' said the court, referring to how he had delayed the introduction of heat treatment and kept knowledge of AIDS from patients.

The court found Allain had tried to steer Dr Garretta in a different direction, but concluded he hadn't done enough. His attempts to sound the alarm showed he knew the dangers of AIDS, but continued regardless:

> Dr Allain collaborated actively in the policy laid down by Dr Garretta. In his capacity as an expert on haemophilia and as a prescribing physician trusted by his patients, he not only supported but substantiated the lie in their minds. He knew better than anyone the danger of the policy that he not only allowed to continue but actually gave decisive public support to.

Allain was found guilty of four counts of fraud and sentenced to four years in prison, with two years suspended.

Dr Roux, director general of health, was found guilty of failing to challenge Dr Garretta but given a suspended sentence because of his ill-health. Dr Netter, head of the French health laboratory, was initially acquitted, but found guilty on retrial and also given a suspended sentence.

Allain lodged an appeal. He succeeded in overturning three of the four counts against him, but the court introduced three new charges and he was found guilty of each of them. In July 1993 his sentence of four years in prison, with two suspended, was confirmed. And the fines against him were increased.

Having had a sense of what was coming that day, Dr Lee wore her most expensive Armani suit and an emerald ring. She went to say goodbye to her husband, who had sweat pouring off him.

'Courage, grace and strength,' she said tenderly, as she gave him a fistful of money. She knew he was going to need fortitude where he was going.

Allain dismissed the idea of becoming a fugitive and was taken to prison. He felt like a scapegoat. During the trial, a member of his defense team had asked the prosecutor why he had been singled out for charges when so many doctors had been treating patients with hemophilia in a similar way. 'It could have been any one of hundreds,' admitted the prosecutor. Allain had been particularly vulnerable having left France and lost the protections of its medical system.

The health ministry had succeeded in deflecting all blame – for now at least. Allain believed the government was trying to diminish the power of the medical profession and using them as a human shield to do so. A source told him the request had come all the way from the top, from President François Mitterrand. 'It was totally political and preconceived,' he maintains, still seething decades later.

In court, Allain insisted he had tried to sound the alarm and protect people but had been ignored. 'My conscience is completely clear, both morally and professionally,' he said. His assuredness and refusal to show contrition infuriated his patients, who said the punishment was inadequate in the face of their own death sentences. They fought for more doctors to face legal action in addition to Allain, Dr Garretta, Dr Roux and Dr Netter. In one protest before Allain's case in March 1992 a hemophilia campaigner stormed the stage at a blood safety conference along with members of the gay activist group ACT-UP. They handcuffed a doctor they held culpable to a radiator, then threw a bucket of red paint in his face.

In Cardiff just over a fortnight after Professor Allain's conviction, on November 12, 1992, Professor Arthur Bloom died of a brain hemorrhage, aged sixty-two. There was a grim irony to his cause of death, given he had spent much of his final decade saying people with hemophilia could die of a bleed in the brain if they stopped taking Factor VIII. To honor his memory, the University Hospital of Wales renamed his unit the Arthur Bloom Haemophilia Centre. In a tribute to the man who had been Britain's leading hematologist, Dr Ian Peake from the University of Sheffield wrote:

> It was with great sadness that we learnt of the untimely death of Arthur Bloom. I had the privilege of being part of Arthur's team in the University Hospital of Wales for eighteen years, and owe him a great deal.
>
> The change from the halcyon days of the late 1970s, when new products were beginning to revolutionize the life of the haemophiliac, to the despair of the mid-1980s, when the full impact of HIV had become apparent, was devastating to all concerned. To provide balanced advice and practical wisdom in such a time of accusation and uncertainty required exceptional talents, and Arthur had them in abundance.

Arthur will be greatly missed by friends and colleagues alike. He
was a kind and gentle scholar.

To his supporters, Professor Bloom had died prematurely, no doubt
because of the stressful toll the AIDS crisis had placed on him. His
mentee Professor Tuddenham believed he had been a great doctor
and rigorous scientist who was thrust into a very difficult situation.
'Arthur Bloom was given a hard rap,' he says. 'He was in a very invidi-
ous and difficult position.' But those hemophilia – in Cardiff and
across the country – came to disagree. Professor Liakat Parapia, who
had thought Bloom 'fantastic' when he trained under him, felt
betrayed by his guidance on the risks of Factor VIII. 'He and Dr
Peter Jones didn't want to cause panic; they were trying to reassure
patients so they continued with treatment,' he says. 'But it was wrong.
You have to be honest and truthful. And you have to give the right
advice.' Parapia believes Bloom's decisions had terrible consequences.
After details emerged of how Bloom had hidden the dangers of
Factor VIII and advised the government to stay the course, survivors
would convince the hospital to remove his name and bust from the
hemophilia center in Cardiff. 'Professor Bloom has been disgraced,'
says Professor Parapia.

In hemophilia centers across Britain, doctors bore the weight of
responsibility for the AIDS crisis among their patients. They had
procured and injected medication that was now killing people.
Many felt as though they had played a part in landing their patients
in terrifying situations. The guilt followed them. Within a decade
of the first AIDS tests in 1985, half of Dr Tuddenham's patients who
were positive for HIV at the Royal Free (around fifty people) would
die. Even though he was no longer working there, he attended the
funerals of the young men and boys whose lives had been cut short.
Many of the services were conducted by Reverend Alan Tanner,
chairman of the Haemophilia Society, whose own son had been
infected with HIV and passed away. If the horror was yet to sink in
for Dr Tuddenham, those memorial services attended by distraught
parents and brothers, who were often infected, too, brought the
sickening reality home. In April 1991, Dr Tuddenham's co-director,
Dr Kernoff, had a heart attack on the path leading to the grey

brutalist hospital. Aged forty-seven, and due to be married a few months later, Dr Kernoff was left with irreversible brain damage, impaired speech and paralysis in his arms and legs. Later investigations showed no signs of an underlying condition that could have led to the heart attack; everyone believed it was caused by intense stress.

As the death toll among British patients climbed in the 1990s, the years became slow and excruciating. People's T-cell counts would start to drop; they would develop infections; and then decline in irrevocable ways.

Ade lost friend after friend from Treloar's: Ray, Simon, Dave and Sean all died. One boy he shared a dorm room with, Chris, had a milder condition of von Willebrand disease, which gave him heavy nosebleeds. Chris only ever had three Factor VIII infusions, one of which gave him HIV. He died in November 1991, aged twenty. Ade reconnected with his biological brothers, Jason and Gary, but the former died from AIDS-related illness and the latter from a hepatitis C–related brain hemorrhage. When the number of friends he had lost reached forty, Ade stopped counting. But he never stopped thinking about them. Ade, like other survivors from Treloar's, was tormented by survivor's guilt. Before Ray and Dave died, he made them both a promise that would come to dominate his adulthood: he would find out what had happened to them and hold the people responsible to account.

Ade's experience was mirrored throughout the country. In Coventry, librarian Suresh Vaghela and his older brother Praful were both diagnosed with HIV and told they had no longer than six months to live. Unable to cope with the news, Praful ran away from home. Suresh stayed healthy longer than his brother and was able to marry. But when his wife became pregnant, doctors urged her to have a termination. Praful became increasingly unwell and died in 1995, leaving Suresh behind as one of the survivors. Suresh and Praful were among at least sixty-five pairs of brothers who were infected with HIV. Around the time his brother died, Suresh went to seventy funerals for friends with hemophilia in one year.

In Norfolk, John Peach lost his two sons, Jason and Leigh, five months apart in the early 1990s. They had both been to Treloar's, where they contracted HIV. Their deaths when they were in their twenties left John feeling insignificant.

In the Farrugia family from east London, two of three brothers contracted HIV from contaminated Factor VIII. The third brother was infected with hepatitis C, as were two more of their relatives. Four of those five died from complications related to their infections. The Farrugias were one of at least six families in which three brothers contracted HIV and hepatitis.

Under horrific circumstances, young children died leaving their parents grief-stricken. Parents passed away leaving their children orphaned. Lee Turton in Cornwall tested positive for HIV when he was four, and passed away at the age of ten. Lauren Palmer became an orphan when she was nine after her parents, Stephen and Barbara, died eight days apart in August 1993.

Gary Cornes was the first brother in the Cornes family from Birmingham to contract HIV. He sobbed as he told his five siblings that he was going to die. Gary's doctor told him there was a 50 percent chance he would infect his wife if they tried for a baby. They tried regardless – and she, too, became HIV positive. Gary passed away in 1992; his wife died in 2000, leaving behind a young son.

Roy was the second brother to discover he had HIV, a month after Gary was diagnosed. The press discovered Roy had unwittingly infected his girlfriend, who died while he was still alive, and started a smear campaign against him. Hazelwell, their hometown near Birmingham, was nicknamed AIDS-elwell. Photographers from the press hid in bushes at Gary's funeral. When Roy passed away in 1994, people threw stones at his grave and someone spray painted 'SHIT' on it.

Gordon received his diagnosis a couple of months after Roy. Having watched two of his brothers die from AIDS, he passed away in December 1995. The remaining three Cornes siblings, including John and Alan, were infected with hepatitis C. Alan died from a brain hemorrhage on Remembrance Sunday in 2017. John passed away in 2023.

★

Grieving for his best friend, Stephen, Gary Webster went on a mission to destroy himself. The burden of seeing his friends die around him, while awaiting the same fate, completely felled him. He found it difficult to care about living anymore. Depression swept over him and he started to drink heavily. One night when he had been drinking, he decided to take desperate action. He drove his car through a brick wall in an attempt to kill himself. The bonnet crumpled and his ankle snapped. Gary had broken a bone, but he survived.

Within a few years, Gary was seriously ill. Just as Stephen had been, he was hospitalized with pneumonia and diagnosed with 'full-blown AIDS.' Life and his infections were finally catching up with him. But luckily, the treatments were improving. In 1995, with twenty-five thousand people living with HIV in the UK, the FDA approved an antiretroviral drug that worked by preventing the virus from copying itself. Saquinavir was the first protease inhibitor. Within a year, two new antiretrovirals were licensed and in 1996 a new treatment for HIV was born: antiretroviral combination therapy. The life span for people with the illness dramatically improved. Gary began to recover, as did his friends with HIV.

'I was around at the right time and it saved me,' says Gary. 'Stephen and a lot of the others, they got ill at the wrong time, before treatments. It was pot luck.'

Meanwhile, Joe and Frankie had fallen into a pattern: they would sit on their white-and-red-checked sofa and talk about trivialities. It was easier to have inane conversations than it was to confront the reality of what was happening to them. They were still young, only in their mid-twenties, but they were grappling with Joe's diagnosis with a terminal illness, financial struggles and the trauma of Frankie's termination. In 1989 Frankie had become pregnant for a second time and again the doctor told her to have an abortion, which she did.

Frankie had a secret coping mechanism. Every morning, when she left the house for work, she would take off her wedding and engagement rings and hide them. She didn't want people to know anything about her – it was too risky. If they asked about Joe, she could end up letting slip that he had HIV. What if someone showed an interest in their relationship and asked if they had plans to start a family? When a woman at work had recently had a baby, she couldn't engage with her in case she gave away that she knew how agonizing the contractions of labor were, having experienced them during her first termination. The risk of exposing her secret was too high. Instead, she stopped making friends and avoided even the most mundane conversations with her colleagues. She isolated herself from her family, too, feeling unable to tell her parents and brothers that Joe had HIV. It would bring them too much shame. As she withdrew into herself, she became adept at lying. The trauma caused her personality to change. The once uninhibited teenager had become a taciturn and untrusting woman.

Joe, meanwhile, was sinking further under the weight of his illness. His life had taken a different shape from the one he had planned, and he couldn't find the motivation to look after himself. He had lost an opportunity to take a dream job in Las Vegas because his HIV meant that he couldn't get a visa. He bounced from job to job, trying and failing to get back on his feet. If he didn't change something about his lifestyle soon, stop drinking and seek medical help, he could contract a fatal infection. His self-destructive behavior was causing his T-cell count to drop and his HIV progressed to AIDS. He had orchitis and was losing weight fast. But he refused to get help. He didn't trust doctors anymore, so he would go to the hospital as infrequently as possible.

Frankie was slowly breaking down psychologically. She was over-stretching herself to make ends meet, working four jobs to keep herself and Joe afloat. The pressure meant she had been neglecting herself for years. Although she desperately wanted to save Joe, she realized she couldn't fix him. As long as they had each other to rely on, they were both going to keep dragging one another down. So, in 1998, at the age of thirty-two, Frankie made the second most difficult decision of her life. She packed her bags and left Joe. She had to leave, so he would start looking after himself again and so she could prioritize her own health. 'I felt like I was drowning,' she says. 'It was either sink or swim.' Leaving her life behind, Frankie returned to her mum.

It had been a grueling week for Joe when Frankie walked out. Over the weekend, his car had stalled as he drove through a flooded underpass. The doors locked shut. Joe was stuck. He had to clamber out and wade through the floodwater. Abandoning the car, Joe had struggled to a nearby pub and spent the night there in clothes borrowed from the landlord. The car didn't survive the experience. Joe was unwell and became increasingly reclusive as he mourned the end of his marriage. Around the same time, he lost his job at a German engineering company. Within a few weeks, a nurse who visited him at home convinced him to go to hospital. He had esophageal candida, which was a sign his health was spiraling downwards.

'You've probably got about three months to live,' said the hematologist. But there was a silver lining. Joe had so far refused to take any medication for HIV or AIDS, which meant he was a blank canvas as a patient. There were new HIV drugs available that weren't as kill-or-cure as straight AZT had been. He agreed to try Nevirapine and then Delavirdine.

On New Year's Day 1999, around nine months after she left Joe, Frankie went to her friend's house for their annual party. Newly single, she wanted to try and enjoy the day surrounded by people. But she started to feel unwell. Walking home through the streets where she had grown up, a wave of nausea overwhelmed her. Unable to hold it in, she threw up violently. Food poisoning, she thought.

Frankie carried on with her life, going to work at the beginning of January and trying to get back on her feet. But she lost her appetite and had to keep running to the toilet to vomit. She went to the doctor to ask for help and they said it sounded like a stomach ulcer. Despite treatment, the problem persisted. For the next three months she went back and forth to the hospital, trying to find out what was wrong. The doctors were puzzled; Frankie hadn't put two and two together. She grew so weak that she went to sleep one day only to have her brother wake her up saying, 'I need to take you to hospital.' She had been out of it for seventy-two hours without eating or drinking.

At the hospital, the doctor examined her with a grave face. She weighed four stone.

'You've got one of two things wrong with you,' said the doctor. 'You've either got cancer – or you've got AIDS. Do you know anybody that could have AIDS?'

The dots connected. Her T-cell count was just fourteen, compared to a healthy count of five hundred to twelve hundred. She hadn't been tested for HIV for a decade, not since her second termination in 1989; doctors had advised her against it, and the Macfarlane Trust had warned that she and Joe could lose their mortgage and wouldn't be able to get a new one. So she had lived in ignorance. But now she finally knew: she had AIDS. And she had probably been HIV positive for the past ten years. A dark part of her felt like she deserved it. Her brother was out of the room when she received the diagnosis. When he returned, she kept it to herself.

Joe went to the hospital that night to be with Frankie. They weren't together anymore, but he could still be there for her. He contacted the Macfarlane Trust and applied for another ex-gratia payment, this time for infected partners. As he sat by her side, fighting AIDS himself on his new antiretroviral regimen, Joe wondered if life would have been easier for Frankie if she had never met him.

Slowly, with the help of combination therapy, Joe and Frankie started to recover. Living on his own, Joe finally found the impetus to care about his health. His T-cell count was climbing and his infections began to wane. With time, AIDS receded sufficiently that he returned to being HIV positive. Like other survivors across Britain, as he felt better, Joe was able to look beyond his own predicament for the first time in many years. He met other people who had also been infected with HIV and hepatitis C. As he got to know these new friends, they told him their shocking theory about how their infections might not have been caused by a terrible accident, as they had been led to believe, but by deliberate policy. Joe no longer trusted doctors and avoided the hospital as much as he could, but what he was now learning made him question authority even more. These friends told him that doctors, politicians and pharmaceutical companies had known much more about the dangers of Factor VIII than they had ever let on. Hearing this for the first time, Joe decided that he wanted to fight.

PART TWO

The Truth

8.   Mother's Curse

Karen Cross refused to believe the answer her son's doctor had continually given her.

She wanted to know how Brad had come to be infected with HIV. But every time she asked Dr Abe Andes at Tulane Medical Center in New Orleans, he would tell her the same thing.

'It was an act of God, Karen,' Dr Andes said.

'I just can't understand why *God* would do this to me,' Karen said with disbelief.

Karen was barely five feet tall and had the candid manner of a Catholic woman from the Deep South. She was a fourth-grade teacher in Baton Rouge, Louisiana, and her daughter would always say, 'Everybody loves Karen.' But the obstinacy of Dr Andes was trying even her patience.

Karen had grown to accept her son's severe hemophilia A, as had her husband, Gary, a Southern gentleman who counted Brad as his best friend. From six months old, Brad had worn knee pads to protect his joints as he crawled. When he went to school, teachers nicknamed him 'Knee-Pad Brad.' Thanks to the protective layer, his joints were surprisingly healthy for a child with hemophilia. In fact, the Crosses were proud to say Brad never had a bleed in his knee – until he became bedridden with AIDS-related illness. He was a joker who loved playing basketball and going fishing with his dad. His cousins would accuse him of cheating when they played cards but his parents always defended him, retorting, 'He's just a little boy.' When his sister Jennifer was born, he treated her as gently as if she were a doll.

The Cross family discovered Brad had AIDS after he asked his doctor outright when he was ten, having heard the word from friends. Dr Andes had a policy of only telling patients their AIDS diagnosis if they inquired about it. Rather than sharing the news with Brad, Dr Andes had told Gary that his son and his nephew Paul, who also had hemophilia, were both positive – a fact that should be kept within the family. Paul's sister later tested positive, too. Dr Andes warned them not to tell Brad's pediatrician, dentist or school. If the school found out, Karen could lose her job. Paul had begged Karen to keep it from his parents, too.

'You can't tell my momma,' implored Paul, who was nineteen. 'And you can't tell my daddy. *Nobody* can know about this.'

Understanding the stakes of an AIDS diagnosis and the associated stigma, Karen agreed to keep her nephew's secret. Months down the line, when Paul's health was faltering, she couldn't maintain her silence any longer. Karen's sister had quietly hoped that Paul was one of the lucky few who hadn't contracted AIDS, but there were no lucky ones in the Cross family.

Dr Andes initially told Karen that having antibodies for HIV meant Brad could be protected against AIDS – a belief held among some doctors and researchers at the time. But it soon became clear that wasn't the case. Their brown-eyed boy, whom they liked to say 'knew how to smile as soon as he opened his eyes in the morning,' was dying.

By 1991 AIDS was encroaching into their daily lives. Before Brad became ill, Gary had worked as a buyer for Shell, which had a plant outside Baton Rouge. After he decided to be honest and open up to his supervisor about Brad's condition, the company said it was transferring him to Mississippi. Gary knew it was because of the prejudice towards AIDS. He had a choice: move or resign. Given Brad's medical needs, the family couldn't leave Louisiana, so he resigned in protest. Gary sued Shell in a case that cost him thousands of dollars and went all the way to the state Supreme Court, where the judge ruled against him. After losing a second job due to Brad's illness, Gary received a call from someone at a chemical company, which had a manufacturing plant near Baton Rouge. The person said they had heard about his situation and wanted to interview him. When they offered him a job, Gary was enthusiastic: he needed a stable wage and medical insurance to support Brad. But there was a catch.

'This is going to sound funny – and don't take it the wrong way,' said someone in the company's human resources department. 'But as long as your son's alive we can't hire you.'

The terms had a cruel edge, but Gary had been blindsided by his previous two employers and knew how challenging it would be to find work given Brad's condition; at least this company was being up front. Appreciating the honesty, he agreed to wait for his family's situation to change before starting full-time. In the meantime, he worked for them as a contractor.

Brad's health declined as he entered his teens. One day, the school called Gary and said Brad was completely unresponsive – could he pick him up? The family had kept his diagnosis secret from the school for fear Karen could lose her job if people found out. But when Gary went to pick Brad up, the teachers left him to carry his son to the car as they watched without helping. When one family did learn about Brad's diagnosis, they panicked about their children swimming in the same pool.

Brad started to have seizures, which slowly eroded his motor function. With each one, he lost his ability to walk and speak, becoming mentally younger as the years passed. Gary and Karen later learned that HIV progressed to AIDS more quickly in children, because their immune systems weren't fully developed. For his part, Brad was generally uncomplaining. But one night, when Karen went to his bedroom to say goodnight, he opened up to her.

'Mom, we beat hemophilia, didn't we?' said Brad.

'Yes, we did,' replied Karen.

'I don't think we're going to beat this,' he said.

'We don't know that,' said Karen, trying to reassure her son.

'I don't know if I'll ever get married, Mom,' said Brad.

Karen tried comforting him again. 'You don't know that either, Brad. It will be whatever God wants it to be. And we just have to keep going.'

But as hard as Karen tried to keep going, she couldn't align Brad's AIDS diagnosis with her religious beliefs; to think that God had willed this on her family was too cruel. And it wasn't just their family.

Brad was part of a Louisiana summer program founded by parents of children with hemophilia called Camp Wounded Knee. In 1982 they took a photo of forty-five happy kids wearing shorts and baseball caps, including seven-year-old Brad. Attending these meet-ups from the mid-1980s, Karen and Gary discovered they weren't the only family whose children had contracted AIDS. In the following decade, many of the children from Camp Wounded Knee became ill and died. To Gary's knowledge, just one of those forty-five kids survived. There were more than 180 people treated for hemophilia at Tulane Medical Center, the majority of whom were infected with HIV and only a few of whom survived. Karen's niece was among the long-term survivors.

The Cross family were on their way home from Disney World, the last trip they would take together as a family, when Brad developed a high fever. Karen and Gary drove straight to hospital, where Brad was kept in for a month while fighting off an infection. In that time, Karen and Gary made a decision: they had to find out how AIDS had infiltrated their family. They needed a lawyer.

It would be a battle with a lot to lose, even more so than their earlier fight against Shell. But Gary was too angry about what had happened to Brad to be scared of the repercussions. He wasn't one to talk about his feelings. Instead, he wanted to let them out by going after the people who had made his son ill. For Karen, the drive was different. Her genes had given hemophilia – some even called it the 'mother's curse' – and she felt an overwhelming sense of guilt. She needed the truth so she could deflect that guilt away from herself.

The legal practice Mull & Mull lay in the quaint town of Covington, Louisiana, on the other side of Lake Pontchartrain from New Orleans. Its owners, Tom and Lorraine Mull, were a peppy couple who would joke that they didn't have time for breakfast; that was for wimps. They split their time between New Orleans and Hawaii, which offered a mental escape with its vast ocean views and sandy beaches. Tom was a 'cutup' to people from Louisiana, but his time with the US Air Force in Vietnam had left him with post-traumatic stress disorder. One minute he could be joking, the next he was overcome with emotion.

Regardless, his steely, penetrating eyes revealed something of the dogged investigator in him. Tom was tall and blond; Lorraine petite with long brown hair. She was the more levelheaded of the two, approaching law with an analytical mindset and a warm, motherly disposition. Lorraine worked behind the scenes while Tom took the floor in court.

In March 1991 four members of the Cross family – Gary, Karen and her niece and nephew – came to Covington to see them. Gary and Karen seemed earnest as they described how their son, Brad, had contracted AIDS. Hearing how ill their child was becoming, Tom and Lorraine felt deeply moved (like the Crosses, they, too, had a boy and a girl).

'If this was an act of God, I can accept that,' said Karen. 'But if it wasn't, then I want to know who did this – and I want them to pay for it.'

'I will find out,' said Tom, promising that if he didn't think there was a case, he would be honest with them.

Karen's niece was particularly quiet throughout the meeting. She had kept her HIV status a secret from all but close family members; the outside world was hostile. She was terrified that if the news spread to the town in northern Louisiana where she and her husband had their own business, they would be ostracized. Tom and Lorraine had heard stories about young boys like Brad and understood the bravery it had taken for the Cross family to come forward.

One boy in particular, Ryan White, had become a poster child for the discrimination against people with AIDS in the US. In December 1984, aged thirteen, Ryan had been one of the first children with hemophilia to receive an AIDS diagnosis. Having been told he had a death sentence, Ryan had recovered enough within a year and a half to want to return to school. But Western Middle School in Kokomo, Indiana, banned him, saying he had to listen to lessons over the phone. People in his town believed he might infect his classmates and grew concerned about catching it from his paper route. But Ryan's mother, Jeanne, refused to let prejudice spoil the remainder of her son's life and took the school to court. People said Ryan must be gay and that his illness was 'God's punishment,' but he eventually won the right to return to school. The White family moved to a more accepting town, where Ryan got his first weekend job in a skateboard shop and went to prom. He died on April 8, 1990, a month before he would have graduated from high school. Elton John performed at his funeral, which drew more than fifteen hundred mourners, including Michael Jackson and First Lady Barbara Bush. That summer, President George H. W. Bush signed the Ryan White CARE Act, the largest federal program on HIV, which funded treatment for people from low-income backgrounds who didn't have medical insurance.

Tom and Lorraine decided to take on the Crosses' case in a knee-jerk kind of way: they were angry and devastated for the family and wanted to help. The benefits of running their own firm meant they didn't always have to act prudently – and could move fast when they wanted to. They would be taking on the case at their own risk, having to front the costs, and would be paid only if they won. They had recently worked on two successful lawsuits on behalf of patients who contracted HIV from a blood transfusion, so they understood some of the issues at stake. But this was different. Factor VIII was a manufactured blood product and the defendants were part of big pharma: a formidable legal foe. To help, Karen had kept detailed records of every batch of Factor VIII they had injected into Brad. The records immediately caught Lorraine's interest: if they could identify the batch that had infected Brad and find out how it had come to be contaminated, they could be onto something.

Within a couple of months, Tom and Lorraine had filed their first hemophilia case. On May 21, 1991, Brad, Gary and Karen Cross sued Bayer's Cutter, Armour, Brad's doctor Dr Andes and Tulane Medical Center for alleged negligence when making Factor VIII, for failing to warn them about the dangers, and malpractice. Brad knew his parents were taking legal action, but they were careful not to burden him with the details. If news stories about AIDS came on the television, they would casually change the channel. They didn't want him to be consumed by it in the way they increasingly were. He was just a teenager, and they wanted to protect him.

As Tom and Lorraine built the case, they wanted to get more people involved. Size would give them a better chance of having an impact. Tom asked Karen if she knew any other families who might want to join the legal action. She was an active member of the Louisiana chapter of the National Hemophilia Foundation and would regularly attend its HIV support groups, so she could think of at least fifty families to start with. She approached them with news: what had happened to their children wasn't an act of God; someone was to blame. Word spread throughout the community and before long scores of people were approaching the Mulls.

Within a couple of years, the Mulls were representing more than four hundred families from across the US. Among their clients was the Committee of Ten Thousand, a group named after the number of people with hemophilia in the US who were thought to have contracted HIV. (The estimate wasn't far off. Figures vary, but the number of those infected turned out to be some eight thousand of the country's twenty thousand people with hemophilia.) The Committee of Ten Thousand was co-founded by Jonathan Wadleigh, who learned he had been exposed to HIV in 1984 and had lost his brother to the disease within a year. Drawing on the civil rights movement, he had formed it with Tom Fahey in 1989. Tom and Lorraine represented two of its key members: Corey Dubin and Dana Kuhn.

Corey, a radio host in Los Angeles, had been in the newsroom in 1983 when the story broke that people with hemophilia were at risk of contracting AIDS from Factor VIII. Having had one of the first ever injections of it in the late 1960s, he feared his fate was already sealed before he received his own diagnosis.

Dana contracted HIV from his first dose of Factor VIII in 1983, after tumbling over in a charity basketball game in Tennessee and breaking a bone in his foot. He was thirty, married with two children, and was studying at a seminary with the aim of being ordained as a Presbyterian minister. Despite asking for cryo for that first infusion, having heard about the dangers of blood products, he had been given contaminated Factor VIII made by Armour. Dana came down with non-A, non-B hepatitis, then HIV. He wasn't tested for and diagnosed with HIV until 1986, by which time he had already passed the virus to his wife. She died from AIDS-related illness in 1987.

★

Early in their investigation, Tom and Lorraine made a fortuitous discovery. A friend in Hawaii, Charles 'Chuck' Kozak, another lawyer and retired marine, was also working on a hemophilia case. Chuck was representing one of his best friends who had contracted HIV from Factor VIII, and was happy to share his initial research with the Mulls. His sense was that the pharma companies hadn't intentionally killed their customers, but he did believe they had been negligent, particularly when it came to how they collected plasma. If Tom and Lorraine wanted to build a case, Chuck said, their focus should be the source of Factor VIII. He could help with a starting point, too. Through a different case in Hawaii a few years earlier, he had met someone who was willing to become a whistleblower.

Dr Thomas Drees had been the president of Alpha in the critical years when the AIDS epidemic emerged. Alpha was the US division of Green Cross, a leading Japanese pharmaceutical company founded after the Second World War by doctors who had led the country's notorious germ warfare research at Unit 731, where thousands of prisoners of war were experimented on and subjected to surgical procedures before being killed. Dr Drees was far removed from that, as an American with a sharp suit, metal-framed aviator glasses and a PhD in the business of blood banking. By the time he met Tom and Lorraine, he was ready to give up everything he knew and become their first star witness.

Dr Drees believed the start of the wrongdoing could be pinpointed to November 1982, when Dr Bruce Evatt of the CDC had spoken with representatives from the four companies making Factor VIII – Alpha, Armour, Baxter and Bayer. At a meeting of the American Blood Resources Association, Dr Evatt had shared the CDC's findings on AIDS: the illness was always fatal, cases were doubling every month and the CDC believed it was transmitted through blood and blood products. Dr Evatt had suggested the companies could limit the danger to patients by screening out high-risk donors and finding ways to kill viruses in Factor VIII by pasteurizing it with heat or chemicals. That month, the CDC also advised healthcare workers to treat the blood and fluids of patients with AIDS as infectious. Despite Dr Evatt's certainty, none of the companies had put an AIDS warning on their products.

Dr Drees had taken Dr Evatt's warning back to Alpha and immediately tried to implement some of his suggestions. He told his colleagues to start asking donors if they had been to Haiti in recent years or had used intravenous drugs. If they were male, were they gay? Alpha encouraged doctors at plasma centers to look for lymphocytosis, an increased white blood cell count, and started researching how to heat-treat Factor VIII.

On January 4, 1983, the CDC had called another meeting in Atlanta at the government's request, to discuss the transmission of AIDS through blood and blood products. Delegations from the four companies attended, along with the Red Cross, the National Hemophilia Foundation and the FDA. The CDC reiterated Dr Evatt's message about screening. Despite his November warning, Armour, Baxter and Bayer were yet to take serious action. A representative from Alpha said it would screen 'aggressively,' which caused 'a great hue and cry' from the other companies, who said asking such prying questions would violate donors' rights to privacy over their sexuality. Gay activist groups, meanwhile, said screening would be discriminatory towards their members. Someone from the American Red Cross told Dr Drees that Alpha was being 'overzealous.' Attendees demanded more data before they took action. The only people listening in earnest were the few with hemophilia, who asked the manufacturers to try to exclude people who could have AIDS from donating blood. But rather than screening out high-risk donors, the other three companies decided to merely give donors the choice to opt out.

The CDC also made a strong case for the companies to test donors for hepatitis B as a 'surrogate' test for AIDS. The epidemiology of AIDS was similar to hepatitis B in terms of who was contracting it and how it was spreading. Testing donors for that virus could therefore find those most likely to contract AIDS. But the companies were reluctant, concerned about losing too many donors – and the additional cost. Cutter was the only company to start running these tests in the middle of 1983, but within a few months it had stopped without explanation, which Dr Drees attributed to the fact that none of its competitors was doing so. Tom saw that as a clear red flag.

At that meeting in Atlanta in January 1983, Dr Don Francis, an epidemiologist at the CDC and head of its AIDS task force, had lost his temper. He had a gravelly voice and thought of himself as a quiet scientist who had dedicated himself to the fight against Ebola in the 1970s, then AIDS. But the manufacturers of Factor VIII had raised his blood pressure. He slammed his fist on a table and shouted, 'How many people have to die? How many deaths do you need? Give us the threshold of death that you need in order to believe that this is happening, and we'll meet at that time and we can start doing something.' As a public health agency, the CDC didn't have the power to compel the companies to act. And the FDA, which regulated blood products, chose to offer guidance rather than directives, such as advising them to temporarily pause plasma collection from gay men.

Before the year was over, Dr Drees had been forced out of Alpha. His superiors at Green Cross said he was too aggressive in screening donors. Dr Drees told Tom that when he left Alpha in November 1983, no Factor VIII manufacturer had put a warning about AIDS on its products, nor had they educated doctors and sales forces about the risks. Dr Drees believed warnings should have been issued immediately in late 1982.

Hearing about that critical meeting in Atlanta, Tom and Lorraine knew who else they needed as a witness: Dr Francis. He had helped them with their earlier transfusion cases, so they had an in. Dr Francis had led the CDC's AIDS research from 1981, when the first signs of gay-related immune deficiency emerged. Along with his CDC colleague Dr Evatt, Dr Francis had been one of the first people to state that AIDS was transmitted by an infectious agent in blood. From July 1982, on seeing those first three cases of PCP in people with hemophilia, they had believed AIDS was blood-borne. Right then, Dr Francis said, they had agreed that 'if our children had hemophilia, we would not have given them Factor VIII at all, but would have gone back to cryoprecipitate.' Having left the CDC to focus on HIV vaccine research, Dr Francis was now free to testify in trials. And he was scathing of the four companies who made Factor VIII. He believed they had been reckless – and that the AIDS epidemic in the hemophilia community was preventable.

Tom and Lorraine went to San Francisco to meet Dr Francis at the offices of O'Connor, Cohn, Dillon & Barr, the lawyers representing Cutter. He tried to stay calm throughout, but there was one moment when the mask slipped. Looking at the defendants' lawyers, Dr Francis said:

> I wouldn't be involved in this if I thought that the companies represented here were aboveboard in trying their best to maximize the safety of their product – and minimize the risk of AIDS transmission. I see it as important, maybe for me personally, to be critical of them when there are obvious steps they could have taken, which they did not take, and which were not huge steps in terms of cost.

Following the meeting in Atlanta in January 1983, Dr Francis said he had urged everyone to act. He wrote a letter to all parties saying he felt there was a 'strong possibility' there would be many cases of AIDS in people who had been treated with Factor VIII in the next two years. His summation was stark: 'For haemophiliacs, I fear it might be too late.' If the T-cell counts of people with hemophilia were an indication, then as many as a third to half of them may have already been exposed, even though only eight cases had so far been confirmed. 'Despite this grim picture among haemophiliacs, we should do our utmost to prevent further exposure,' wrote Dr Francis. He suggested pharma companies should exclude all potential donors who were intravenous drug users, sexually promiscuous, had had sexual contact with someone from either of those two categories in the past two years, had lived in Haiti in the past five years, or had tested positive for hepatitis B. He said they might lose 5 percent of donors, but there was 'good evidence' this screening could eliminate over three-quarters of those who had AIDS. It would add around $5 to the cost of each unit of blood and plasma. 'These seem to be small prices for preventing a serious disease and a potentially dangerous panic,' he said. In the meantime, Dr Francis advised, people with hemophilia should *only* be treated with Factor VIII made from the blood of less than a hundred people – or return to cryo.

'I understand these recommendations will be controversial and that there will be objections by industry and blood bankers,' wrote Dr Francis. 'However, to wait for their approval of our recommendations will only endanger the public's health.'

His suggestions were not heeded by the companies or the FDA, which regulated them. And people with hemophilia were left in ignorance. It wasn't until February 1984 that all the companies had finally put AIDS warnings on their products. Most patients were never told about the potential risks or given the option to change treatment.

Dr Francis now told the lawyers that the problem had gone all the way to the president. Ronald Reagan's administration was 'terrible' in its handling of AIDS – 'and we all know that,' he said. Reagan had only mentioned AIDS publicly for the first time in September 1985, allowing Congress to finally approve $190 million for research into the disease. As reticent about addressing the epidemic as Thatcher, Reagan gave his first speech about AIDS in May 1987. Dr Francis was willing to testify that under Reagan's free market capitalist ethos, the FDA had given pharma far too long a leash to self-regulate the safety of its products. Although the CDC had advised the FDA to force companies to screen donors and introduce hepatitis B testing, it hadn't done so. The regulator had been toothless and left the responsibility solely with the industry. And even though the companies had known Factor VIII was infectious, first with hepatitis then with the virus that caused AIDS, they hadn't taken steps to screen donors or kill viruses.

Speaking directly to the lawyers for Cutter and Armour, Dr Francis added that their clients had been 'very narrow-sighted and ultimately led to not only a lot of death and misery, but a destruction of your customers.' (Dr Francis maintained this view, later calling them 'doofuses' and 'the evil people.' 'The thousands of people who died really without any reason are just a negative tribute to their dullness and lack of response,' he said in 2017.)

During Dr Francis's six-hour deposition, the opposing lawyers accused Tom of 'trashing it up' and denigrated the other employees who worked with the Mulls as their 'sidekicks.' Tom and Lorraine were two years into their eleven-year fight against the pharma behemoth, and they were already getting used to the adversarial stance of the defense lawyers, who saw their small-town outfit as beneath them. But with the pivotal testimonies of Dr Drees and Dr Francis, they now had evidence that Cutter and Armour had neglected to make their products safe by failing to exclude high-risk donors and introduce hepatitis B testing. And they had a date to which they could pin their case, from when they could argue the negligent behavior had begun: late November 1982, after the meeting with Dr Evatt at the American Blood Resources Association.

Among the wealth of documents Dr Drees shared with Tom and Lorraine was a videocassette. Its contents would form the centerpiece of the puzzle they were starting to piece together. The film was rough and gritty, but Tom could see it was revelatory. For the first time, he was looking inside a factory where Factor VIII was manufactured. The video showed Alpha's whole process from start to finish. Bottles of plasma were loaded onto a conveyor belt, which was lined with workers wearing protective clothing that made them look like astronauts. The tops of the bottles were sliced off as they traveled down the belt, then their contents emptied into a massive stainless-steel barrel. One by one, thousands of plasma donations were poured into the same barrel, which could hold around five thousand liters. The liquid looked like pond scum, thought Tom, with its greenish tinge.

The plasma was spun at a high speed to separate the cryoprecipitate, which then went through a process called fractionation to divide it into its constituent parts: the layers of proteins that all had different properties. There was albumin, immunoglobulins and clotting proteins. Albumin was a protein made in the liver, which could be used to treat low blood volume and help people with burns, major injuries and liver disease. Immunoglobulin is another word for antibodies, or proteins that the immune system needs to fight off viruses and infections. Some people are deficient in these and require plasma products to boost them. The final layer was the clotting proteins, which included factor VIII. As part of the manufacturing process, the factor VIII was packed together in the shape of a cake and freeze-dried, which gave it a powdery consistency. The powder was bottled into glass vials, labeled with stickers and placed into medical boxes.

Another whistleblower from Alpha shook her head when she saw the video and said to Tom, 'High-school science. Nothing but high-school science – and they couldn't even get that right.'

She told Tom a batch of Factor VIII could be made with plasma from around five vats, each of which contained some five thousand donations. So any one Factor VIII injection could contain the blood of twenty-five thousand people. But Dr Drees said there was, in fact, a much bigger range, with small-batch Factor VIII containing the blood of ten thousand people, all the way up to the FDA's limit of one hundred thousand donations. Only one donor needed to be infected for the whole batch to be contaminated.

Watching the footage, Lorraine grew scared for herself. She had received multiple injections of an immunoglobulin product called RhoGAM, or anti-D, when she was pregnant with their two children. It was a standard procedure given her blood was rhesus negative to prevent her body from attacking the fetus. But albumin and RhoGAM were some of the last proteins to be extracted, by which point the plasma had been treated with chemicals that killed viruses. Factor VIII was in the first fraction – and it wasn't pasteurized with heat or chemicals.

If Tom and Lorraine had had a wall chart with arrows connecting the different parts of their investigation, this video would have gone in the middle. Tom had expected the process of making Factor VIII to be clean and sanitary, but this video made it look sloppy and dangerous. The vats were open-topped and unprotected. He could see so much room for abuse. But the detail that was most revealing to him was the hazmat suits worn by the workers. Those had been adopted in the early 1970s after fourteen workers in one plasma processing plant contracted hepatitis B from their work. 'They thought it was dangerous enough to put their employees in moon suits,' says Tom. 'That was shocking to me.'

Dana Kuhn, one of Tom and Lorraine's clients, had been widowed after his wife died from AIDS-related illness in 1987 and was left to raise his two children alone. Before reaching his mid-thirties he had moved back to Richmond, Virginia, so he could be near family for help. He found a job in the local hospital as a clinical counselor for people with hemophilia, many of whom had HIV. Being HIV positive in the American South wasn't easy, and he was grateful to have found a community where he could be honest without facing stigma.

It was through this work at the hospital that Dana would discover how he had come to contract HIV and hepatitis C in the first place. He was in his office in 1991 when a doctor he worked with placed a box of documents on his desk.

'If you're going to be counseling people, you probably need to know the story behind it,' said the doctor.

Dana already knew an obvious mistake had led to his and his wife's infection with HIV. On March 4, 1983, the CDC had said blood products 'appear responsible for AIDS among hemophilia patients.' Three weeks later, on March 26, Dana had his basketball accident and asked to be treated with cryo. But the hospital had given him Factor VIII contaminated with HIV and hepatitis C. It had then failed to offer him a test until 1986, by which time he had passed HIV to his wife. But with the documents in this box, which contained the doctor's detailed records of the AIDS crisis in hemophilia as it had unfolded, Dana would learn there was a much more complicated story behind their infections.

Dana took the records home with him. He was often unwell in those days because of the new treatment he was taking for hepatitis C, Interferon Alfa, which was notorious for its side effects. On sick days, he leafed through the documents. Placing them into chronological order on the floor of his living room, he started to learn exactly what doctors, the government and the National Hemophilia Foundation had known – and when.

In 1981 the foundation had declared bankruptcy and been restructured so that 45 percent of its funding came from the companies that made blood products. It had then continuously downplayed the dangers of AIDS to people with hemophilia, telling them to keep using Factor VIII even as the evidence against it mounted. The foundation had published its first patient alert in July 1982, a week after the CDC reported on three cases of PCP in patients with hemophilia, but it had spurned the opportunity to raise the alarm, instead using the alert to say that the risk was 'minimal' and people should continue with their treatment. When Baxter issued its first recall of Factor VIII in August 1983, the foundation had reaffirmed that nothing should change. The advice continued in 1984 when 72 percent of a sample of people with hemophilia tested positive for HTLV-III, and again in 1985 when further recalls occurred.

Throughout that time, the FDA had been equally impotent. Dana found evidence of a revolving door between Factor VIII manufacturers and the FDA: there were people from pharma who served on FDA and blood advisory committees; some of those now regulating had worked in the industry; and there were a few who had promises to return to the companies after their stint in government. Dana thought this must explain why the companies had never lost their licenses to make and sell unheated Factor VIII, even after the dangers became clear.

As he dug deeper, Dana struck up a correspondence with Dr Michael Rosenberg, an activist in California who had co-founded the Hemophilia/HIV Peer Association and who had more evidence of pharma company neglect. Between them they collected enough material to understand the oversights that had caused their infections. Completing the timeline that had started on his living-room floor, Dana concluded that all parties knew what was happening – the companies and the National Hemophilia Foundation had blatantly lied in order to convince people Factor VIII was safe long after they had evidence to the contrary. The FDA had failed to force the companies to withdraw their contaminated products from the market and let them continue selling a dangerous version of Factor VIII when safer ones were available. They had all traded lives for profit, manufacturing high-risk Factor VIII while keeping the dangers from patients; the government, pharmaceutical companies and National Hemophilia Foundation had all been part of the conspiracy. He put together a 350-page document titled *The Trail of AIDS in the Hemophilia Community*. The story revealed how avoidable the infections were, as well as who was responsible. He hoped it would be the catalyst for a government investigation and ultimately new safeguards 'to ensure that this iatrogenic catastrophe never happens again.'

Dana printed and bound ten copies in 1993 and sent them to members of Congress. But first, he shared his findings with the National Hemophilia Foundation, where he was on the board of directors.

'How can we sit here and do nothing?' he asked the other members.

But they were reluctant to hear him out, not wanting to draw public attention to the link between HIV and hemophilia because of the stigma surrounding AIDS.

That year, Dana became the third person with hemophilia in the US to go public with his HIV diagnosis. Ryan White had been the first, Ricky Ray the second. Ricky had been diagnosed with HIV alongside his two brothers, Robert and Randy, in Florida. The three boys, all under ten, were shunned by their church and banned from Memorial Elementary School after people found out about their diagnoses. The Ray family sued DeSoto County School Board over the decision to keep their children from school. They endured threats from people in the community. Ricky won the court battle at the age of ten, but a week after he returned to school his family home was burned down in an arson attack. Luckily they were out at the time, but they were forced to move. Ricky died in December 1992 of multiple organ failure, aged fifteen; Robert died a few years later, aged twenty-two; Randy lived until 2023, when he passed away, aged forty-three.

Dana's life had blown up after his wife had died, leaving his children without a mother; he felt like he had little left to lose by revealing his illness, especially since his colleagues at the hospital already knew he was HIV positive. On National Public Radio, he shared what he had discovered. 'I want the truth to come out,' he said.

After he had been on the radio, Dana's phone didn't stop ringing. Some callers were abusive, some – not least the National Hemophilia Foundation – were angry. But Dana found support in unlikely places. One day his children were on the school bus when some kids said, 'You can't sit next to them; you'll catch it from them.' The driver pulled over and spent a couple of minutes educating the kids about HIV.

'I never want to hear this mentioned on our bus again,' the driver said.

With the National Hemophilia Foundation unwilling to help, Dana got in touch with Corey Dubin at the Committee of Ten Thousand and asked for its help in taking the evidence he had amassed in 'The Trail of AIDS' to Congress. Their efforts got the backing of the chair of the Senate Health Committee, Ted Kennedy, and Secretary of Health and Human Services Donna Shalala, triggering a two-year investigation by the National Academy of Sciences' Institute of Medicine. By then, Ricky's mother, Louise Ray, had begun lobbying politicians in Florida for a bill to support people with hemophilia who had contracted HIV. The two campaigns collided productively, creating momentum for a federal law called the Ricky Ray Hemophilia Relief Fund Bill, which would recognize the harm caused by the so-called 'wonder treatment.'

By 1992 Brad Cross was bedridden and his parents had to feed him through a tube in his stomach. Gary and Karen were used to injecting him with Factor VIII, but giving him three meals a day via a syringe felt degrading for both him and them. They set up an at-home hospice in their den, which was next to the kitchen, so Brad could remain at the center of their lives. He had a mechanical bed that filled with air to regularly alter his position in the hope of preventing bed sores, but he still developed painful sores on his hip and coccyx. At any given time, there were a dozen drugs laid out on the coffee table next to him, including the high dose of AZT he was taking. For Gary and Karen, caring for Brad was full-time work on top of their jobs. They would go to sleep at 1 a.m. and wake up around four hours later because of the stress of looking after their sick child – a habit they are stuck with today. On the rare occasion when they slept through the alarm on Brad's feeding machine, his eleven-year-old sister, Jennifer, would turn it off herself so her parents could sleep. When the sun was shining, Gary would carry Brad to the garden and cradle him as the sun beat down on them. Brad's muscles had wasted away, his thin teenage body wrapped in an adult diaper.

Brad was mostly unresponsive, because of how AIDS had attacked his brain. Sometimes he moaned in pain and Jennifer would sit with him for comfort. Medical staff tried to encourage Gary and Karen to move him to a nursing home for their own sake, saying he didn't know where he was, but they knew that wasn't true. They could see Brad's eyes follow them around the room. When they told him they loved him, they saw it reflected in his eyes. There were times when he cried and they knew he was in agony. One day, Gary and Karen were discussing the things they needed to put in order before the day they were all dreading came. When Gary next looked over at Brad, he had his middle finger in the air. 'It was like he was saying, "I'm not ready,"' says Gary.

Tom and Lorraine Mull met Brad for the first time when they were passing through Baton Rouge. Seeing their first client lying in the den, consigned to his mechanical bed, brought tears to Tom's eyes. He must have been expecting to see Brad sitting up and talking, thought Gary, not lying in the fetal position. Until then, Brad had been a four-letter word in their mountain of paperwork, ripe for projection.

'Oh my God,' said Lorraine. 'We are so sorry.'

'Brad, we're going to do what we can for you,' said Tom, before turning to his parents. 'Karen, I wish I could say I'm gonna come back and visit, but I can't. I can't ever see Brad like this again.'

Tom might not have been able to cope with seeing Brad again, but meeting Brad strengthened his and Lorraine's resolve to work around the clock. They went on to visit their other clients at home, many of whom were in similar situations. Because of the healthcare costs and the limits to what insurance companies would cover, many families ended up putting hospital beds in their living rooms and caring for their children themselves. Family life played out under the shadow of death. 'They slowly waste away in front of your eyes, day by day,' says

Tom. 'And it takes a year; it's not just a few weeks or months. And this just blew us away.' With a sharp exhale, he adds, 'Still does.'

On April 16, 1993, Brad was struggling to breathe. His carer called an ambulance and his family made their way to the hospital. They were joined by friends who wanted to see Brad one last time. His pediatrician came in his golf clothes, having left the course as soon as he heard the news. Brad held on until his sister, Jennifer, joined them from school. Karen and Gary told their son how much they loved him, then let him know it was OK for him to go. As he took his final breath, aged seventeen, his parents held him. Brad had been 5ft 6in tall when he was first laid in the mechanical bed; he was around 6ft when he left it for the last time. A teenager who had kept growing even as life escaped him.

A week after Brad's death, Gary started the full-time job he had been promised at the chemical company. He was grieving, but he needed to earn money for his family. Work would have to fill the space left by his son.

Karen decided it was time to be honest about Brad's battle with AIDS after he had passed away. She wasn't ashamed of her son and she wanted the world to know how a medical treatment had ripped a hole in her family. The majority of teachers and parents at her and Brad's school were supportive, but there were a few who were angry: she should have told them because of the risk.

'I'm sorry,' Karen replied. 'I didn't think it was that important to you. You didn't have any contact with my son.'

To this day, she feels guilty that Brad didn't receive the support that should have been afforded to a child dying from a vicious illness. 'If he'd had cancer, oh my gosh, he would have been treated wonderfully,' she says. 'There wouldn't have been any questions. People would have been like, "What can we do?" We didn't have that support. That was one of the hardest things.'

Six months after Brad's death, the Cross family joined the Mulls at the Civil District Court in downtown New Orleans for the first day of their trial against Cutter, Armour, Tulane Medical Center and Brad's consultant there, Dr Abe Andes. The case now included alleged wrongful death. To Gary and Karen, it felt like their son had been murdered.

Tom and Lorraine knew the odds weren't in their favor and it would be a feat to achieve the closure the Cross family were desperate for. They wanted to learn how their son had come to be infected, and to seek retribution. At that point, at least eleven similar cases had gone to court and people with hemophilia had lost all but one, which was then overturned on appeal. Karen and Gary's case was one of a ballooning number of lawsuits. Over a thousand cases would end up being filed against the pharma companies, with some seven and a half thousand people with hemophilia taking legal action. Many states had laws that shielded manufacturers of blood products from no-fault liability claims, meaning those suing would have to prove the companies had taken risks that made their products dangerous or defective, not just that their products had contained viruses. They needed to show that Alpha, Armour, Baxter and Bayer had failed to act when they could have to make their products safer (by testing donors for hepatitis B, screening out those at high risk of AIDS and introducing heat treatment). But to win, they would also have to identify the specific batch and brand of Factor VIII which had given them HIV. That was incredibly difficult when there were multiple brands and most patients had infused Factor VIII hundreds of times.

The National Hemophilia Foundation warned its members in 1989 how difficult it would be for them to win lawsuits. Someone with mild hemophilia had just won a case against Cutter by proving they had been infected by a batch of its Factor VIII that was recalled after a donor died from AIDS-related illness. The jury found Cutter at fault, because it hadn't screened out high-risk donors after January 1983, and awarded the family $1.6 million. But the judge overruled the jury's verdict, saying Cutter hadn't needed to start screening until March 1983, when the FDA had mandated it, and that the person could have contracted HIV from another company's Factor VIII. The National Hemophilia Foundation cautioned its members: that case had been unusually strong because the person had mild hemophilia and had only infused Factor VIII on a handful of occasions.

And yet they had still lost. People who had infused many times would find it even more difficult to prove.

Lorraine still believed the facts were some of the most outrageous she had seen. How could such a strong case not be winnable? Gary secured their trial with a plea to Judge Max Tobias. 'Brad was my best friend,' he said.

On October 4, 1993, the courtroom was packed with supporters and other affected families. Outside were a gaggle of journalists who had come to report on this significant AIDS case. But Judge Tobias quickly silenced the Cross family, agreeing to a gag order that prevented them from speaking to the press until the case concluded. The only way to raise awareness for their cause was for other families to share their stories.

Ever since her son's death, Karen had worn a red ribbon made from rhinestones pinned to her breast. Cutter's lawyers argued that Karen and her family shouldn't be allowed to wear anything reflective of AIDS; it could influence the jury. To Karen's amazement, Judge Tobias agreed and she had to turn the pin around, hiding its significance. Throughout the trial, people with hemophilia came to court to support the Cross family whenever they were in New Orleans for treatment at Tulane Medical Center. When someone entered the courtroom on crutches, the defense lawyers objected. The absurdity peaked when a boy with AIDS was made to remove his T-shirt, because of the message printed on it: I WON'T BE SILENT ANYMORE. I HAVE AIDS. AND I WON'T GO QUIETLY. The T-shirt was scanned into the court record. The boy was also one of Tom and Lorraine's clients and later died from AIDS-related illness. 'I grew up with all these boys,' says Jennifer. 'And then they all just died.'

Tom and Lorraine's case hinged on the negligence of the defendants. Cutter hadn't screened out donors or tested them for hepatitis B. And it had then exacerbated the risk by collecting plasma from high-risk sources and pooling thousands – in many cases tens of thousands – of donations.

Cutter's lawyer, Duncan Barr, defended the company by saying hardly anything was known about AIDS before Brad seroconverted in December 1982. It hadn't known AIDS was caused by a virus, let alone that it could be transmitted in Factor VIII. The product was 'unavoidably unsafe'; the company couldn't have improved it and its benefits outweighed the dangers. 'This was a tragedy that happened through no fault of anyone,' said Barr.

The case ultimately boiled down to a narrow question: Had a specific batch of Cutter's Factor VIII infected Brad with HIV? The Mulls would have to prove it had for Cutter to be at fault. A gay man in Austin, Texas, had sold his plasma forty-eight times from November 1982 to September 1983, when he developed AIDS. Tom argued the blood bankers should have known the man was at high risk of contracting the illness and stopped him from donating. Cutter had recalled the batches of Factor VIII containing this man's blood in November 1983, which for Tom was an admission of a problem. Before it was recalled, Brad had infused it on six occasions. Tom argued it was one of those infusions that infected Brad. But Cutter's lawyers said retrospective tests of Brad's blood showed he had already seroconverted with HIV by December 1982, long before he infused that contaminated batch.

What was supposed to be a two-week trial dragged on for six weeks, becoming the longest civil court case in Louisiana at the time. Gary took unpaid leave from work, which crippled his family's finances. At the start of the trial, believing it would be a short trip, the Crosses stayed in the second most expensive hotel in New Orleans, which had a white-columned entrance and Grecian statues. In the second week they downgraded to a Sheraton, then a Holiday Inn, before ending up in a $39-per-night 'fleabag' hotel near the airport by the end of the trial. In the courtroom, Gary and Karen endured a painful revisiting of history, grueling questions and an attempt by the defense lawyers to accuse them of 'contributory negligence' for allowing Brad to have the experimental AIDS treatment AZT.

Tom persisted. With the help of his witnesses, he laid out the facts of what was known about AIDS in the crucial year when Brad was infected, and how Cutter had failed to take action to make its product safer. But he couldn't go into as much detail as he wanted. Judge Tobias accepted the defendants' objection to Dr Drees as a witness:

his PhD was in business, not science, so he couldn't be used as an expert witness on the making of Factor VIII. He could only speak about the business side of Alpha, and he couldn't hypothesize about how Cutter had acted. In keeping with the companies' hopes, Dr Drees's testimony became so narrow that it missed the crux of the wrongdoing.

Cutter called on prominent hematologist Dr Louis Aledort to highlight how little doctors had known about AIDS before the virus was isolated and a test became available in 1984. Dr Aledort had been a hero during the golden age of plasma products, according to Michael McLeod of the *Orlando Sentinel*. He was medical director of the National Hemophilia Foundation and had successfully lobbied the government to provide more funding for hemophilia centers. He had also been 'closely aligned' with Cutter, which had given him funding for research and paid him for many years to edit a monthly journal for people with hemophilia. Dr Drees said Alpha had also paid him $25,000 a year for research. Dr Aledort was one of those doctors who had forcefully downplayed the AIDS risk. In May 1983 he had said the danger was 'completely unclear' and there was 'no evidence' AIDS could be transmitted in Factor VIII. Two months earlier the CDC had concluded that blood products appeared responsible for cases of AIDS in people with hemophilia.

'Hindsight is great, but we had to make logical decisions based on the information we had at the time,' Dr Aledort later told McLeod.

In the 1990s, Dr Aledort became a regular expert witness on behalf of pharmaceutical companies in the trials against them; and was on a 'shame list' of doctors the hemophilia community believed had betrayed them. The list's author, Dr Rosenberg from California, called Dr Aledort the Josef Mengele of the 'haemophilia holocaust.' An outraged Dr Aledort retorted that a mob mentality wouldn't help anyone. Gary believed that Dr Aledort had been bought out, plain and simple. By the end of the decade, the doctor had earned hundreds of thousands of dollars as a consultant and expert witness for Alpha, Armour and Cutter. Tom had evidence they had paid him $320,000 from 1991 to 1994, with him receiving more consultancy fees every year until 1999. In 1993 alone, Cutter and Armour paid him a total of $130,000. Karen started to think the doctors had been more financially driven than even the pharma companies.

In the trial, Dr Aledort testified that it was reasonable to discuss a possible link between AIDS and blood products from December 1982, but the benefits of Factor VIII had outweighed the risks. He said medical consensus of how AIDS was transmitted hadn't come until 1984, when HTLV-III was discovered. When Cutter recalled the batches of Factor VIII in November 1983 containing the Austin donor's blood, which could have infected Brad, Dr Aledort claimed the company couldn't have known for sure that the product was dangerous.

For Dr Francis, claiming that the risk of AIDS hadn't been known until the discovery of HTLV-III constituted willful ignorance. The Pasteur Institute in France had found LAV in late spring 1983, and although it had taken a year to establish it was the virus that caused AIDS, the CDC had evidence as early as July 1982 about the risk to people with hemophilia, when the first three patients had developed PCP. The spread among those with hemophilia quickly mirrored the overall epidemiological curve, Dr Francis said.

The trial had not gone to plan for the Cross family. Judge Tobias issued a directed verdict that dismissed Armour from the proceedings. Brad had infused two lots of its Factor VIII that were later recalled, but there was no evidence they contained HIV, he said. When the jury eventually reached its verdict, they found that Cutter was not responsible for Brad's infection with HIV and Dr Andes had not breached care standards in his treatment of Brad. Tom and Lorraine had failed to convince the jury that Cutter's negligence in allowing the man from Austin to give plasma despite being a gay man at high risk of AIDS had led to Brad's infection.

The Crosses were devastated. Karen was too numb and exhausted for tears, but her sister and the dozen other mothers of sick and dying children who surrounded her all broke down. That moment was the first time Jennifer saw her dad cry. After the verdict had been delivered, Gary and Karen noticed one member of the jury laughing. 'It was such a disappointment to find our legal system was so corrupt and could be manipulated so easily,' she says.

One of their mistakes, Karen and Gary later reflected, was suing Tulane Medical Center. It had a reputation of caring for the people of New Orleans, so targeting it had worked in Cutter's favor. Years later, after Tom and Lorraine uncovered more evidence about how the pharmaceutical companies had behaved, Brad's doctor, Dr Andes, realized he had been deceived about the safety of Factor VIII and agreed to help with their next case. But Karen and Gary remained angry with him. 'He knew us, he watched our children grow up,' says Karen, and yet he hadn't warned them about the risk of AIDS. Gary wanted Dr Andes to go to jail or have his medical licence stripped. Neither happened, but when Dr Andes was offered a job at another hospital, Gary phoned them and explained how many children had died at Tulane under his watch. He still got the job.

The Cross family returned home with their grief, to the empty space Brad had left behind.

Tom and Lorraine might have lost their first case, but the trial had set off a chain of events that would ultimately unravel the line of infection that had killed Brad – and thousands like him.

9.   Poisoned Lines

In the course of the twentieth century, plasma gained a nickname: 'liquid gold.' Thanks to a boom in advanced surgery and medical treatments, the trade in this human resource became so profitable that plasma was more valuable than gold and oil. By the 1990s, the contents of a 160-liter barrel of processed crude oil would have been worth $42. The same amount of blood, divided into constituent products including plasma and the proteins within it, was worth $67,000. As a result, the plasma industry was worth more than $18.5 billion each year.

The industrialization had begun during the Second World War. As blood was shed on the battlefield, the Allies had a secret defense strategy. Dr Edwin Cohn, a researcher at Harvard University, discovered how to separate plasma into its constituent parts. One of these was albumin, which was stored as a powder that could be mixed with water to help soldiers recover from trauma injuries. The Allies quickly realized it carried a risk of hepatitis after outbreaks in the field, but it nevertheless became a savior of wounded soldiers.

After the war, the commercialization of blood took off. Plasma and its products became vital for medical advancement. New plasma treatments, including Factor VIII for hemophilia, brought increased demand. And so began the plasma boom. American blood bankers were allowed to pay donors for plasma and they went in search of ever more lucrative supplies. The largest center was in Nicaragua, nicknamed the 'House of Vampires,' which collected plasma from up to a thousand people per day. In 1978 the press connected the death of a donor there to dictator Anastasio Somoza, sparking the Nicaraguan revolution. These were the 'wildcat days' of plasma. Blood bankers collected plasma in Haiti, Nicaragua, Mexico, Colombia and the Dominican Republic, then shipped it back to the US. With this, the US became 'the OPEC of plasma.' 'We were supplying the world with plasma,' says Douglas Starr, author of *Blood: An Epic History of Medicine and Commerce*. According to the president of one pharma company, there was a time when the US imported more plasma than bananas from Costa Rica.

Within a few short decades, this natural fluid within the human body had become a vital commodity. Plasma was a billion-dollar industry and the people who dealt in it became rich. But with money came an all too common by-product: exploitation. As the AIDS crisis developed, the World Health Organization stopped one company from opening a new plasma plant in sub-Saharan Africa, where cases were ballooning.

'It was a giant moneymaking industry,' says Tom. 'And God, they just didn't want to give it up.'

In the years after losing Brad's case in 1993, Tom was left chewing over a detail Dr Drees had given him about where the pharma companies had sourced their raw material. Dr Drees had said companies that made Factor VIII, including Alpha, had collected plasma at Louisiana State Penitentiary, known colloquially as Angola. From his earlier work as a public defender, Tom was well acquainted with the notorious prison. In court, Cutter had insisted its plasma came from safe sources. The company's former president Jack Ryan said they had sourced a small amount of plasma from prisons, but not in Louisiana. Then Gary got a new lead. At church, someone told him about something similar to what Dr Drees described: that blood was being collected from inside Angola. Around the same time, a local news story revealed a hunter had found a collection of needles and plasma bags buried near the prison.

Tom decided there was only one way to find out who was telling the truth: he would have to go there himself. He drove to Angola with an initial plan of speaking with the editor of the prison newspaper and the guards. He was shocked by what they told him, even though he had been investigating this issue for years. Inside Angola there had been a plasma center where prisoners could give plasma twice a week in exchange for cash to spend in the canteen. Plasma donation was popular among the inmates, who exceeded five thousand people, because it gave them a day off from their arduous jobs in the field as well as good money. At $15 per bleed, or $30 a week, plasma donation was a lucrative business. A carton of Camel cigarettes cost around $6, meaning bleeders had easy access to this valuable prison currency. Elsewhere in the prison, people were paid just a few cents per hour to farm cotton, corn and other vegetables, as well as make coffins in the prison workshop, clean the dormitories, or cook for their peers.

Tom was alarmed to learn that what Dr Drees had alleged was true: pharma companies had been collecting plasma from people in prison. He wanted more details, such as who ran the center, what safety measures they had in place, and whether its donors were more high risk than those on the outside. But the guards were reluctant to speak on the record, let alone testify – they were scared of losing their jobs.

Returning home, Tom knew he had barely scratched the surface of what sounded like an industrial operation inside the Louisiana prison. When he told Lorraine, she felt the color drain from her face. Cutter had insisted under oath that its plasma was safe and that it didn't collect blood in prisons.

Tom was able to pry small nuggets of information from the prison guards, but what he really needed was to speak to inmates who had donated plasma and were willing to go on the record. Thanks to the prison newspaper, *The Angolite*, word had been spreading that Tom wanted information for a case he was working on. One day, he received a letter from Camp C.

'Dear Sir,' wrote David Grillette. 'While reading my paper I ran across an article about tainted donations of blood plasma from Louisiana State Penitentiary.' David explained that he had used intravenous drugs since he was young and that he had contracted hepatitis B sometime around 1983. At the time, he wrongly thought he had been sick with hepatitis A, an acute but short-lived form of the illness. It wasn't until 1991 that he discovered his blood contained antibodies for hepatitis B. Throughout that time, David had been a plasma donor. Although he was not aware he had hepatitis B, staff in the prison and its plasma center had known from the time he started donating, because it was in his medical records.

'My point is, they knowingly let me donate blood plasma with hep B,' said David. The staff also knew about his drug use, 'which makes the plasma people that much more at fault. If someone has become ill because of it, I feel awful, even though it was beyond my knowledge.' By the time he was writing to Tom, David knew he should have never become a plasma donor. But back in 1983 those who understood the dangers had failed to warn or stop him.

Soon after that letter to Tom, another followed. David had shared news of the legal case with fellow inmates. 'I'm writing on behalf of the lawsuit you are putting together,' wrote Richard Vincent. He explained he had been one of Angola's 'bleeders' – the hundreds of men who gave plasma twice a week in the prison – and knew how it worked because he had briefly had a job in the center. He was willing to share his experiences. 'Let me know what I've got to do.'

Tom sought permission from a judge to return to Angola to speak with Richard. Within a couple of months, he was driving to Angola again with his associate Fran Phares. In the prison, Tom and Fran were led to a private room, surrounded by armed guards. Richard was brought in, handcuffed. He had a strong brow and eyes that were more likely to scowl than smile. The hours spent working in the exposed sun had tanned his skin. Richard told Tom and Fran he had first been imprisoned in Angola in the late 1970s, aged twenty-one, after being convicted for burglary. His young adult life had been a revolving door of sentences in Louisiana's prisons and jails. He would be released, then wind up back inside for another burglary. Twice he had managed to escape from prison; on one occasion hiding out for over a year.

Tom asked Richard to run him through the process of donating plasma in Angola. To start with, Richard explained, you had to get an inmate who was already a bleeder to put you on a list of donors in the plasma center. Then, you had to have a short physical exam. 'If it took four minutes it was too long,' said Richard. The doctor asked two questions: Had he had a tattoo in the past six months and had he ever had hepatitis? He answered no to both, even though he did have a number of tattoos, including a peacock, a skull and a spider. They had the rough style of penitentiary tattoos.

'What are penitentiary tattoos?' asked Tom.

'You make a tattoo gun with a motor, a tape player, an ink pen and a guitar string,' said Richard. 'And you get the tattoo ink and somebody who knows how to put tattoos on.'

It didn't sound very hygienic.

'Did you give plasma during the time period when you were receiving these tattoos?' asked Tom.

'Oh yeah. When I went and took my physical, I had got a spider over here,' he said, pointing to his right arm. But the doctor 'didn't never see it, because he never made me take my shirt off.'

Richard wouldn't test positive for hepatitis B and C until years later. But even if he had known he had those viruses at the time, he could still have become a bleeder. He knew people who had turned yellow, then carried on donating. One way was to bribe the inmates who worked in the plasma center with cigarettes.

On his 'plasma day' – when he was due to bleed – Richard would get a 'call out' along with scores of other inmates who would be joining him. Security guards checked their names on a list, then they boarded a bus that would amble across Angola's sprawling grounds to the plasma center. That day, they got a break from working in the fields. The center was in a concrete building with a tin roof. Inside, there were metal hospital beds where the bleeding would take place, as well as bathrooms, a waiting area and a holding cell. Around the room, people in prison uniforms busied themselves. When Richard and the other bleeders arrived at the center, an inmate would check their identification cards against names in a folder. They would then join the long line of people waiting for their turn on one of the metal beds.

Before donating, Richard went through the rigmarole of having his blood pressure taken by an inmate. Those who were 'cool with the guys' who worked in the plasma center didn't have to go through the routine. 'It was just checked off that you was all right,' said Richard.

'You referred to the guys who worked in the plasma center,' said Tom. 'Who were these guys?'

'This is inmates,' replied Richard, without hesitation.

'Inmates actually staffed the plasma center?' Tom asked.

Richard nodded. 'Inmates pricked your finger, inmates gave your blood pressure, inmates pulled your record, inmates cleaned the thing on your arm where you was going to get stuck,' he said.

The whole operation was run by inmates with no medical training. A civilian would insert the needle into the bleeder's vein. After that, incarcerated people – who were easily corruptible by fellow inmates – took the blood, placed the bag on the plasmapheresis machine to separate the amber plasma fluid from red blood cells, returned the red blood cells to the donor for reinfusion, then put the bags of plasma in storage freezers. For this work, they were paid around $3 per day.

In one bleed, inmates filled two bags, which were sized depending on their weight. Richard was a slight ten stone, so he gave two small bags. Open from early morning into the evening, the plasma center would collect donations from as many as a hundred inmates every day. The process was uncomfortable – a journalist writing for *New York Magazine* in the 1970s said it felt like being impaled with a car antenna. He wrote that he got an electric ping in his heart and then felt every beat as the blood was sucked out of his vein.

Nevertheless, plasma day was a welcome reprieve for those in Angola lucky enough to become bleeders. On the bus and in the center, bleeders could socialize with friends who were housed in other blocks of the prison, briefly escaping Angola's regimentation and the prying eyes of security guards. Some used the opportunity to take drugs; others got into fights. Richard told Tom he had seen people shooting intravenous drugs while they waited to donate, safe in the knowledge that no one would check them for track marks. He didn't personally inject drugs – he preferred snorting heroin and cocaine, or smoking marijuana. But drugs weren't the only plasma center vice.

'It wasn't nothing to see people in the bathroom having sex before they go on the table to bleed,' said Richard.

'In the plasma center?' asked Tom.

'In the bathroom, yes,' said Richard. 'They're having oral sex and anal sex, then five minutes later they're on the table giving blood.'

If the guards caught people having sex in the plasma center – in what was known as the 'honeymoon suite' – they would remove them from the donor list. But it was an open secret that they could easily bribe their way back in if they were friendly with the inmates who worked in the center.

Seriously concerned by what Richard had told him, Tom quizzed the guards again. They confirmed the account. At one point, the plasma center had become so lawless they had removed the doors from adjoining bathrooms so it wouldn't be abused so readily. Still, sex and drug use had continued. It was one of the few places in the prison where inmates could get away with it.

Each day, Angola's plasma center collected a couple of hundred bags of plasma. Inmate workers placed these into large storage freezers until the fortnightly collection, when they would be loaded onto a truck. From that point, Angola's inmates had no idea what happened to the plasma. As Tom spoke to Richard and David Grillette, he realized they had been kept in the dark about how their plasma had been used. When they found out it had harmed people on the outside, they were devastated.

'They told us the plasma was being used for cosmetics for women,' said Richard. 'Never that they're making this kind of pill or whatever. It was never told to us. It was about makeup, eye shadow, mascara and stuff for ladies.'

'Had you at any time been told that this plasma you were selling was being used to make a product that young children would infuse into their veins, would you have sold your plasma for that purpose?' asked Tom.

'No, I wouldn't have,' said Richard.

'Why not?'

'Because I don't want to hurt no one, not thataway,' he said. 'I've hurt people by stealing from them and I feel the pain. So I can imagine what it is for someone to lose their child or their husband or their wife thinking that this doctor is helping them – and the whole time the doctor is killing them. I wouldn't do it.'

After he was released from Angola, Richard was jailed in a smaller Louisiana prison that didn't have its own plasma center. But that hadn't stopped him from donating: the prison ran a regular bus service that would transport inmates to a plasma center in the nearby town. Throughout the 1980s, Richard had continued to donate. When he was imprisoned at Angola again in the early 1990s, he became one of the lucky ones who worked in the plasma center.

When Tom relayed all this detail back to Lorraine, she felt physically sick. The idea that companies had been taking plasma from Angola to make a medical treatment was unconscionable. Their clients had been so courageous in the face of this enormous tragedy that had befallen them. And yet here was evidence the companies had been totally reckless with their lives, then lied about it. 'It changed my whole view on pharmaceutical companies,' says Lorraine. 'The sheer greed of it, corporate profits above the safety of these kids.' For Tom, it was outrageously irresponsible. They were furious on behalf of the Cross family and their other clients.

Tom learned the center at Angola was run by a private company called Louisiana Biologics, which turned over millions of dollars in profit by selling plasma collected from inmates in Louisiana, Tennessee and Florida. When plasma left Angola, it was taken to a manufacturing plant in Glendale, California, which was owned by Baxter's Hyland. In the early 1980s, up to a quarter of the plasma processed at Glendale came from prisons. It was then used to make Factor VIII and sold around the world.

Angola was far from being the only prison in the US where private companies harvested plasma. There were FDA-licensed plasma centers at prisons in Arizona, Arkansas, Florida, Mississippi, Nevada and Tennessee. Bayer's Cutter paid the state of Arizona $12 per week for each inmate who worked in the plasma center in its main prison. The center was open for twenty years before finally closing in 1987.

In Arkansas, a blood banking company called Health Management Associates sold bags of plasma collected at the Cummins Unit prison for $50 each, having paid inmates $7 per donation, according to the *Encyclopedia of Arkansas*. The operation was mired in corruption and poor supervision, which allowed people with HIV and hepatitis to donate plasma. Two investigations in 1985, one of which was initiated by Governor Bill Clinton, found Health Management Associates had violated its state contract in dozens of ways. Some inmates had been paid for donations with drugs rather than money.

But even after the results of that investigation were released, Health Management Associates kept its license for another year, in part thanks to its president Leonard Dunn's successful lobbying of Governor Clinton. In 1990 Dunn worked on Clinton's gubernatorial reelection campaign, revealing just how much political influence he had earned as a blood banker. When Arkansas finally closed its prison plasma center in 1994, it was the last state to do so. A year later, in 1995, the FDA formally recommended all companies stop the collection of plasma from inmates, by which time it had already been brought to an end voluntarily.

The dangers of prison plasma were evident in the high rates of hepatitis and HIV behind their barbed-wire fences. Intravenous drug use, penitentiary tattoos and sex between inmates all increased the spread of viruses. In 1997 an inquiry in Canada revealed just how lethal prison plasma was: Factor VIII made with plasma collected in Arkansas prisons had infected more than a thousand Canadian people with HIV and some twenty thousand with hepatitis C. In France, where blood was also collected in prisons, donations from incarcerated people accounted for 0.37 percent of transfusions, but were responsible for 25 percent of HIV infections.

Viruses from inside Angola's walls traveled down the road to Baton Rouge, and thousands of miles away to the British countryside, infecting people indiscriminately. As Tom learned more about the lines of infection, he started to look at Factor VIII in a whole new light. He now thought of it as a 'fatal poison described as medicine.' Life expectancy for people with hemophilia in the US had plummeted from fifty-five in 1982 to forty in 1990.

When Tom and Lorraine told their clients what they had discovered about Angola, the words they heard back were unrepeatable. Parents screamed, cried and cursed. 'They were angry beyond belief,' says Tom. But there was a small comfort: they now knew that what had happened to their children wasn't their fault. There was nothing they could have done to protect them. 'The guilt these poor mums had was just impossible,' says Lorraine. 'It was such a head snap to have given this genetic problem to their children, then infused them with poison. This wasn't drunk driving; it was like a mass shooting.

It was so egregious. So when we found this out, it gave them a place to put their guilt and anger.'

Karen felt her preconceptions shatter when she heard how pharma companies had been collecting plasma inside Angola. She had thought the blood for Brad's Factor VIII was collected through donation drives at churches and local grocery stores, from conscientious citizens who wanted to help. *Stupid me,* she thought, even though she could never have predicted the truth. Both she and Gary were haunted by the fact they had injected such a toxic treatment into their son.

Tom and Lorraine continued to dig and they soon found the low cost of prison plasma wasn't the only reason it was so valuable.

Mull & Mull was being held together with duct tape and chewing gum; Tom and Lorraine had to mortgage their home twice to fund their investigation, under a near-constant threat of bankruptcy. Everyone around them was dedicated to the operation, with clients themselves helping dig through documents and contact potential witnesses. But they needed deeper pockets and more hands on deck, so they decided to enlist another law firm to work alongside them.

Michael Baum might have won multimillion-dollar legal battles against large corporations, but he was still the type of Californian who preferred to wear a beaded necklace and unbuttoned shirt. One of the partners at Baum Hedlund Aristei & Goldman, he had resources the Mulls were desperately lacking: a large team and plenty of money.

The new team agreed to divide the workload. Tom and Lorraine had leads to follow in Louisiana, while Michael would focus on plasma collection elsewhere. If they were to prove negligence and fraud, they needed to show not just how companies had taken risks in making and distributing Factor VIII, but also exactly how that behavior had caused the death of at least one of their clients. The second part was where previous cases had fallen down.

Michael knew about plasma collection on Skid Row in Los Angeles. It was common knowledge that blood bankers had recruited people living in poverty to become regular donors. Court documents had shown some centers allowed people with track marks to donate if employees believed they hadn't used intravenous drugs in the past six months. And he had heard gay men were reliable donors because of the community's sense of civic duty. But he discovered companies had taken mobile plasma trucks into cities like Miami, New York, and LA then parked outside gay nightclubs and encouraged people to donate in the middle of the night. Some had bought recovered plasma from sexual health clinics in those same cities. 'It was as if all these haemophiliac kids and adults who were depending on Factor VIII were sharing needles with intravenous drug users and prisoners during one of the worst epidemics of blood-borne diseases in history,' says Michael.

Reading through documents from the pharma companies, Michael's team saw a reference to adverts that had been used to attract donors. It gave one of their clients with hemophilia, Charlie Bryant, an idea. What if the companies had explicitly advertised in magazines whose readers included high-risk donors? Charlie and his wife, Kay, were happy to go and find out. They traveled the US and combed through copies of local newspapers and magazines from the early 1980s held in library archives. They eventually hit a treasure trove in San Francisco: a back catalogue of *The Advocate*, a premium national magazine for the gay community. In the middle of each issue were a few pages of classified adverts that contained listings for things like sexual hypnotherapy, colorful underwear, poppers, screening for sexually transmitted diseases – and plasma donation. They saw an advert from Alpha, surrounded by phone numbers for sexual health clinics, which asked for healthy adults to donate plasma to help trauma patients and people with hemophilia.

But Charlie and Kay soon spotted a different pattern. One advert contained a sketch of a man's flexed, muscular arm, and a call to readers:

We need a few good arms!
Have you ever had hepatitis? Have you ever been in contact with hepatitis?
Now you can make it pay as much as $650 extra each month. And at the same time, you'll be helping to contribute to the health

and welfare of other gay men. HOW? Your blood plasma contains various amounts of antibodies or antigens which are used in research and the production of a new vaccine against hepatitis. A simple hour and a half procedure, whereby we'll extract your valuable plasma, is all it takes to not only put money in your pocket, but help other gay men as well.

SO, DO YOUR SHARE!

The advert contained details for a donation center run by Trimar Hollywood Inc., located on Sunset Boulevard, LA. Michael later discovered that that center had collected some of the most lethal plasma in the world. Charlie and Kay found similar adverts posted from 1980 until December 1982, after Dr Evatt had his first meeting with the companies about AIDS. Gamma Dynamics offered free hepatitis and syphilis testing as part of its drive to find people who were positive for hepatitis. Baxter's Hyland said, 'Give life, give plasma, help stamp out hepatitis B.' But Alpha's adverts were the most explicit:

CHANCES ARE, YOU'VE GOT HEPATITIS – OR WERE EXPOSED TO IT

If you're an active gay, you have an extremely high chance of getting hepatitis. This disease can cripple you for months. It can hurt you, and everyone around you for a lifetime. It might even kill you. Yes, hepatitis is a serious disease. But now there is something you can do to stop it.

HELP DEVELOP THE ANTI-HEPATITIS VACCINE

At Alpha Plasma Centers we are collecting plasma for use in the hepatitis vaccine that may one day stop hepatitis dead in its tracks. You or anyone you know who's had hepatitis can help in our research.

Charlie and Kay photocopied the relevant pages and took them back to the offices of Baum Hedlund Aristei & Goldman. Seeing them, Michael realized the pharma companies hadn't just taken a chance that their donors could have hepatitis B; they had actively recruited people who had tested positive for the virus, because they wanted their antibodies for vaccine research. And at the same time as these adverts ran – as the pharma companies went to STI clinics and nightclubs to collect plasma – the first signs of a new illness were beginning to appear: gay-related immune deficiency, or GRID. Michael knew that meant the plasma was highly likely to contain not just hepatitis B, but also HIV. He needed to find out if this infectious plasma had been used to make Factor VIII – and if the companies had taken additional risks with safety once they learned about AIDS in 1982.

Michael had a line to Dr Drees, who had been head of Alpha when these adverts had run. Dr Drees said plasma from the gay community had been used to make hepatitis B immunoglobulin, an antibody treatment that could protect people from the virus in the short term, which had been chemically treated so it didn't contain live virus. The plasma wasn't meant to be used to make Factor VIII, said Dr Drees, but it had been. Because when the level of hepatitis B antibodies in a donor's blood had dropped too low to be useful for immunoglobulin, that person was added to the general pool of donors. Alpha had knowingly collected plasma from people with hepatitis B antibodies and poured it into those stainless-steel vats Tom and Lorraine had seen in the factory video, infecting not just patients but also lab workers. 'To make it cost effective and make a profit, they dumped all these donors into the same vat,' says Michael. 'Those viruses were going straight into the arms of hemophiliacs.' The company knew doctors accepted hepatitis as a risk of the treatment. But it quickly emerged those donors with hepatitis B had the highest risk of contracting AIDS – and by the time the danger became clear, many of them would already have been HIV positive.

Confirming what Dr Drees had said, Michael found an internal Cutter letter from the end of August 1982, which described how it used this high-risk plasma to make Factor VIII. John Hink, Cutter's director of plasma procurement, wrote, 'Until recently Cutter's [hepatitis B antibody positive] plasma (all collected from centers dealing predominantly with homosexuals) has been used in the manufacture of coagulation products,' which included Factor VIII. He added that their competitor Hyland sold its hepatitis B plasma to Alpha, rather than using it to make Factor VIII.

Michael noticed something else surprising in this letter. A month after the CDC had published its report in July 1982 on the first three cases of PCP in the hemophilia community, Dr Dennis Donahue, director of blood products at the FDA, had asked Cutter and its competitors to 'voluntarily exclude plasma collected from known homosexuals' from Factor VIII. Dr Donahue had not based 'this request on scientific concerns that such plasma transmits AIDS,' Hink reported to his colleagues, but because he believed 'the action is a political necessity to prevent national adverse publicity and undue concerns in the haemophiliac population.'

Here Michael could see Cutter had discussed the dangers of high-risk plasma with Alpha and Hyland as early as the summer of 1982, and that they had together agreed to temporarily exclude donors with a history of hepatitis from their Factor VIII, 'for political, moral and liability reasons,' according to Hink. Cutter and Alpha asked the FDA to make the commitment voluntary because a formal request could 'have political repercussions, could be difficult to amend, and would ultimately create concerns and problems with both the homosexual and haemophiliac populations.' With that small concession, the companies succeeded in keeping the situation under wraps. Five months later, when they met with the CDC in Atlanta, those same companies refused to start screening out high-risk donors and testing them for hepatitis B. Michael believed this was evidence that Cutter hadn't been interested in making Factor VIII safer, but merely in protecting its reputation. And the risks the companies took with hepatitis had continued as the AIDS crisis emerged, though with more deadly consequences.

In another internal memo from December 1982, Cutter's head of regulatory affairs Steven Ojala said the company had reviewed its use of prison plasma. He stressed that Dr Donahue of the FDA had told him 'the actual risk was less important than the perceived risk.' At the start of 1983, an employee responsible for buying plasma for Cutter, including from prisons, wrote a note saying there was 'strong evidence to suggest that AIDS is passed on to other people through plasma products.' By March Cutter had paused the use of prison plasma in Factor VIII, but it continued to spread confusion about

AIDS. In June it had told the UK's Department of Health it was 'unclear' whether people with hemophilia had contracted AIDS and that it was 'only an assumption' it could be transmitted 'by certain blood products.'

Even as companies stopped using plasma from prisons, sexual health clinics and AIDS hot spots to make new batches of Factor VIII, they continued to sell that which had already been manufactured. 'They had a lot of plasma in warehouses that they didn't want to give up using, because it was expensive,' says Michael, referring to stocks collected before 1983. 'If you imagine taking thirty thousand donors from San Francisco during the height of the AIDS epidemic, a few of them are going to be HIV positive no matter how much screening you do – and they knew that.'

When Michael told Tom and Lorraine about the adverts and letters from Cutter, something clicked. This was evidence of negligence: Cutter and Alpha had known their product was dangerous because of hepatitis, had targeted high-risk donors, then sold it without a warning to customers. 'That was the big "Aha!" moment,' says Lorraine. 'I've always thought it was criminal that they were using this plasma source without doing anything to remove the viral load in it.'

Dr Kay Noel struggled to remember the exact moment it dawned on her that she needed to leave the plasma business. It might have been when she sat at the kitchen table of a family who had just lost their child to hepatitis as they asked her to pay $1,000 towards the cost of the burial. Or it could have been the successive occasions when other families made the same request. Dr Noel had rarely faced anger from these bereaved parents; they just wanted support and to know Alpha cared. But every time marketing manager Dr Noel requested the money, it was denied. Ultimately, it was Alpha's culture of indifference towards hepatitis in Factor VIII that had given her the push she needed. No matter how many times she raised concerns about the virus with her colleagues, they had been noncommittal. They claimed it wasn't possible – or necessary – to remove hepatitis from their product. The risk was both inevitable and accepted. In her mid-thirties, Dr Noel turned down a career-defining offer to become vice president at one of Alpha's rivals, and moved into biotech.

Dr Noel had joined Abbott Laboratories in her twenties, in 1974, as a researcher looking at the first hepatitis B test and immunoglobulin treatments. Within four years, Alpha acquired the division she worked in and Dr Noel moved away from the laboratory and into marketing, frustrated by a lack of interest in her research. Dr Noel was remarkably outspoken in the pharma business; if she saw a problem she would raise it with her colleagues. She thought of herself as a fearless busybody, which made for a volatile combination once she concluded her colleagues were neglecting their customers' safety.

Her initial concern was hepatitis B. 'The companies wanted to use every drop of plasma for every product they could,' says Dr Noel. 'And therein was the problem.' She believed Alpha should warn its customers of the hepatitis risk in Factor VIII and be transparent about where they were collecting plasma. But her colleagues disagreed. They were knowingly putting people at risk and it didn't align with even basic moral standards.

Dr Noel's concern had deepened with the emergence of another strain of hepatitis. From the mid-1970s, hemophilia doctors had noticed their patients were contracting a new form of the liver-attacking illness, known as non-A, non-B hepatitis, which appeared to be more virulent and chronic. Dr Noel thought Alpha should invest time and money into killing viruses in Factor VIII, given how prevalent they appeared to be. After all, other plasma products went through pasteurization with heat and chemicals. When her suggestion was met with resistance she sent papers about non-A, non-B hepatitis to people high up at the company, but they ignored her. There was consensus among her peers and bosses that the factor VIII protein was too unstable to withstand high temperatures: the process would kill too much of it. Some research showed as much as half of the proteins would be destroyed by heat. Alpha wanted its research to improve yields, not reduce them. Added to that, her colleagues said, their initial studies had shown heat wouldn't kill non-A, non-B hepatitis. And given that their customers – the hemophilia doctors – continued to believe the benefits of Factor VIII were greater than the risks of an unidentified virus, Alpha and its competitors were able to maintain the status quo.

Dr Noel decided that she couldn't be associated with this any longer. The companies knew they had a problem with their product, but weren't interested in fixing it – and she couldn't sit across the kitchen table from any more bereaved families.

Dr Noel left Alpha in 1981, the year that the first cases of GRID appeared. Hearing the early reports in people with hemophilia, she thought AIDS must be transmitted through blood. Her attempts to mitigate the catastrophe had failed, because her colleagues refused to listen to her.

When Michael Baum contacted Dr Noel more than fifteen years later to ask if she would assist with the case he was working on, she was willing to lay it all out. As a disillusioned insider, she could help in two ways: she had important background on how the companies had reacted to hepatitis, and she had the key to unlocking their legal case.

Case after case was being fought – and lost – across the US. The avenues of investigation were plenty. Tom, Michael and Lorraine were working on the 'dangerous donor theory,' which they believed showed the four companies had been negligent. In New Jersey, a lawyer called Eric Weinberg was constructing a case around 'bad science,' looking into how they had underinvested in killing viruses in Factor VIII before AIDS emerged. The sluggishness that had incensed Dr Noel was just a fraction of what Eric had found.

Eric's case had begun in much the same way as Tom and Lorraine's, when a woman walked into his office in 1991 and told him she had recently lost her husband to AIDS-related illness after contracting the virus herself. Eric spent the first year poring over books and research papers to gain a detailed understanding of the science behind Factor VIII. He constructed a timeline that showed how pharmaceutical companies had known about the viruses in plasma products more than twenty years before Factor VIII was first released – but still hadn't done anything to make it safer.

In July 1945, as the Second World War was coming to an end, Captain Emanuel Rappaport from the US Army noticed a pattern in soldiers who had developed jaundice after battlefield transfusions. Those treated with plasma that contained blood from up to fifty donors had a far greater chance of developing hepatitis, which caused liver damage and could be deadly. Captain Rappaport said there needed to be immediate research into pasteurizing blood products, and that donors should be screened. After the war, Dr Edwin Cohn found that albumin could be heated to 60°C in a water bath for ten hours with a stabilizer to protect the proteins. The process killed the viruses in it.

When Dr Edward Shanbrom, medical director at Hyland, created Factor VIII in the late 1960s, it wasn't put through a similar process. 'For a long time, nothing was done,' said Dr Shanbrom when Eric first made contact with him. 'I feel responsible for that.' Eric flew from New Jersey to California to meet Dr Shanbrom, who had a white moustache and wizened look, but came across as self-assured. Dr Shanbrom told Eric that, when he first developed Factor VIII, Hyland had decided it wasn't necessary for him to try heating it. The factor VIII protein was more fragile than albumin and they believed it might not survive heat. When Hyland applied for a license for one of its clotting factors in 1968, the National Institutes of Health (which regulated blood products until 1972, when the FDA took over the responsibility) said it was 'deeply concerned over the risk of hepatitis with this product' and asked the company to do 'thorough clinical evaluations.'

'We do not understand the concern expressed about hepatitis,' replied John Palmer, vice president of Hyland. He said it was 'unlikely' hepatitis could be removed from Factor VIII and that 'the product is needed in spite of its risk.'

Explaining this to Eric years later, Dr Shanbrom said people with hemophilia had already been exposed to hepatitis. 'There wasn't a compelling need to kill hepatitis in clotting factor, because it was in cryoprecipitate and they were infected anyway,' said Dr Shanbrom. 'That's what we thought at the time.' With the National Institutes of Health having the same toothless approach later adopted by the FDA, Hyland managed to convince it that hepatitis was an 'unavoidable risk.' It received the first license for Factor VIII without having to inactivate viruses in it.

This regulatory oversight enraged some researchers. Dr Joseph Garrott Allen, the blood expert at Stanford University who urged Britain to stop importing 'extraordinarily hazardous' American Factor VIII in the mid-1970s, said there was 'no valid reason' for it to have been licensed before Hyland had found a way to kill viruses in it. Especially since it was made from paid-for, pooled plasma. 'Large pools are highly profitable, but they are medically bankrupt,' said Dr Garrott Allen. Throughout the 1970s, conscientious experts echoed this argument, including the World Federation of Hemophilia which said manufacturers should kill viruses in Factor VIII 'for future generations of persons with haemophilia.' But with the Factor VIII boom underway, the regulator and doctors were happy to accept a risk of hepatitis, thereby allowing the companies to ignore these calls.

Within a year of Factor VIII's release, people with hemophilia who already had antibodies for hepatitis B became ill with what appeared to be a similar illness. Workers in the laboratories contracted it, too, from exposure to the toxic plasma. Concluding Factor VIII had the potential to transmit viruses they didn't yet know about, Dr Shanbrom wrote to the higher-ups at Hyland in 1970 laying out the hazards of their new product. He expressed fears about collecting plasma from Angola penitentiary, where he had heard hepatitis was rampant and the fields were fertilized with human waste. But the executives weren't interested. 'They're more concerned with how they look to the board of directors,' Dr Shanbrom told Eric. Following his complaint, Dr Shanbrom was demoted to consultant. Within two years, Baxter had let him go.

Despite the setback, Dr Shanbrom continued his research and by 1980 he had patented a method to kill viruses with a detergent. The process was applied to plasma before it was fractionated, making all products safe. Dr Shanbrom approached the four companies with his findings, but again, Alpha, Armour, Baxter and Bayer weren't interested. When the CDC reported on the first three people with hemophilia to contract PCP in 1982, there was a paragraph that floored

Dr Shanbrom: all patients treated with Factor VIII or cryo had developed not just hepatitis B, but also non-A, non-B hepatitis. His detergent process would have inactivated these dangerous viruses.

A picture soon emerged that the quartet had sealed an echo chamber around the assumption that Factor VIII simply couldn't withstand viral inactivation. Heat destroyed up to 90 percent of the factor VIII proteins, they said, making it more expensive to produce much less. And it wasn't clear if heat would kill hepatitis. In 1972 Cutter ran heat experiments on Factor IX, a plasma treatment for hemophilia B, but didn't use the stabilizers that had worked for albumin and didn't run trials on Factor VIII. Baxter looked into viral inactivation in 1977, but didn't make it a priority, so the research soon ground to a halt. Armour only started similar experiments on its Factor VIII in 1980, while Alpha never researched heat treatment throughout Dr Noel's time there, despite her protestations. One researcher, Dr Frank Putnam, believed there was 'convincing evidence' heat-treated Factor VIII could have been released as early as 1973 if the research had actually been conducted.

In May 1981 German company Behringwerke was granted the first license for 'heat sterilized' Factor VIII, which had been warmed to 60°C for ten hours with sucrose and glycine as stabilizers. It was ten times more expensive because heating had indeed reduced the amount of factor VIII protein by 50 percent, but it was safe from hepatitis. Only in the face of this competition did the US companies start to seriously consider making their own heat-treated versions. Internal memos from Baxter show it believed hepatitis was having 'a negative effect on sales and profits' at the start of 1982 and there was a 'business need' to conduct research into viral inactivation, particularly if it was to stay competitive in Germany. By the end of the year, Baxter had created a heat-treated version of its Factor VIII and obtained a license to sell it there. It applied for the first FDA license for heat-treated Factor VIII in June 1982, which was granted in March 1983. But its safer product was still prohibitively expensive.

The attitude that viral inactivation was an issue of sales and profit rather than safety was commonplace in other companies, too. Alpha began researching how to kill viruses in Factor VIII in the middle of 1982 after a directive from its marketing department. Within four months, Dr Charles Heldebrant, Alpha's sole researcher into heat treatment, had managed to kill hepatitis B by heating Factor VIII at 60°C for twenty hours. If he had been given the funding, he said, he could have developed this method anytime from 1979, after Professor Tuddenham and his colleagues isolated the factor VIII protein.

When Baxter's licence for heat-treated Factor VIII was granted, Bayer waged a campaign against it. In its laboratory, Cutter was working rapidly to produce its own safe Factor VIII, but publicly it said there was no proof that heat could kill hepatitis and encouraged its customers to continue to use its cheaper, unheated version. When France halted imports of Factor VIII in May 1983 because of the AIDS threat, an internal marketing plan showed the company wanted to 'give the impression' it was improving its product without making any promises about heat treatment. As part of its misinformation campaign, Cutter sent a letter to distributors saying that 'AIDS has become the center of irrational response in many countries' and that there were 'unsubstantiated speculations' it could be transmitted through Factor VIII. Bayer was the last company to receive FDA approval for its heat-treated Factor VIII at the end of February 1984. It continued to manufacture the older, unsafe version until August, and kept selling it for another year until the summer of 1985.

During the years of underinvestment and delay in killing viruses in Factor VIII that the companies presided over, some forty thousand people with hemophilia around the world contracted HIV.

In autumn 1984 the CDC and *The Lancet* confirmed HIV was killed by heat – proving just how much safer the new generation of Factor VIII was. The National Hemophilia Foundation recommended doctors stop prescribing unheated Factor VIII. Although a vocal minority of American people wanted all unheated Factor VIII to be recalled, the switch was gradual. There was no apology or investigation. By then, around half of the country's hemophilia population had contracted HIV.

Rather than revoking the four companies' licences for the older, unsafe Factor VIII, the FDA let its collegiate attitude prevail and trusted them to transition all their customers onto the heat-treated version. When Dr Harry Meyer, head of biologics at the FDA, realized in May 1985 that the companies were still selling dangerous Factor VIII, he wrote to them asking them to stop. They had all been granted licenses for a safer version well over a year earlier. In a summary, Cutter wrote, Dr Meyer 'did not want any attention paid to the fact that the FDA had allowed this situation to continue for so long,' and would 'like the issue <u>quietly</u> solved without alerting Congress, the medical community and the public.' And still the companies tried to push back, saying they had extensive supplies of the old product in their inventories.

Finally, Dr Meyer insisted, 'no one anywhere in the world should be allowed continued exposure to HTLV-III.' The companies conceded and in the summer of 1985 said they stopped selling unheated Factor VIII. They also agreed to add warnings about non-A, non-B hepatitis to the product.

Debate persists over whether heat treatment could have been introduced earlier, and therefore have prevented people with hemophilia from being infected with HIV. Today, Professor Jean-Pierre Allain is on one side, saying researchers couldn't have known heat treatment killed HIV before 1984, when Baxter's heat-treated Hemofil was proven to put a stop to patients seroconverting. He says the method hadn't initially worked against non-A, non-B hepatitis, so it had not appeared to be safer right away, and it required more plasma to make a batch. But Dr Francis from the CDC insists companies should have heat-treated Factor VIII years earlier. During a court case he said that doing so 'would have inactivated HIV and we would not be sitting here today.'

As lawyer Eric Weinberg developed the 'bad science theory,' he concluded that, with everything the companies had known about hepatitis, there was a legal and ethical duty for them to have killed viruses earlier. But the production of Factor VIII had been profit-driven ever since Baxter received its first license and the American Red Cross contracted it to supply the country's needs. With a lack of regulation from the FDA, profits had superseded patients' safety. Eric and his co-author, Donna Shaw, later surmised that people with hemophilia had been 'severely impacted by a perfect storm of events: the commercialization of blood products, the emergence of a deadly virus, and a regulatory system too weak to handle them.'

Perhaps the most telling document unearthed in the many lawsuits was the minutes from an October 1985 meeting at Armour's parent company, Revlon Healthcare. Eighteen months after HIV was defined as a blood-borne retrovirus, Armour's executives discovered a problem. Dr Albert Prince at the New York Blood Center found that even after their Factor VIII was heat-treated it still contained some traces of HIV; unlike the other companies, Armour's viral inactivation method was not completely effective. If it didn't fix the problem quickly, it would be at risk of losing $6 million in sales. 'The issue is not one of regulation, but rather marketing,' said Dr Mike Rodell, vice president of regulatory and technical affairs at Revlon Healthcare. He was less concerned about whether Armour's heat-treated Factor VIII could infect people with HIV than he was about how customers would react to the news if it leaked. Dr Rodell and his fellow executives contemplated telling the FDA that their heat-treated product could still transmit HIV, but they already had a license and didn't want to rock the boat unnecessarily. They decided neither to recall the product nor tell the FDA. Instead, they threatened Dr Prince that if he released the results of his research he would be in breach of the confidentiality clause in his contract.

In February 1986, Dr Jones in Newcastle disclosed that he knew of four patients who had contracted HIV from Armour's heat-treated Factor VIII. The company wrote to him denying that live HIV had ever been found in its safe product. Seven months passed before Armour alerted the UK Department of Health. In that time, the product infected two more children in Birmingham with HIV. Armour finally withdrew its defective heat-treated Factor VIII from Britain in October 1986, but continued to sell it in the US and elsewhere until 1987, when six Canadian patients tested positive for HIV after being treated with it.

★

In the years Donna Shaw reported on this story, she saw that the behavior of Alpha, Armour, Baxter and Bayer mimicked a business-school lesson from the University of Pennsylvania called the Panalba Role-Playing Case Study. Based on a real case from before the AIDS crisis, students would act out a scenario as executives in a pharmaceutical company who had discovered one of their most profitable drugs was lethally dangerous. The 'chief executive' and 'chief scientific officer' had to decide how to react to the developing situation. To add to the tension, one of the 'board members' would threaten to tell the newspapers everything if they didn't pull the drug from the market. The students considered whether to (a) keep selling leftover supplies, (b) continue to supply the drug to doctors who requested it but stop their marketing of it, or (c) carry on with no changes until the regulator banned it.

Over hours of discussions, the student groups nearly always came to the same conclusion: keep selling the product. Donna says she found that 'disturbing on so many levels. It says a lot about human nature, and that once we get into that corporate environment, our own individual morals and ethics fall aside for the sake of money and for the sake of profit.' Donna herself once took part in this case study and a student in the class made an even more startling choice: assassinate the person who was threatening to whistleblow.

Author Douglas Starr interviewed people from across the plasma business and found none was so hardened as to say, 'The hell with it, I made money and I don't care who got sick.' Those he spoke to felt they were in the medical industry to make money *and* help people in an effective way. Like the doctors who prescribed Factor VIII, those at the companies who manufactured and sold it told themselves they were helping people with hemophilia by providing them with this miracle treatment. Even as the evidence piled up that it could contain fatal viruses, they were so enamored with their own creation and the good they believed they were doing that they were blind to its faults. It was a fiction, but a stubbornly attractive one. Those who would ultimately suffer were kept at an abstract distance. Robert Massie, a political activist with hemophilia and professor in business ethics at Harvard Divinity College, was less forgiving than Douglas. 'It was clear to anyone who looked at the system that it was absolutely per-verted, with little concern for safety, driven by the search for cheap plasma and the desire to maximize profit,' he told the *Orlando Sentinel*.

When Michael Baum shared some of the internal company memos he had found with whistleblower Dr Noel, she lost the little faith she had left in her old industry. There were documents that showed the companies had colluded to protect their reputations, and calculations for how the AIDS crisis might financially impact them. She realized how they had placed a low value on the lives of people with hemo-philia and decided that it wasn't cost effective to act. In this light, Dr Noel's former colleagues seemed callous. 'They were very cold,' she says. 'One of the problems with capitalism is the profit motive. Somehow, we've lost heart.'

Dr Noel had insight she believed could secure a victory for people with hemophilia, but it would be time-consuming. Michael, Tom and Lorraine had set themselves a daunting goal for their next case: to bring one suit against all four companies. For it to succeed, they would need to prove all of them had played a role in killing their cli-ent Ken Dixon, who had died in 1995, aged twenty-eight. To do this, they would have to look at the plasma that went into every batch of Factor VIII he had infused throughout his life. With her insider knowledge, Dr Noel could help them do just that. She told Michael to subpoena plasma pooling records. In the days before digital records, these were a literal paper trail that would show how Ken came to be infected with HIV. Each record showed where the thousands of plasma donations that went into an individual batch of Factor VIII had come from, both in terms of the center's location and the people who had donated. The lawyers could narrow their search by first looking at batches that were made with plasma from AIDS hot spots such as San Francisco and New York. The records were also stamped with the results of a screening test for hepatitis B; those positive for the virus were highly likely to be contaminated with HIV.

The court ordered Alpha, Armour, Baxter and Bayer to hand over thousands of records to Michael and his team. Within them were the lot numbers of every Factor VIII treatment Ken had infused from January 1982 until his death. With dozens of members of staff working intensively for years, Michael and his team started to piece together a list of high-risk donors. They typed the records into a spreadsheet so they could identify batches that contained blood that had come from prisons, sexual health clinics, and areas with a high prevalence of HIV, as well as those which contained the blood of a donor who had died from AIDS-related illness.

At long last, they could draw a line from donors who were at high risk of AIDS to Ken, via the Factor VIII he had infused. They could see Ken had injected Factor VIII containing plasma that had come from Arizona State Prison and the Northern Nevada Correctional Center, as well as the plasma centers that targeted donors with hepatitis B. It became clear that almost every batch of Factor VIII Ken had infused from 1982 contained blood from a donor with AIDS. Ken, like so many other people with hemophilia, had reinfected himself with HIV every time he had injected his 'life-saving' medical treatment.

Michael was certain they had a strong case. They had evidence of dangerous behavior from inside Angola and in the advertisements from *The Advocate*. He believed they could prove deception, fraud and negligence on the part of the four pharma companies – they just needed to persuade a jury.

10.   The Trial

Prison wasn't as awful as Professor Jean-Pierre Allain had imagined it would be. Yes, he was fifty and incarcerated alongside people convicted of murder in Europe's largest prison, Fleury-Mérogis, a formidable grey mass in the southern suburbs of Paris that looked like a 1960s housing development. But he was in a wing reserved for those who would be at risk in the general prison population, most of them professionals. The prison had a notorious reputation of being an overcrowded 'monster.' Built for a maximum of just under three thousand inmates, its population had mushroomed to around five thousand, including some of France's most infamous violent criminals. Allain and twenty others – including lawyers and police officers convicted of drug possession, money laundering and murder – had their own corner of the 450-acre estate. Outside their cells was a small courtyard covered with an iron grid.

Allain's fellow inmates fascinated him. He taught them English, painted their portraits and learned their stories. To make the thirteen months he spent inside productive, he did a master's degree in clinical psychology, studying the characters around him for his dissertation. One man had murdered his lover after he was rejected by him; another was a police officer who had accidentally killed someone he was interrogating. Allain listened carefully to their stories, all the while thinking his own sentence unjust. Routine helped the days pass. Once a week, he would write a long letter to his family describing his fellow inmates and the scenes he had painted. He compiled these into a short book so his grandchildren could understand why he went to prison, which he called, *Contre mauvaise fortune, bon coeur* (*Against Bad Luck, Good Heart*) – a French proverb.

While he was in prison, Allain was variously demonized and absolved by his peers in the medical community. 'When you are in deep-shit trouble you find out who your true friends are,' he says.

The French doctors and researchers who had been among his closest colleagues maintained their critical view of him, including Professor Montagnier. Other friends refused to support him because they thought it would be detrimental to their own careers. And there were his former patients who believed justice had been served, and wanted more doctors to join him in prison. But the beleaguered professor found support in unlikely places. Unlike her research colleague, Professor Barré-Sinoussi remained Allain's friend and advocate. In July 1993 – a month into his sentence – *The Lancet* ran a supportive feature about his 'trial and tribulations' and called the French court 'Palais d'Injustice.' Diana Brahams wrote: 'The outside observer surely cannot escape the conclusion that Professor Jean-Pierre Allain has been made into a scapegoat on the dangerous principle that he was there and was knowledgeable and somebody must be held to blame.'

Allain's colleagues at Cambridge University supported him, too. Before his conviction, fellow hematologist Professor Robin Carrell had traveled to Paris twice from Cambridge to meet the judge in Allain's case and explain he had behaved ethically. When Allain later thanked his colleagues for their continued loyalty, they replied that they didn't do it for him; they did it because Cambridge University needed to be on the right side of history. They believed Allain had done the best he could in the face of a moving health crisis and had tried to warn his colleagues about the dangers of Factor VIII. 'They understood science, they understood the virus, and they were wise enough to see the rabid reaction of the French government,' says his wife, Dr Helen Lee. 'They had the wisdom and clarity of thought and the strength to go against the prevailing wind.'

Once Allain was imprisoned, Professor Max Perutz, who had won a Nobel Prize in 1962 for his research into the structure of hemoglobin and myoglobin, petitioned thirty-two other Nobel winners to sign a letter to President Mitterrand calling for Allain's exoneration and release. Separately, fifteen hundred doctors and researchers who were part of the International Blood Transfusion Society appealed for the convicted French doctors to be pardoned. 'The verdict on these doctors was delivered after an unprecedented "trial by media" where sensationalism dominated to the detriment of accuracy,' said the letter. But more than three hundred people with hemophilia in France had died from AIDS-related illness and President Mitterrand chose to ignore the appeal.

Throughout Allain's time in prison, Cambridge University continued to pay his professorial salary, defending the decision in the press. 'The circumstances of this case were unprecedented,' said Sir David Williams, vice-chancellor of the university. Those wages, along with most of Allain's assets, went to paying his legal fees and the Fr15 million (£1.7 million) fine he had received. The East Anglian Regional Blood Transfusion Service, where Allain was also director, initially suspended him on full pay while he was in prison. An internal inquiry found him fit to continue holding the post, but after coverage in the press, the NHS fired him.

On August 7, 1994, after thirteen months in prison, Allain was released. But he couldn't visit his wife in Chicago, or return home to Cambridge. Because, on the same day he had been freed, he and Dr Garretta had been placed under investigation for a new charge: poisoning. They were forbidden from leaving France.

Within a month, more than thirty French doctors were similarly accused, including pioneering AIDS researcher Jean-Baptiste Brunet and notable biologist and former government adviser François Gros. Former French prime minister Laurent Fabius and two of his ministers, Edmond Hervé, who led the health department from 1983 to 1986, and Georgina Dufoix, of social affairs, were also indicted for conspiracy to poison, later increased to manslaughter. The ministers were accused of delaying the introduction of HIV testing in 1985 to favor the Pasteur Institute's test over the American ELISA test. Abbott Laboratories had applied for a license for the ELISA test in France in January that year, but French officials didn't grant it approval until July, a month after the French test was licensed.

British doctors looked at the situation of their French peers with horror. 'These are colleagues just like people sitting in this room, who I know perfectly well behaved just as we did at that time,' said Dr Peter Jones from Newcastle at a seminar with fellow hematologists in 1998. 'Young physicians are reluctant to treat people with hemophilia because they are frightened they will be embroiled in litigation.' But

in Britain there would be no such charges against doctors or politicians. Unlike in France, where politicians started pointing fingers at
doctors in order to protect themselves, the British establishment
locked down around the defense that it couldn't have done anything
differently; it was all a big accident. By uniting around one story, they
protected one another. Reflecting on the experiences of his French
peer decades later, Professor Edward Tuddenham says, 'He was really
taken to the cleaners and it wasn't him at all. He was very much on
the side of getting to the bottom of it.' But there were survivors with
hemophilia in Britain who wished their country's justice system had
been as heavy-handed as France's.

After four years of living under the shadow of further charges,
Allain's phone rang in June 1998. Finally, news he had been waiting
for: France's Supreme Court had dismissed the poisoning case. That
evening he dined at The Four Seasons hotel to celebrate with his wife
and some friends. With the case over, Allain returned to his quiet
academic career in Cambridge, where he and Dr Lee eventually settled down. Dr Garretta, finding his reputation in tatters after years in
prison, vanished from the public eye and went to work in recruitment. In 1999 former prime minister Fabius was found guilty of
manslaughter, but received no sentence. His colleagues Hervé and
Dufoix were acquitted.

Professor Allain once told his wife he would rather try to change
the system from the inside than resign in protest over his peers dragging their feet. But having failed to prevent disaster and then been
sent to prison for his actions, Allain developed a stubborn and divi-
sive view of the events of the 1980s. He believes the contaminated
blood affair doesn't constitute a scandal; that everyone acted as
quickly as they could with the knowledge at hand; doctors and politicians weren't negligent; and that the truth was lost in the French
legal cases. To this day, he is unflinching in his final summation of his
conviction: 'It was all fabricated,' he says. Dr Lee agrees: 'There is
really no scandal per se. There was a lot of medical and scientific
ignorance, but no one in the system – particularly in medical circles –
would want to treat anything other than the best with what they
know.' This conclusion conveniently forgets that she once castigated

Dr Garretta, saying he would be responsible for ten to fifty HIV infections per month if he didn't start importing heat-treated Factor VIII. Douglas Starr estimates there were an additional seventy to three hundred and fifty HIV infections among France's hemophiliacs because of the delays.

The repercussions of Allain's conviction strike when he is least expecting it. There was a recent time when a colleague invited him to give a lecture at the French Society of Blood Transfusion. Within twenty-four hours he was disinvited because someone took umbrage with his involvement. Another time, a student approached him after he had given a lecture at the London School of Hygiene and Tropical Medicine and called him a murderer. He replied that they were mis-informed; France's Supreme Court had dismissed the case.

At the opening of Professor Allain's original trial, Dufoix had given a statement on television about '*l'affaire du sang contaminé,*' which became infamous in France as a slogan for evasion of justice. 'I feel deeply responsible,' she said. 'However, I do not feel guilty.'

In America, with more than a thousand cases underway across the country and some seven and a half thousand plaintiffs, contaminated blood had become the most sprawling legal battle in the country's history. In an attempt to bring the fight to one court, Jonathan Wadleigh of the Committee of Ten Thousand filed a class-action lawsuit that everyone with hemophilia could join. But the judge he went up against was known for his joint specialism in not just law but also economics, and he had a reputation for deciding whether to take cases forward based on the economic impact they could have. In this case, the judge decided, the potential damages against the pharma companies were far too high: they could 'hurl the industry into bankruptcy.' And so he threw out Wadleigh's efforts. Separately, hundreds of cases were combined in a federal court in Chicago, including those being brought by Tom and Lorraine Mull and Eric Weinberg. Between them, they had unearthed enough evidence of negligence that the companies were open to settling. People with hemophilia, who were dying at a rate of one per day, were keen to avoid a lengthy court battle. In 1996 Alpha, Armour, Baxter and

Bayer made a joint offer: they would pay $640 million to settle all the cases, amounting to around $100,000 per person who had been infected with HIV. The companies would divide the burden based on their market share from the 1980s, with Bayer paying 45 percent; Baxter and Armour 20 percent each; and Alpha 15 percent. Some 6,900 people accepted the offer.

Six hundred rejected it, more than half of whom had pending lawsuits. One of those was Dana Kuhn, who accepted the $100,000 on behalf of his deceased wife, but refused to take it for himself. 'I knew they were plumb guilty,' he says. 'They were guilty as sin.'

Dana and his fellow campaigners in the Committee of Ten Thousand, including Gary and Karen Cross, as well as Corey Dubin, Jonathan Wadleigh and Louise Ray, were angry that the US government had failed to do anything to support people with hemophilia. Nearly every other country they looked to had done something, but the government at the epicenter of the crisis was immovable. Year after year they traveled to Washington, DC, to picket outside Congress, some limping, others on crutches or in wheelchairs. At the end of a day's campaigning, they would go to a gay bar in DuPont Circle, where they would be accepted with their red AIDS ribbons.

A breakthrough came when the Institute of Medicine released the results of its two-year investigation in a damning report that contained visceral accounts of how HIV had devastated the lives of people with hemophilia. Drawing on Dana's 'The Trail of AIDS,' the report said there had been a 'failure of leadership' at the FDA over AIDS and blood products. It found the government should have mandated recalls of contaminated Factor VIII, insisted upon heat treatment and made the companies screen out high-risk donors earlier. Both the government and companies had been negligent by not erring on the side of caution when the public health risk emerged, and had failed to inform patients and doctors. As a result, Newt Gingrich, Speaker of the House of Representatives, agreed to shepherd the Ricky Ray Bill through Congress. 'The federal government did not do the right thing,' he said. 'This bill is a matter of simple justice.'

Eventually in 1998, six years after Ricky died and after a tireless campaign from the Committee of Ten Thousand, Congress passed the Ricky Ray Hemophilia Relief Fund Act. Separate to the legal settlement of the same amount, Congress would provide compassionate payments of $100,000 to everyone infected with HIV by Factor VIII, as well as any partners and children who had also contracted it. By then, more than 4,700 people with hemophilia had died in the US since 1979, with AIDS the main cause of death. But lobbying from big pharma meant the payments would be delayed while the lawsuits continued.

With all the evidence Tom and Lorraine had gathered, they were willing to represent the people who rejected the settlement. They knew their clients weren't interested in money; they wanted justice – and a guilty verdict in court. And the Mulls were set on getting it for them.

Leo Dixon had taken some convincing from Gary to join the legal action with the Mulls. He was a laid-back churchgoing man from the Deep South, with a calm voice and genial temperament. Gary thought him one of the sweetest people you could meet, having spent years getting to know him at Camp Wounded Knee, where their children became friends. A forgiving man, Leo hadn't initially wanted to join Gary's fight against the pharma companies. But after hearing how badly they had behaved – and being cajoled by Gary and his own son – Leo had agreed.

Leo, his wife, Shirley Dixon, and their two sons, Kenneth and Tyrone, both of whom had hemophilia, moved to Youngsville, Louisiana, from Alabama in 1981. Ken was more outgoing than his brother, behaving as if everyone was his friend as soon as he met them. He liked to draw, spending the weekends sketching portraits of his family, which were framed around their home. He enjoyed basketball and pool, but his goal was to be an artist. Tyrone, meanwhile, wanted to be a cook and could make delicious blackened fish and other Cajun classics.

Ken had never liked Factor VIII. Whenever he had a bleed, he would quietly take himself to his bedroom with an ice pack to avoid injecting himself with it. But his doctors, pressured by their suppliers, had encouraged him to inject Factor VIII again and again prophylactically, even when he wasn't having a bleed. On moving to Louisiana, Tyrone discovered he had an inhibitor to Factor VIII, meaning it didn't work as well for him, so in January 1982 he was switched to an alternative treatment normally used for hemophilia B. Ken tested positive for HIV, but Tyrone avoided infection. Before Ken developed symptoms, his cousin with hemophilia had died from AIDS-related illness. 'They were just dying at a tremendous rate,' says Leo. 'It was very hard for my boys.'

In his final year, Ken was burdened with opportunistic infections. He had thrush, PCP and wasting syndrome. His body felt itchy all over and he would wake up in the middle of the night sweating with a fever. As his organs failed, Ken started to have double vision and would feel faint when he walked. He was also plagued by hallucinations. Leo and Shirley watched as their son's body weight retreated to seven stone. One day, when he was seriously unwell, Ken confessed to Leo, 'I'm not going to be able to finish this fight [against HIV and the pharma companies], but I would like for you all to finish this. Please do that for me and for the others.' Leo and Shirley agreed to continue the battle on behalf of Ken and all his friends who had already passed away. A few days later, on June 3, 1995, Ken died from AIDS-related illness at home in Youngsville. He was twenty-eight, and had spent his last months being looked after by his parents as though he were a young child again.

The end of the twentieth century was approaching, and still the pharmaceutical companies continued to thwart their accusers, winning virtually every case that went to trial. There were a handful of exceptions that gave Tom a glimmer of hope. In 1997, a jury in Indiana had found Bayer negligent for its use of high-risk donors and its failure to put an AIDS warning on Factor VIII after December 1982. The family received $2 million. In Missouri, a jury awarded another survivor $1.4 million, but the decision was reversed on appeal. Tom, Lorraine and Michael had greater ambitions with their next trial. They wanted a jury to find Alpha, Armour, Baxter and

Bayer responsible for Ken's HIV infection and wrongful death – and by extension get a conclusion for all of their clients.

The case opened in November 1998 back in New Orleans with Judge Max Tobias once again presiding. Shirley, Leo and Tyrone were there, along with Gary and Karen. The small courtroom was packed, with supporters and lawyers spilling into the hallway. In the five years since Tom had stood before Judge Tobias and litigated for the Cross family, he and his colleagues, who included lawyers from three other practices, had unearthed a catalogue of new evidence. Added to their arsenal since the Cross trial were the advertisements from *The Advocate* proving pharma companies had purposefully collected plasma from people who had antibodies for hepatitis B, the interviews with inmates from Louisiana State Penitentiary, including Richard Vincent, and the lot records of the Factor VIII that Ken had infused, which they had traced back to infected donors. Tom was feeling confident as he started his hour-long opening address.

'This is a vial of Factor VIII,' said Tom, holding up a glass bottle the size of a saltshaker. 'It looks like cocaine. But it is much more dangerous than cocaine. The evidence will show you that it's deadly, that it kills those who use it.' The small vial was worth around $1,000 and it contained the plasma of as many as forty thousand people. Within were all the viruses those people had, including hepatitis and HIV.

Tom outlined how the four companies had taken risks with Ken's life. Some of them had collected plasma in prisons and advertised for donors with hepatitis B. He alleged they had conspired together to hide the dangers of Factor VIII; strategized on how to respond to the growing risk of AIDS; perpetuated the message that patients should 'infuse, infuse, infuse' rather than switch to cryo or limit their exposure; ignored their own lawyers' advice to add a warning about high-risk donors to Factor VIII; chosen not to introduce hepatitis B testing; and continued to sell unheated Factor VIII after a safer version was available. Between them, they had only ever recalled about 1 percent of Factor VIII throughout the AIDS crisis.

'The evidence will show you that the defendants covered it up,' said Tom. 'It was their big secret until recently.' And because of that secret, Ken had become infected with HIV. If he had known the dangers of Factor VIII, he would have switched his treatment like his brother had done. 'Tyrone doesn't have HIV. Tyrone is going to walk in here just like you and I walked in here, straight as an arrow, sad but alive.'

By 1998 AIDS had become the most common cause of death in people with hemophilia. And the four companies, said Tom as he pointed to their representatives in turn, were to blame. 'Kenneth Dixon never had a chance,' he added.

The companies defended themselves in the way they always had, saying Ken's death was a terrible but unpreventable tragedy. There was no conspiracy, because they hadn't known about the dangers of AIDS. By the time Ken became HIV positive in July 1982 (according to retrospective tests), just three people with hemophilia had developed a rare form of pneumonia.

Philip Beck, lawyer for Alpha, had some astonishing figures that showed how rapid and vicious the spread of HIV through the hemophilia population had been. Tests on frozen blood samples had shown the first infections happened in 1978, when 450 people with hemophilia were positive for the virus. By the end of 1979, 1,300 people had contracted it. The number increased year-on-year until there were 4,500 cases in 1981. At that point, 'not a single hemophiliac had come down with symptoms, so they didn't know anybody had the disease,' said Beck. By the end of 1982 – when the CDC had reported seven cases of AIDS among the twenty thousand or so Americans with hemophilia – 7,775 had already contracted HIV. 'Most of them were infected before anybody knew the disease existed, much less had any way to combat it,' Beck concluded.

The figures were convincing, thought Tom, but they ignored the fact that the AIDS crisis within the hemophilia population could have been prevented in the first place if the companies hadn't been so blasé about hepatitis; if they had recruited healthy donors rather than those more likely to be carrying blood-borne viruses; and if they had invested in heat treatment a decade earlier.

'The fault here is with this terrible disease that crept into our blood supply like a thief in the night and infected it before anybody realized what happened,' said Bayer's lawyer Terry Tottenham, who had a thick Texan drawl. To think researchers could have prevented the hemophilia AIDS crisis by addressing hepatitis was pure fiction, he explained. For one thing, HIV behaved differently from hepatitis: a positive antibody test was a sign of infection rather than immunity (he ignored the fact both were blood-borne viruses with similar epidemiology). In the 1970s, Tottenham said, the risk of hepatitis had been accepted because of how great the benefits of Factor VIII were. Ken's uncle had died at the age of ten from a tooth extraction, because he lived in a time before Factor VIII existed. Ken, by comparison, had been able to play basketball and rappel down mountains. The companies all contended that they had their patients in mind when developing the hepatitis B immunoglobulin. Some had tried deactivating hepatitis in Factor VIII, with little success.

As Tom had expected they would, the companies complained that being lumped together in one case was unfair. They weren't an amorphous collective, but separate businesses with competing products. To use the line that had won them so many previous cases, they said Tom and his team could not prove whose Factor VIII had infected Ken, or when it had done so.

Beck explained Alpha had only come into existence in 1978, after people with hemophilia had already been infected with HIV, and that Ken hadn't used its Factor VIII until after he was HIV positive. Alpha had been the first to say it would screen high-risk donors, but it had caused uproar. 'Congressmen made speeches on the floor of the House of Representatives condemning us because we were discriminating against homosexuals,' claimed Beck. 'The American Civil Liberties Union threatened to sue us. Doctors' groups said we were overreacting.' (In his research, Tom had found infected donors would have been more than willing to screen themselves out.) Baxter's lawyer Charles Albert said Ken had infused its product on only two occasions, and that it had been the first company to introduce heat treatment and add an AIDS warning to its product back in December 1983. Armour's legal team said Ken had not infused its Factor VIII until 1984, two years after he contracted HIV and by which time its packaging contained a warning about the AIDS risk. Bayer's lawyer Tottenham said it hadn't collected plasma in Los

Angeles, San Francisco or Miami and it had complied with every
FDA regulation.

But Tom could come back against all four of them with ease. Alpha
was responsible for most of the ads calling for donors with hepatitis
B; Baxter was the main company to use blood from Angola; Armour
kept selling its defective heat-treated Factor VIII after Dr Prince had
found it contained traces of live HIV; and Bayer had lied about collecting blood in prisons.

With the assuredness of someone who's undeniably right, Tom
called one of his star witnesses, Dr Kay Noel. She was nervous as she
took the stand, seeing those on the pharma side of the courtroom stir
at her public betrayal of them. Although she felt ready to share the
things she had seen inside Alpha, she was facing people who considered her a traitor, who had made her feel ostracized. Dr Noel steeled
herself by thinking back to the nonchalance of her colleagues, how
none of them had cared about the hazards of non-A, non-B hepatitis.
But no sooner was she sworn in than her efforts were frustrated. Tom
asked Dr Noel a question and the lawyers from the pharma side
objected. Over and over, the companies intervened before she could
answer; Judge Tobias upheld their objections. Dr Noel had wanted to
tell her story, but was restricted to sharing technical scientific details.
By the end of a dispiriting day on the stand she felt as if she had done
little more than share her name.

The continuous objections from the pharma companies' lawyers
began to frustrate the jury. Amid devastating testimonies from Leo,
Shirley and Tyrone, the legal wranglings appeared callous. Tom
hoped the jury would see how flagrantly irresponsible these companies were, and just how unwilling they were to accept any responsibility for fatally infecting Ken.

The open hostility and invective from both sides made the case feel
more like a barroom brawl than a trial. More than once, in the hallway outside the courtroom, Gary had to separate Tom from the
opposing lawyers after he found them pushing and shoving one
another. Tom and Michael thought their adversaries, whom they
had been fighting for years, were arrogant and aggressive. On the
final day of hearings in December, before proceedings were adjourned

for the holidays, Tom leaned over to Michael and said, 'Watch me shove a Christmas tree up Phil Beck's ass.' He stood up and presented evidence that Alpha had used recovered plasma from a sexual health clinic in a batch of its Factor VIII, which it had denied doing. Tom and Michael watched Beck storm down the hallway as the day finished. They knew they had him.

Tom's turn to become incensed came when Dr Louis Aledort, the leading hematologist from New York, took the stand in defense of the pharma companies. Tom had a particular gripe with Dr Aledort for having turned so completely on his patients, testifying against them in virtually every court case and earning tens of thousands of dollars for the privilege. The companies said Dr Aledort had advised them back in the early 1980s to ditch plasma only if they discovered it was contaminated before they had made Factor VIII with it. If it was already in the product, he told them they should not recall it, because he was concerned about a lack of supply. (In 1983 he stepped down as medical director of the National Hemophilia Foundation after his peers disagreed with this view.) Following FDA rules and Dr Aledort's advice, the companies had only recalled batches of Factor VIII when doctors reported that a donor had died from AIDS-related illness.

Dr Aledort had stepped down as head of hemophilia care at Mount Sinai Hospital in New York years earlier, a move he had always said was a personal choice. But Tom had new evidence for this trial. He had found a letter from the president of the hospital that said Dr Aledort was removed because of his alleged conflicts of interest in receiving research money from pharma companies and numerous investigations into him, including one by the New York attorney general (of which he was found not guilty). As Tom questioned Dr Aledort about this, the doctor was obstinate: the letter proved nothing. Tom became increasingly angry and eventually paced to the back of the courtroom, turning his back on Dr Aledort while questioning him.

Judge Tobias sanctioned Tom. 'I understand the emotions in this case, believe me,' he said. 'The histrionics, the jury has seen it. This ain't television. There's no camera in the courtroom. I'm not Judge Judy. I'm just a little bitty judge, gaining weight – not that little – sitting down here in a little southern town on the banks of the Mississippi River, just trying to make a living.'

'Sir, I accept your criticism,' said Tom. 'It was unprofessional. I would apologize to everyone in the courtroom – except Dr Aledort.'

'That's inappropriate right there,' said Judge Tobias. 'That's a contempt. Twenty-five bucks payable to the Judicial Expense Fund.'

Tom was so angry with Dr Aledort he would have paid $1,000.

For Leo and Shirley, it was something else Dr Aledort told Tom that was more ruinous.

'Virtually all, if not all, of the Factor VIII manufactured and available for sale in 1982 and 1983 was infected with the HIV virus – is that correct?' asked Tom.

'Highly likely,' replied Dr Aledort.

'More likely than not?' pressed Tom.

'Yes,' said Dr Aledort. 'Highly likely to be all infected.'

Every single little vial of white powder that had been injected into Ken's veins was infected with HIV and hepatitis C after 1982. Leo went into the trial wanting the companies to admit they had done wrong – and here Dr Aledort had given him the final conclusion he needed. 'They knew it was all infected but they kept pushing it,' says Leo.

Over 90 percent of US patients with severe hemophilia who had infused Factor VIII from 1982 to 1983 had contracted HIV, said Dr Aledort. By 1999, when he was on the stand, more than half had developed AIDS and around a third had died.

'I took care of these people my whole life,' he said. 'I took care of them from the day they were born, hundreds and hundreds of them. This great tragedy killed my children.' Like other hemophilia doctors, he spoke of his patients as though they were family.

But Tom didn't buy the expression of regret; Dr Aledort had testified against patients in cases up and down the country for over a decade. Now he had a chance to put it right, to admit he knew Factor VIII was 'defective.' But Dr Aledort refused to be drawn, because saying the product was defective would have implied the companies were at fault.

'You're stating that a product that is contaminated with a virus that causes AIDS and death is not defective?' said Tom.

'Defective means that it doesn't work,' said Dr Aledort. 'It worked. It was effective. However, there was a tragic, horrible thing that happened. It had viruses in it.'

Tom and Michael were certain they could prove Ken's death wasn't just a tragic accident; the companies had taken risks with dangerous donors, fraudulently misrepresented their products and failed to make them safe. It was time to present the adverts from *The Advocate*. On seeing them, Dr Don Francis, formerly of the CDC, said he would have gone straight to the surgeon general and the head of the FDA to report the companies had he known they were targeting high-risk donors at the time. And he would have advised patients to return to cryo.

But the real concession came from one of the companies' key witnesses: Dr Meyer, head of blood products at the FDA. Dr Meyer had always maintained he had done a good job of regulating the companies as AIDS emerged, but his perspective changed when confronted with this new evidence. As Tom showed Dr Meyer one advert after another, reading out the details of plasma centers that called for donors to 'help develop the anti-hepatitis vaccine' and 'make it pay as much as $650 extra each month,' Dr Meyer was visibly shocked, his mouth falling open.

'Do you think it would have been good manufacturing practice for the defendant pharmaceutical companies to target, advertise and solicit plasma from high-risk gay men for use in the production of Factor VIII as late as December 6, 1982?' asked Tom.

'No, I don't think that would have been good practice,' said Dr Meyer. 'Had I been aware of it, it might have led to discussion as to whether this could be construed as a violation' with regards to safety.

Trying to defend themselves, the companies turned on the FDA, saying they had followed its regulations at all times and any delays were because it had been slow to make recommendations. From Skid Row to prisons, their plasma centers had licenses, they said, and they had stopped collecting in prisons long before the FDA mandated it. Some delays were out of their hands as they waited for guidance and approval from the regulator, which hadn't wanted to spark a plasma shortage. Beck said Alpha had requested approval for an AIDS warning for its Factor VIII in May 1983, but the regulator had rejected its request saying there wasn't enough evidence. Baxter said it had applied for a license for its heat-treated Factor VIII in June 1982, before the first cases emerged, and the FDA had taken nine months to grant it.

But Tom wasn't going to let them get away with pushing the blame back on to the FDA. How could the regulator have made an informed decision about the safety of Factor VIII when the companies had neglected to tell it about their dangerous plasma collection practices? Dr Meyer had been shocked by both the adverts in *The Advocate* and the details of the plasma center in Angola. And he had accused Alpha, Baxter and Bayer of lying to the FDA, which amounted to negligence (Armour was exempt from this claim because it hadn't recruited high-risk donors).

For the kicker, Michael revealed the thousands of dangerous donations Ken had infused. The 'hottest lot' was from Alpha, which contained plasma from nearly two thousand donors at Irwin Memorial Blood Bank in San Francisco, one of the hotbeds of the early AIDS crisis. Around a third of those donors were gay and a significant proportion had HIV. Ken had injected himself with their plasma in June 1982.

Hearing all this evidence, Ken's local pediatrician, Dr Charles Hamilton, said he would have stopped treating Ken with Factor VIII and moved him onto cryo had he known where the plasma for his treatment was coming from, and how many donations went into each batch.

In the last week of the trial, Tom played his interview with Richard Vincent. From inside Angola, Richard described how inmates had used the plasma center to have sex and inject drugs; how they had been in charge of running the plasmapheresis machines and choosing who could donate; and how the screening process had allowed people with infectious diseases to sell their plasma.

Summing up, Tom told the jury Ken had experienced 'death by a thousand cuts.' Each time he had infused Factor VIII, he was reinfecting himself with HIV. By 1983, Dr Aledort had said, it was 'highly likely' every batch of Factor VIII from the four companies was contaminated. Had Ken not compounded his initial infection, he may have survived beyond 1995, when the first treatments for AIDS became available. Tom urged the jury to therefore find *all* the companies, not just one, responsible for Ken's death.

'A miracle drug turned into an unmerciful killer,' said James Orr, a lawyer who worked with Tom. 'Eighty percent of people who took the miracle drug are [either] dead, HIV-infected or have AIDS.'

The case drew to a close in March 1999, following four months of hearings. After three days of deliberation, the jury concluded Cutter and Alpha had been negligent in their manufacture of Factor VIII. They had both made unreasonably dangerous products, then fraudulently misrepresented the safety, which had caused Ken's death. The Dixon family should receive $35 million in compensation, increased to $56 million when the length of the lawsuit was taken into account. The record sum showed just how high the true damages for people with hemophilia were; and why so many courts had been reluctant to take on these cases.

Leo and Shirley hugged one another, expressing sheer relief and a rare kind of happiness, given everything that had happened. The truth had won out, not just for their family but for everyone with hemophilia. Having weathered many setbacks and losses, the community finally had reason to celebrate. This was a proper and unequivocal victory.

But the Dixon family never received that $56 million. Because after the jury had given its verdict and left the courthouse, Judge Tobias had his own decision to deliver. He opened an envelope and read from a piece of paper: he was overruling the jury's verdict because the statute of limitations had expired. The case should have been filed within a year of Ken contracting HIV, he said. Given that a finding of fraud can negate the statute of limitations in Louisiana, Tom was utterly exasperated, and then furious. It was a pattern they had seen across the country that played right into the pharma industry's hands.

Back in the mid-1980s, when doctors had disclosed their clients' infections, the companies had claimed antibodies to HTLV-III might be a positive thing, a sign patients were protected against AIDS. By the time they became fatally ill and the truth was clear, the statute of limitations had expired. In one fell swoop, Judge Tobias blocked Tom from bringing any more of his cases to court.

Leo and Shirley appealed the decision, but before the Louisiana Supreme Court had a chance to rule, they had accepted a seven-figure settlement from Alpha, Armour, Baxter and Bayer, which would help make life more comfortable for their surviving family. For them, it had never been about the money. No amount could heal their family's wounds. Leo just wanted the truth of how Ken died. The jury's finding of responsibility was the ultimate victory, albeit a partial one.

The ordeal had been grueling for the Dixons. Disgusted by what he had seen in court, Tyrone stopped taking his Factor IX for a time. Three years later, in 2002, he needed a tooth extracted and the doctor couldn't stop him from bleeding. Following so many before him, Tyrone died from loss of blood, leaving his parents grief-stricken and childless. Within a decade, Shirley had passed away from complications caused by diabetes, brought on partly by the stress of losing her two sons.

Having served in Vietnam as a machine gunner in the infantry, Leo thought he had seen his worst days long ago. That was until the AIDS crisis hit. In seventeen years he went from sitting around the dining-room table with his three happy family members to eating alone. Leo lives with PTSD, still waking up with night sweats and flashbacks. Sometimes he dreams of the dirt in Vietnam, at other times of his sons Ken and Tyrone. Yet he still has a broad, welcoming smile and the comfort of his religion. 'My purpose is to be the best person I can and to help any and all people whenever I have the opportunity,' he says.

Tom, Lorraine and Michael were determined not to let their efforts go to waste. Judge Tobias might have thrown their case out, but they wouldn't let that detract from the victory: a jury had agreed that Bayer and Alpha were responsible for Ken's wrongful death. And so, they set in motion a plan to get justice for every single one of their remaining clients.

With the jury's ruling in Ken's case, Gary Cross could at last conclude that his son, Brad, had died because of negligence. In the early years of their legal fight, Gary had rejected the idea of settling on Brad's behalf; he wanted to learn the truth in court. But with everything now out in the open, he softened. He and Karen were one of 124 families who were yet to settle their cases; and he agreed with Tom that a fair settlement would be $1 million per family, a total of $124 million.

Tom and Lorraine started negotiations in secret. They knew Bayer would outright refuse such a high figure, given that it would be responsible for around 45 percent of the cost, proportionate to its market share when the infections occurred. But Alpha, Armour and Baxter were ready to bring the decade of lawsuits to an end. Behind closed doors, over some months, those three companies each agreed to pay their share of $100 million. With a partial settlement secured, Gary and Dana came up with an idea that might bring Bayer on board. They proposed to Tom that they should get the executives from all four companies to sit down with the patients and families, to negotiate directly. Gary and Dana wanted to be in charge of running the negotiation, along with their friend Terry Rice – a trained bio-chemist who had been unable to practise after he contracted HIV from Factor VIII. Once in the room, they would play their trump card: threaten Bayer with a boycott of its products until it agreed to settle. They could use Dana's sway within the hemophilia community to pull it off if they needed to.

'Think that'll work?' asked Tom.

'All they're worried about is money,' said Gary. They needed to talk in the only language pharma understood.

The plan was unconventional, but Tom had maverick tendencies himself and was willing to take a chance with a new tactic. To his surprise, the pharma companies agreed, understanding how hard they needed to work to win back the trust of their surviving customers. A date was set in mid–October 2000 when the families would be able to face the companies whose products had changed their lives – first for the better, then towards disaster.

Those who had been infected and bereaved wanted the companies to know the destruction they had wrought, and to apologize for it. With that in mind, Tom arranged for the first day to be spent with the families sharing their stories with the executives from Alpha, Armour, Baxter and Bayer. More than forty families joined Gary and Karen in the basement of a Los Angeles hotel. A long line of tables divided the room. Across from them were senior representatives from the companies and their lawyers. Gary thought it was like a scene from a film, the good guys pitted against the bad. They were next to a young man in the early stages of AIDS who had come to California on his own. He told Gary and Karen the only people who knew about his infection were his parents. There was also a girl who was carrying a poster of her brother. On one side he was the picture of health; on the reverse, he was dying from AIDS-related illness. Another girl clutched a cuddly toy, which had belonged to her recently deceased brother. 'It's all I have left,' she told the executives. A farmer who had lost his son to AIDS shortly after his wife died asked Gary and Karen what he should say. Karen told him to talk about his son: who he was, how he had died, and the hole he had left behind. She did the same for Brad.

'It was torture,' said Karen, to watch her son in pain and not have any means to make him better again.

'When we brought our son into our den to live and placed him in a hospital bed, he had no dignity,' said Gary. 'When we had to have a hole cut into his stomach and pump liquid food into him, he had no dignity. When he couldn't talk anymore, he had no dignity.'

One by one, the families spoke of the horrors they had experienced following the contamination of Factor VIII. People swore and cried as they discharged fifteen years' worth of pent-up anger, trauma and heartbreak. The executives listened in silence, many of them with tears silently running down their cheeks. Lorraine saw one of them break down in the hallway outside. Another said to her he didn't think he could take it anymore – did she know how hard it was to listen to?

'Yes, I do,' she said. 'This is what we have been listening to for over ten years. It's about time you heard it.'

After everyone had spoken, John Bacich, the president of Baxter, stood up and said, from the bottom of his heart, he was sorry. In an unplanned speech, he explained how he had a family of his own and he couldn't begin to imagine the pain and sorrow they had all experienced. Bayer's senior vice president of sales and marketing, Terry Tenbrunsel, apologized, too. The companies hadn't been diligent enough. Karen thought, if only they had admitted to the problem with Factor VIII and apologized two decades earlier. 'I don't think these people had any idea what they were doing and how bad it was,' she says. They may now have understood the suffering they had caused, but it was all too late.

Following the emotional release, Gary, Dana and Terry were ready to start negotiating. Gary was forthright about being the one who should talk, not Tom or any other lawyers. He was a businessman, after all, and this was now the time to discuss money. Dana was respected in the plasma industry, so he would play the good cop, friend of the companies. Terry could be his own fiery and defiant self, not afraid to swear and hammer home what the companies should have done to make Factor VIII safe. In their first meeting, Terry stood by having once called Bayer's Tenbrunsel a 'motherfucker': 'I meant what I said.' Tom nicknamed them the Three Amigos, men who had inadvertently become activists and lawyers as they sought justice for themselves and their families.

Early in the negotiation it became clear the lawyers for the pharma companies were going to continue with the combative attitude they had maintained for the past decade.

'You attorneys, both sides, get the hell out of here,' said mediator Eric Galton, a Texan in cowboy boots. 'Let the three people representing the community and the company executives negotiate.'

There was uproar among the lawyers, who protested that they were needed. But for some reason the executives acceded to Eric's demand and chose Bacich from Baxter to represent them all. The next day, just five people would return to the negotiating table: the Three Amigos, Bacich and the mediator, Eric.

That night, Gary woke up in the small hours of the morning with an idea. The Ricky Ray Act had been held up in Congress by a few members of the Senate Appropriations Committee who were blocking the approval of its finance. Gary knew it was really the pharma companies, with their lobbying influence over some senators, who were standing in the way. They had been against the bill from the start, because if the federal government paid compensation it could imply fault and impact their legal cases. Gary was in Los Angeles to negotiate for a small group of people, but if he could secure funding for the Ricky Ray Act he could help more than seven thousand families just like his. He nudged Karen.

'I know how to beat them,' said Gary.

'What?' mumbled Karen, barely awake.

'We make them call all their little contact people in Congress and get our money approved. To show good faith. And we won't do anything until they do that.'

The next morning, before the mediation began, Gary made the request.

'We know that you have enough pull in Congress that you can get this money approved,' he said. 'Show us and our community good faith.'

Bacich conferred with his fellow executives before asking for a couple of hours to make some calls. By the afternoon, when they reconvened, the companies had removed the block and Congress had released some $750 million for every person infected with HIV by blood products, or their surviving family members, to receive $100,000. Gary believed Brad had sent him the idea as he was sleeping – and that the money for around seven and a half thousand people might never have been approved without the help of his son. The Cross family, like many others, would use it to pay off exorbitant medical bills.

With the negotiation finally underway, and $750 million already won, the pharma companies were initially obstructive. Dana thought they were being asinine by competing rather than acting on the supposed remorse they had shown just days earlier. In a rare outburst, he lost his temper, slapping his hand on the table.

'These families are all messed up, because of what you have done,' he said. 'You can live with that on your conscience for the rest of your life. You can live knowing you will go to sleep every night seeing those families that you heard give testimony and the pictures of their dead children, until you settle this fairly.'

As the companies continued to bicker among themselves, Eric's nerves frayed. At one point, he stormed out of the room swearing like a sailor.

Gary decided to use their trump card. He pointed at his comrade and said, 'Dana Kuhn is known throughout this country. He will get every hemophiliac to quit buying products from those of you who don't settle and we'll start buying it from the other companies.'

The tactic worked. Bayer agreed to provide its share of the $100 million. Terry thought they should take it.

'Hell no,' said Gary, who was still aiming for $124 million.

'Tell me what the hell's going on,' said Tom with a genial tone when they caught up during a break. 'You've got everybody over there going crazy.'

'The stupid son of a bitch just turned down a hundred million dollars,' said Terry.

'We're not settling for that,' said Gary. 'I can get more.'

Tensions were rising among all parties. Save for Tom, who had thrown his trust behind Gary, the other lawyers for the victims were exasperated – they wanted to close at $100 million. Eventually, Dana struck a deal with the companies. They would accept the offer if the lawyers on both sides agreed to cover the outstanding medical expenses for the 124 families, which in some cases exceeded $1 million. The result was unprecedented. Never had litigation been settled so directly with the victims and company executives facing one another. Gary wrote out the final settlement on a piece of paper, including medical expenses, and handed it to Tom.

But Tom wasn't as pleased as he might have been. For one thing, he believed they could have pushed the companies up to $124 million.

And those medical expenses terrified him. The agreement said his firm, along with the others representing the plaintiffs, would split the millions of dollars' worth of medical expenses with the lawyers for the pharma companies. With some hard work, Tom's associate Fran Phares managed to negotiate those expenses down so they became minimal.

Finally, the case came to an end. 'Those 124 people were, quote, "adequately compensated" compared to the other people,' says Tom. 'But not compared to any other sense of justice – how do you replace a loved one?'

The settlement brought a forced peace between the US hemophilia community and the pharmaceutical companies. But it wasn't without consequences. The decade of animosity had been grueling and the high stress of the negotiation had taken its toll. Soon after, Gary needed a triple heart bypass, Dana developed an infection that almost killed him and Terry contracted pneumonia. All three recovered slowly.

For Dana, they had achieved the best justice available in America. Others had wanted criminal convictions or a congressional hearing – they told Dana they would never be able to forgive those they held responsible. 'The manufacturers, the FDA, and everyone who had a hand in this got away without criminal indictments,' says Dana. 'They stood by and watched our population die.' But not wanting to let resentment become a prison, he told himself he would move on. He used the settlement money to pay off his mortgage, put his children through college and invest for his retirement. There was a portion he held back for altruistic purposes. Four of his friends had experienced devastation in their lives, having lost their husbands and children to AIDS-related illness. They accepted the initial $100,000 settlement but later found themselves struggling. Dana created a fund for each of their surviving children so they could go to college.

Tom and Lorraine tried to get criminal proceedings off the ground in the US. They reported their findings to the FBI and the US attorney general. As Tom traveled the country, meeting clients and speaking to witnesses, he would go to each local police force, but the authorities never pursued the allegations. Tom found it frustrating and eye-opening. Despite his superhuman efforts, no one from the companies would face a trial in the US.

Brad Cross was seventeen when he died. To his parents he might have been an intelligent boy with an IQ of 140 and a promising future ahead, but in the calculations of how the $100 million settlement would be divided, he was among those with the lowest worth. He hadn't finished high school, let alone been to college. 'They put a value on my son, even at the end,' says Gary. It made him feel sick. Justice was always going to have a bitter taste to it.

With the fight against the pharma companies now over, Gary and Karen could at least put their worst days behind them and try to build a future for themselves and their daughter, Jennifer. They moved to a new home, where they could focus on happy memories of Brad, rather than thinking of him lying in his mechanical bed every time they passed the den. They also bought a plot of land on the river in Louisiana's bayou, near Morgan City. Amid the dripping Spanish moss, bald cypress trees and alligators floating lazily in brackish waters, they could find a kind of peace. As Gary cast his fishing line, he would think of his son who had so enjoyed fishing alongside him. A wooden sign at the entrance to the land still says 'Camp Bradley.'

Michael Baum had time to decompress after the mediation. But even as he dusted himself off, something kept niggling at him. In his office, he had a few boxes of internal Cutter documents Bayer had disclosed during the lawsuit. He had been waiting for a time to go through them, as he knew they contained information about the company's international distribution of Factor VIII. Over the summer of 2001, Michael picked his way through the material. He was familiar enough with the behavior of the pharma companies to understand where their priorities had lain; but reading the documents, he realized he had enough evidence for another case.

In the boxes, Michael found Bayer's Far East marketing plans for 1984 and 1985. The company had received an American license for its heat-treated Factor VIII in February 1984. Within a couple of months, it was teaching its international sales representatives about the new product. But Bayer had continued to make unheated, dangerous Factor VIII for six more months, in part because it had fixed-price contracts in place and the older product was cheaper to make. In its 1984 plan, Bayer said it would not do any major product recalls in the Far East, because it could lose $2 million worth of sales. One by one, countries were banning unheated Factor VIII, first in the US, then Europe. The marketing team said the 'lustre' had fallen out of Bayer's international sales because New Zealand had rejected its AIDS-riddled product. As the company looked to 1985, it realized it would have 'excess' supplies of the unsafe version. Bayer's solution: sell that product to countries where low prices were the priority. The company predicted, 'AIDS will not become a major issue amongst Asian haematologists during 1985.' If 'hysteria' did take hold, it could reduce sales of unheated Factor VIII by as much as $400,000.

The reason those at Bayer believed AIDS would not affect its sales in Asia was 'because the region has so many other health hazards of greater, more common concern.' Hepatitis B was prevalent, the authors explained, particularly in Taiwan, where 16 percent of people were carriers of the virus. 'With these considerations in mind, we have no immediate plans to introduce Koate-HT or Konyne-HT [heat-treated products]. If we see a need for a heat-treated product in the Far East, we will react to the demand swiftly. Otherwise, we will try to continue to dominate the markets with low-cost, standard Koate and Konyne.'

The company planned to expand sales in Hong Kong, Taiwan, Singapore, Malaysia, Indonesia, the Philippines and Thailand, introducing heat-treated products in each country only 'if necessary to defend against fear of AIDS.' It would also continue to sell the older product in Latin America.

Michael read that, in February 1985, Bayer had wavered over the ethics of selling unheated Factor VIII that it knew could contain HIV. A company task force asked, 'Can we in good faith continue to ship non-heat-treated coagulation products to Japan?' But in another document, it considered trying to get Japan to delay the approval of its heat-treated Factor VIII so it could dump older supplies there. Bayer later said it didn't follow up on that plan. But in the first three months of 1985 it exported more than five million units or twenty thousand vials of unheated Factor VIII likely to contain HIV and hepatitis C to customers across the globe.

By May 1985 there was a furor among doctors in Hong Kong, panicking about a health emergency after their patients started testing positive for HIV, who accused Bayer of having dumped dangerous Factor VIII there. Bayer's marketing manager for the Far East told the distributor in Hong Kong that there was little they could do. Regretfully, they could not switch the country's Factor VIII orders to the heat-treated version for another few months, because stocks had been 'depleted' by high demand in the US. The marketing manager outlined how doctors in Taiwan, Singapore, Malaysia, Indonesia and Japan were still primarily using the original unheated Factor VIII, while countries in Latin America, as well as Spain and Portugal 'appeared to be in no rush to convert.' They had to prioritize the countries that were refusing the older version, such as the US, UK, Germany and Italy.

'Be assured there is no severe hazard from the regular Koate Factor VIII concentrate now being supplied in Hong Kong and numerous other countries,' said the marketing manager for the Far East. 'It is the same fine product we have supplied for years.' They did, however, concede that the heat-treated version was safer and 'should be substituted at the earliest possible date.' They apologized to the Hong Kong distributor for any anxiety caused by the delay and said Bayer could provide some supplies of the safer product for the 'most vocal patients.' All this, despite an internal memo acknowledging a month earlier that a leading hematologist had told an international conference 'no non-heat treated concentrate should now be used' and 'AIDS may soon exceed haemorrhage as the major cause of death in haemophiliacs.'

Reading these documents, Michael knew he had enough for another case. He pieced together the dates and realized that when Dr Meyer at the FDA had told the companies to stop selling all unheated Factor VIII in May 1985, Bayer had been rapidly trying to use up the HIV-contaminated stocks in its warehouses. At the end of July, after Bayer realized there were no countries left in the Far East where it could 'expect to sell substantial quantities' of unheated Factor VIII, it announced that it would stop selling it altogether – eighteen months after it had US approval for its safer heat-treated version, and nine months after heating was found to definitively kill HIV. From February 1984 to July 1985, Bayer had successfully exported $4 million worth of unheated Factor VIII, around one hundred thousand vials. In September, it wrote to its distributor in Taiwan to say it would do a free exchange of any stocks of unheated Factor VIII for the heat-treated version.

Michael got in touch with doctors and patients in Taiwan and Hong Kong with his findings. They were outraged to think the company had treated patients differently based on whether they knew about the dangers of the old product, and the racism inherent in treating those in the West first. Bereaved mother Li Wei-chun from Hong Kong, who lost her twenty-three-year-old son to AIDS in 1996, told the *New York Times*, 'They did not care about lives in Asia. It was racial discrimination.' The documents made a mockery of the Hong Kong government's commission into tainted blood, which had concluded the tragedy was unavoidable. Bayer told the paper it had 'behaved responsibly, ethically and humanely' when it sold unheated Factor VIII abroad, defending itself that some countries had been slow to grant licenses for the heat-treated product and that there were doctors who initially believed it was not as effective. But Michael agreed with Dr Sidney Wolfe, from the Public Citizen Health Research Group, who concluded, 'These are the most incriminating internal pharmaceutical industry documents I have ever seen.'

Michael filed additional lawsuits against Bayer on behalf of new clients in Taiwan and Hong Kong, but the ultimate result was disappointing: a US judge ruled that even though the defendants, experts and evidence were all based in America, the cases should be tried locally. In Taiwan, a court decided the statute of limitations had expired. 'There were tens of thousands of people worldwide who were HIV infected from their Factor VIII and these decisions, which were unjust decisions, let the companies off the hook,' says Michael.

From the heart of the plasma industry in the US, contaminated Factor VIII was pumped to Europe, Asia, Africa and Latin America, infecting almost everyone who used it with hepatitis C and more than forty thousand people with HIV. The hemophilia population was decimated. In Germany, almost three thousand people contracted HIV from Factor VIII; by 2020, just 343 survived. In the US, where an estimated eight thousand people were infected, 719 were still alive. And in the UK, of the 1,250 people who contracted HIV, there were 258 survivors. Meanwhile, the nations that became self-sufficient in blood products and didn't import from the US avoided the full scale of devastation. In Belgium, where cryo was the main treatment, just 7 percent of people with hemophilia were infected with HIV.

No two countries responded to the crisis in the same way. There were governments who were up front about the disaster, launching investigations and compensating victims. Others left it to survivors to fight lengthy court battles and wage public campaigns before addressing the injustice. Some are yet to recognize their citizens whose lives were destroyed by blood products contaminated with HIV and hepatitis C.

Canada's response was comprehensive and swift, with the government paying people infected with HIV $120,000 (roughly £65,000) in humanitarian aid in 1989. The provinces later added lifetime annual payments of $30,000. Still angry about how their infections had occurred in the first place, and scared history could repeat itself, survivors pushed for a public inquiry. The government conceded in 1993 and launched the Commission of Inquiry on the Blood System in Canada, led by Justice Horace Krever, to establish how contaminated blood had given over a thousand of its citizens HIV and tens of thousands more hepatitis C. Justice Krever spent four years combing through the evidence, hearing from almost every victim or family and gathering a million pages of documents. His first witness was Dr Don Francis, who spoke for three days about how the CDC should have pushed the FDA to regulate and even control the pharmaceutical companies in the early days of the AIDS crisis. Released in November 1997, the Krever Report offered a scathing critique of Canada's slow response to HIV, which lagged behind that of the US with fatal consequences. The government, doctors and the blood system had rejected 'an important tenet in the philosophy of public health,' said Justice Krever. 'Action to reduce risk should not await scientific certainty.' He made fifty recommendations, including an overhaul of Canada's blood system and the adoption of a precautionary approach to infectious threats. His first recommendation was no-fault compensation for all victims 'without delay.' The government acted upon the reforms immediately and provided compensation for people infected with HIV and those who contracted hepatitis C between 1986 and 1990. In 2006 it announced a further $1 billion for five and a half thousand people who had contracted HIV and those who contracted hepatitis C outside of those dates.

Following Justice Krever's report, the Royal Canadian Mounted Police brought thirty-two criminal charges against organizations and individuals for negligence and endangering the public. Among them were the Canadian Red Cross, its former director, senior researchers at Health Canada, Armour in the US, and its head of regulation Dr Mike Rodell. The Canadian Red Cross was found guilty of negligence and distributing contaminated blood. It was fined $5,000, told to contribute $1.5 million to the University of Ottawa, and stripped of its rights as the country's main blood collector. In a series of trials concluding in 2008, the other defendants were all exonerated. 'There was no conduct that showed wanton and reckless disregard,' said Justice Mary Lou Benotto, ruling that everyone had acted as well as they could with the knowledge to hand. 'The events here were tragic. However, to assign blame where none exists is to compound the tragedy.' With that, the only possibility for criminal convictions in North America against the companies was closed.

Germany's pharma laws meant patients didn't need to prove companies had been negligent in making Factor VIII in order to receive compensation, just that the treatment had caused them harm. By as early as December 1988, pharmaceutical companies had paid a total of DM100 million (around £30 million) to around twelve hundred people, with payments reaching DM350,000 (roughly £110,000). In 1994 an investigation by the German government found that all parties – the government, pharma, blood donor service, doctors and hospitals – had failed to safeguard the blood supply. The report said the risk of AIDS had been clear by 1983 and Behringwerke's heat-treated

Factor VIII should then have replaced all other products. As a result, the government announced full compensation: federal and state governments would provide DM150 million (£67 million), while Bayer, Immuno, Baxter, Behringwerke, Armour and Alpha were made to contribute DM90.8 million (£40 million). People with AIDS received DM3,000 per month (around £1,300).

Japan, like France, was draconian in its response, bringing criminal charges against former government officials and executives at Green Cross, which owned Alpha, for the HIV infections of some two thousand Japanese people with haemophilia. The battle started in 1989 with two cases of negligence against the pharma companies and agencies that regulated them. Yoshiaki Ishida, one of the few public faces of those with HIV, gave an emotional plea in court for the matter to be settled quickly: his T-cell count felt like an hourglass counting down his life. 'Each day I can watch the sand falling,' he said. 'When there are only a few grains of sand left, that would mean I am about to reach the state of death.' He died in 1995, before a settlement was reached.

The cases had been underway for more than five years when the new health minister, Naoto Kan, released a swath of documents that his department had previously said were 'lost.' These revealed grave errors, such as the Japanese government failing to license heat-treated Factor VIII until July 1985, some eighteen months after it had first become available in the US. Green Cross had continued selling unheated Factor VIII well into 1987. There was evidence that the relationship between government officials and pharma had been far too close, contributing to a dangerous situation for people with hemophilia. As a result, the Japanese government agreed to settle both cases in 1996 with compensation of around $430,000 per victim (roughly £280,000), as well as monthly payments for life and future medical expenses. The government would cover 44 percent of the costs; pharmaceutical companies the rest. The Japanese government formally apologized 'for the heavy damage inflicted on many innocent people' and Green Cross expressed 'deep regret' that its products had caused such pain.

'Lives were at stake!' shouted one victim's mother. 'If it was your child, do you think a casual apology like that would be enough?' She demanded *dogeza*, a ritual in Japan that involves a person kneeling on the ground to express sincere apology and deference.

The president of Green Cross, Takehiko Kawano, stepped forward, knelt down and pressed his forehead to the floor. His colleagues joined him in the nationally televised act of shame and apology. Representatives from Baxter and Bayer also apologized, but were reluctant to accept responsibility in case it bolstered lawsuits in other countries. Wolfgang Plischke, president of Bayer, said he was sorry 'for the suffering of haemophiliac patients and their family members, who are unwitting victims of a terrible tragedy.'

The apology didn't mark the end of the matter in Japan. Police raided the offices of Green Cross and arrested its former president, Renzo Matsushita, and two of his colleagues. In 2000 the three executives were found guilty of negligence for having 'put a priority on profits and ignored the dangers.' Matsushita, who had previously been a senior official in the health ministry, was sentenced to two years in prison, while his fellow executives Tadakazu Suyama and Takehiko Kawano were sentenced to eighteen and sixteen months, respectively. Dr Takeshi Abe, Japan's former leading hemophilia adviser, and his colleague Akihito Matsumura, the former head of blood products, were also remanded in custody while awaiting charges of professional negligence. Dr Abe, by then in his mid-eighties, was exonerated, while Matsumura was found responsible for the death of a patient who contracted HIV from unheated Factor VIII in 1986 and given a one-year suspended sentence. Victims said the punishments were too lenient. Doctors and health officials in Iran and Portugal also faced criminal charges.

In contrast, Saddam Hussein's regime in Iraq locked away those who had been infected with HIV in sanatoriums with barred windows. Some managed to escape, because guards were too scared to touch them. The 189 people who contracted HIV from Factor VIII there were forced to sign a pledge vowing they would not marry, work, or use public services including schools, doctors' surgeries, swimming pools and barbers. Violating the agreement – or telling anyone about their condition – carried a death sentence.

By the late 1990s, over twenty countries had established support schemes for people who had been infected with HIV, and in some places hepatitis C as well.

No charges or civil lawsuits against the pharmaceutical companies have been brought in the UK. In 2003 some three hundred British survivors joined a US lawsuit filed on behalf of people from several countries. Among the plaintiffs were Frankie and Joe, who traveled to Chicago to give evidence. For permission to travel, they had to go to the US embassy in London, where their passports were stamped to say they were HIV positive. Frankie faced a room full of defense lawyers who grilled her about her two terminations and her morals. She found the process painful and humiliating. Ultimately, the American judge ruled that British authorities were more responsible than the pharma industry for infections in the UK, but ordered the companies to pay £20,000 to each plaintiff with HIV and £5,000 for hepatitis C. Frankie thought it was so inadequate as to be insulting. The other thousand or so British people with HIV who were not involved in the case – like Clair and Richard – never received a penny.

Just as safety had been a lottery depending on where people with hemophilia lived, so justice was haphazard, piecemeal and dictated by the chance of geography. Alpha, Armour, Baxter and Bayer ultimately paid well over a billion dollars to people infected by their products. But only a fraction of the total number of victims were compensated, and in amounts that varied drastically. To receive any money, victims had to fight exhausting legal battles that dragged on for years, at a time when they were getting weaker and weaker from their illnesses. Through it all there was no guarantee that justice would be served. Their lives had been permanently contorted by contaminated Factor VIII – and no court case would undo the damage.

11. 'We Accuse'

Joe was standing outside a building in Paris with a scarred exterior in the early years of the new millennium. The area next to the front door, where the letterbox should have been was blackened by fire damage. The office had been firebombed. Joe had been brought here in secrecy, without being told the final destination. The people in the organization he was meeting didn't know if they could trust him, and they wanted to make sure no one discovered where they were based. This building with the scorched facade was the head-quarters of a militant French hemophilia campaign group. And Joe needed their help.

Since his separation from Frankie a couple of years earlier, Joe had become vengeful; he wanted to see British doctors and former government ministers punished like they had been in France. Along with other British people with hemophilia, he was concocting a plan to capture public attention and spark action against those he held responsible for his infections. The plan would involve criminal damage in a busy area of central London. They were going to dye a fountain blood-red. Joe was willing to risk arrest if it attracted atten-tion, but he had heard this French organization had developed an antidote to red dye, which would allow them to turn the fountain red, then reverse it. It could minimize the extent of the damage – and how much trouble they would be in. He was in Paris to see how it worked.

Joe's recovery from AIDS had been slow and hard-won. After he started antiretroviral combination therapy in 1998, his T-cell count had gradually climbed and his health improved over the next year. For the first time, he was able to think beyond the confines of the house he had once shared with Frankie; the house where he had been wal-lowing for thirteen years since his AIDS diagnosis. As he felt better, Joe had tried to contemplate the future, but he couldn't picture it.

Having married Frankie so young, he had never really dated. Now, he would have the unenviable task of telling any future partner he had HIV. He had grown accustomed to hiding his hemophilia, let alone that he was HIV positive, and he couldn't fathom when would be the right time to tell someone: On a first date, giving them an easy opportunity to leave? Right before they slept together? He certainly couldn't do it afterwards – that could land him in jail. As stories of HIV-positive people being prosecuted for infecting others began to circulate, Joe became acutely aware that to some people his body was considered a weapon. Although those cases involved deception, Joe still found the ethical quandary of new relationships more or less impossible to resolve.

Unable to decide how best to make new connections given his HIV status, Joe decided to seek out others in a similar situation. Most AIDS charities catered to the gay community, with campaigners like Peter Tatchell and the Terrence Higgins Trust vocal in fighting for the rights of gay men with HIV. But people with hemophilia who were HIV positive didn't fit the mold. Many were heterosexual, some married, and the press had created long-standing animosity between them and the gay community by painting them as 'innocent victims.' Gay campaigners took umbrage at that, since it presupposed sexually active gay men somehow 'deserved' to get AIDS. Joe had heard stories of people with hemophilia being turned away from organizations like the Terrence Higgins Trust, shunned both by society at large and by others with HIV. But then someone with hemophilia asked him if he had heard about the Birchgrove Group. He hadn't. They gave him a number to call.

Birchgrove had started as a group of four people in Cardiff back in 1986 in the snug of a pub called The Birchgrove. They had all been infected with HIV while under Professor Arthur Bloom's care and had been devastated by the death of seven-year-old Colin Smith in 1990, who was treated in the same hemophilia center as them. Before long, Birchgrove was sending a newsletter to hundreds of people with hemophilia and hospitals across Britain. As more people joined and they compared notes about their own stories of infection, they started to discover the pattern of mistakes that had been made. Across

Wales – and then London – their stories echoed one another. None of them had been warned of the dangers of Factor VIII. Few had known when they were being tested for HTLV-III. They didn't buy the 'disaster theory' that what had happened to them was an accident, terribly sad and tragic, but ultimately unavoidable. Disquiet began to grow within Birchgrove; members wanted to do something.

By the time Joe called Birchgrove at the end of the 1990s, they had been established for a few years. At the first meeting, Joe felt comforted just from being in a room with other people who had been infected by Factor VIII. For the first time since 1985, he could relax and have a drink without worrying about his big secret. He didn't have to be furtive like he was at work or in his local pub; if he wanted to talk about his symptoms or how he was feeling, he could. Joe's new friends in Birchgrove started to tell him about the evidence of wrongdoing they had discovered. They had been in touch with the Committee of Ten Thousand in America and learned how much longer it had taken Britain to react to the AIDS risk: the CDC had accepted it was probably blood borne in March 1983, when Bloom was only just beginning his public campaign to deny the connection. Joe decided he wanted to join the more radical members of Birchgrove, ready to unleash his pent-up anger at the establishment he believed had disfigured his life. He joined in with plans to run treatment strikes and march in London. He went to Paris for red dye, but never actually turned a fountain red because they couldn't get the right material. One seriously unwell member said he would even consider dying on the steps of 10 Downing Street as Birchgrove delivered flowers to Tony Blair, so desperate were they for the government and public to take notice of their struggle.

Joe became one of hundreds of infected blood survivors in Britain who were slowly adapting to a new reality in which they had to become activists. They had survived the death sentence handed to them in the mid-1980s, and the longer they lived, the more they realized how pitiful the government's ex-gratia handouts had been. The money they had received in the 1991 legal settlement (£23,500 for single people with HIV) hadn't stretched far, and the independence of a working life was now out of reach for many because of their infections.

As people in Britain heard about justice in the US, Canada and Japan, they asked why support at home had been so inadequate. In 2002 they heard how their neighbors in Ireland had been compensated and felt angry. The Irish government's Lindsay Tribunal of Inquiry found that the country's National Haemophilia Treatment Centre had been sluggish in its response to the AIDS risk, which was compounded by continued home treatment and use of unheated Factor VIII after a safer version was available. Doctors had also presided over unacceptable, years-long delays in telling patients about their HIV and hepatitis C results, adding to their distress. Following the report, the Irish government apologized and paid €566 million in compensation to 2,666 victims of infected blood, amounting to an average of £150,000 per person. It also improved hemophilia care and provided victims with access to free health services and bespoke insurance. Following a separate civil case, pharmaceutical companies paid €6.7 million to fifty-nine Irish people with hemophilia. Joe heard all this and couldn't understand why they were still being ignored.

British infected blood campaign groups proliferated in the 1990s and early 2000s. Scotland, Wales and Northern Ireland all had their own organizations seeking equal payments and treatment for people there. The thousands who had contracted hepatitis C from Factor VIII were starting to feel the effects of the disease, developing chronic fatigue and pain, as well as liver cirrhosis and cancer, but the government refused to offer them any assistance. In 1993 an angry faction had broken from the Haemophilia Society to form the Manor House Group, seeking recognition and compensation for hepatitis C infections. The groups weren't all working together – and some had fierce rivalries – but they had common goals. Paramount was to make known the truth about how their medical treatment had become tainted with deadly viruses and to secure justice for themselves and their deceased loved ones. Some wanted compensation as a priority, others wanted an apology, and there were those like Joe who sought revenge in the form of criminal convictions. But achieving these goals wasn't going to be easy, because it would require the government admitting to serious mistakes.

In Newcastle, one group was making progress on revealing wrongdoing in the corridors of Westminster. Peter Longstaff, a former Treloar's pupil, had been co-infected with HIV and hepatitis C alongside his brother Stephen, who died of AIDS-related illness in 1986. When Peter's doctor told him he had hepatitis C in 1994, alarm bells rang, because he had been tested for it without being informed. Peter and his wife, Carol Grayson, who had worked as an AIDS nurse in the early days of the epidemic, went to see the lawyer who had represented him in the 1991 HIV litigation against the Department of Health. They wanted to do something about Peter's infection with this second chronic virus. But the lawyer had bad news: Peter couldn't bring any legal action over hepatitis, because he had signed that waiver crafted by Dr Andrzej Rejman before he or any of the other plaintiffs knew they had hepatitis C. Peter was floored by how underhanded the government had been. Once again, an authority he had trusted had misled him.

Peter then discovered his doctor had tested him for hepatitis C two years before he was given the result. He and Carol started to investigate further, teaming up with other survivors to form Haemophilia North (later renamed Haemophilia Action UK). They encouraged others with hemophilia to request their medical records so they could start to build a clearer picture of when people had been tested for viruses and how long they had been kept in the dark. Many had similar experiences to Peter of having been tested without their consent and not discovering their diagnoses of HIV and hepatitis C for years. In that time, they had missed out on possible treatment and risked passing on viruses to their partners. Some discovered their medical records had mysteriously gone missing, or contained only a fraction of their history.

Peter and Carol's greatest discovery came when their solicitor gave them access to a mound of documents the Department of Health had passed over during the HIV litigation. Sifting through the windfall of material, they saw the government had known about the dangers of American Factor VIII from the very start of the AIDS crisis, but had continued to endorse its use because of the underinvestment in Blood Products Laboratory and on Bloom's dangerous advice. They found epidemiologist Dr Spence Galbraith's letter from May 1983 in which he warned the government to stop importing commercial blood products. By failing to act or warn the public, the government had put Peter and his brother directly in harm's way. They saw swaths of references to non-A, non-B hepatitis going back to the 1970s, long before Peter had signed the waiver. The deeper Peter and Carol dug, the more they came to realize the government had known far more than it had ever let on.

One piece of damning evidence captured it all. Like other Treloar's boys, Peter had an inkling that he had been part of research trials as a child at the school. In a letter from January 11, 1983, two of Britain's top hemophilia doctors explicitly said it would be more cost effective to research the transmission of hepatitis from Factor VIII with humans than it would with chimpanzees. The typed letter was sent from Bloom and Dr Charles Rizza, of the Oxford Haemophilia Centre, to their peers across the country. It said at least four pharma companies were planning to release a version of Factor VIII that had been heated to reduce the risk of hepatitis. They wanted their colleagues to help monitor how safe this new Factor VIII was:

> Although initial production batches may have been tested for infectivity by injecting them into chimpanzees it is unlikely that the manufacturers will be able to guarantee this form of quality control for all future batches. It is therefore very important to find out by studies in human beings to what extent the infectivity of the various concentrates has been reduced. The most clear cut way of doing this is by administering those concentrates to patients requiring treatment who have not been previously exposed to large-pool concentrates.

The doctors were going to use previously untreated patients, whom they called 'pups,' to see if this new Factor VIII gave them hepatitis. People with hemophilia had been 'cheaper than chimps,' thought Peter and Carol. In the letter, Bloom and Dr Rizza said there weren't many of these patients left in the UK, but they could conduct the research with a small cohort, as they were already doing in Oxford. The doctors said they didn't want to follow the conventional route of introducing the new Factor VIII product on a named patient basis before it was licensed, because it would reduce their capacity for research.

'We hope that the companies concerned will collaborate in these trials and will offer appropriate supplies of their concentrate as well as financial support,' they said.

Here was evidence that medical practitioners had not only known about the danger of hepatitis C long before they had told people with hemophilia, but that they had also conducted unethical trials on oblivious patients. The companies who made Factor VIII had been complicit in supplying the treatment and funding the research. As in America, there had been a cozy relationship between some doctors and the companies, who provided funding and materials in return for free trials of their products. It was also proof the doctors had had access to heat-treated Factor VIII as early as 1983.

Peter and Carol took their findings to every institution they could find. They lodged formal complaints with the Haemophilia Society and complained to the General Medical Council about Dr Peter Jones, Peter's doctor in Newcastle, whom they alleged had tested him for hepatitis C without his consent and withheld the positive result. Dr Jones insisted he had given Peter his hepatitis C diagnosis in 1990, after informing him he was being tested. The General Medical Council dismissed the complaint and said Dr Jones had 'appeared to act reasonably.' Peter and Carol went to the police, believing they had evidence of negligence and criminal behavior. But they were bounced between multiple police forces: the Met Police in London said they should report it to their local force, but Northumbria Police didn't understand how it was a criminal issue. Eventually, they went to Dyfed Powys Police in Wales, which had previously handled one of the first corporate manslaughter cases in the UK, but the allegations disappeared down a rabbit hole. It would be nearly impossible to bring a corporate manslaughter case, given the law had only been introduced in 2007 and could not be applied retrospectively.

All the while, the government was silent. 'There was a massive amount of evidence, but the government just didn't want to address it,' said Carol.

Year after year, campaigners came up against brick walls. Just as Thatcher's Conservative government had used a stock answer about the risk of AIDS in blood products in the 1980s, Blair's Labour government repeated itself ad nauseam in the early 2000s: the government of the day had done all it could and there was nothing more to discover.

In the House of Lords, there was a small contingent of dissenting politicians who thought the government was being deceitful. One of these was Lord Alf Morris, president of the Haemophilia Society and longtime advocate for people with disabilities, who believed the only way to uncover what the government and doctors had known about the dangers of Factor VIII was an independent public inquiry. The Haemophilia Society had first called for an inquiry in 1988 with no luck. Again and again, Lord Morris raised the issue of infected blood in the House of Lords, calling it 'the worst treatment disaster in the history of the National Health Service':

> In none of the many parliamentary campaigns I have been closely involved in over forty-five years in Parliament – even thalidomide, vaccine damage, and those nearly forty years ago for statutory recognition of dyslexia and autism – have I had so strong a sense that no campaigning should have ever been necessary to right the wrongs suffered by the haemophilia community. Support for their cause is an issue not of right and left, but of Right and Wrong.

Every time Lord Morris tried to get attention, the government pushed back. In a typical example, Melanie Johnson, parliamentary undersecretary of state for public health, wrote to him and said, 'The government does not accept that any wrongful practices were employed and does not consider a public inquiry is justified, as we do not believe that any new light would be shed on this issue as a result.'

In a particularly galling move for people with hemophilia, the government had announced an inquiry into Bovine Spongiform

Encephalopathy (BSE) two years after the first human death from variant Creutzfeldt-Jakob disease (vCJD), known at the time as 'mad cow disease.' In 2000 the inquiry found the government had given a false impression that BSE wasn't a risk to humans and had presided over unacceptable delays because it was 'preoccupied with preventing an alarmist over-reaction to BSE.' With the failures laid out in black and white, the government agreed to pay £67.5 million in no-fault compensation to families of those who contracted vCJD. Each received around £120,000. Overall, 131 people died from vCJD after eating BSE-contaminated meat.

Tellingly, there were thousands of people infected with HIV and hepatitis C by contaminated blood products. It would have been significantly more expensive to compensate them all – and the government didn't want to foot the bill. So, without holding a public inquiry, it decided after the settlement of the HIV litigation in 1991 that neither the Department of Health nor the NHS had been at fault.

In public, the government maintained this bullish stance, but behind the closed doors of Whitehall there were civil servants who were running scared in the early years of the new millennium – and trying to cover their tracks.

Lord David Owen, by now a life peer, was once again trying to get to the bottom of why his ministerial papers had been pulped. Like Lord Morris, he thought a public inquiry was the only way to uncover the 'gross maladministration' by successive governments in handling the affair. In 2002, with new evidence to hand, Lord Owen wrote to the Parliamentary and Health Service Ombudsman for a second time, asking it to reopen his 1988 complaint. He had found a memo about a March 1973 meeting at the Department of Health in which a group of experts recommended the UK should become self-sufficient in blood products as soon as possible for safety reasons. 'I am now satisfied that your predecessor's conclusion was totally false,' wrote Lord Owen, referring to the previous decision by Sir Anthony Barrowclough that his self-sufficiency plan had been about saving costs. Lord Owen hoped that if his complaint was successful, the government would have to launch an inquiry. If it did, he believed the government wouldn't have a leg to stand on, because he was sure there had been a catalogue of errors.

Lord Owen implored the ombudsman to resolve the injustice. 'A serious wrong has been done to haemophiliacs who caught hepatitis C during the period when Parliament could reasonably expect that we were self-sufficient,' he said. 'You might say it is all a long time ago, but you are really their only hope . . . I am not allowed to look at the departmental files. Only you can do this. I hope very much that you will do so.'

Initially, the thought that the Department of Health could be conspiring to cover up the events of the 1970s and '80s hadn't crossed Lord Owen's mind. But then he got his hands on a staggering memo: an internal briefing meant for John Reid, Blair's secretary of state for health, which civil servants sent to him by mistake. The Department of Health had recently tried to put together a timeline of key events from 1973 to 1985 to show what had happened with self-sufficiency, but so much of the evidence had gone missing it had failed to do so. The reason was laid out in the memo Lord Owen now had a copy of, which said:

> Unfortunately, none of the key submissions to ministers about self-sufficiency from the 70s and early 80s appear to have survived. A search of relevant surviving files from the time failed to find any. One explanation for this is that papers marked for 'public interest immunity' during the discovery process on the HIV litigation have since been destroyed in a clear out. . . . This would have happened at some time in the mid-90s.

As he read it, Lord Owen realized something far more serious was going on: Could a deliberate cover-up have been underway for years? Documents about a critical period of time, when the government had imported a dangerous medicine into Britain that infected thousands of people with lethal viruses, had been destroyed. This on top of the destruction of his own ministerial papers.

Lord Owen wasn't the only former minister to discover papers had gone missing. When Lord Patrick Jenkin, secretary of state for health from 1979 to 1981, found in 2004 that his documents had met the same fate, he went straight to the most senior civil servant in the Department of Health, Sir Nigel Crisp. 'I would very much like to come and discuss this with you and to explore why it was thought right to destroy these files,' said Lord Jenkin. 'They represent, by any standards, a most unhappy chapter in the department's history and I would be very distressed indeed if this was felt to be an adequate reason for their destruction.'

Catapulted into action by Lord Jenkin's letter, Zubeda Seedat, a policy officer in the department, unearthed the results of an internal audit about document destruction, which detailed how records on blood products had been pulped between 1989 and 1998. The first batch went missing just as the HIV litigation was being negotiated, and as Professor Allain and Dr Garretta were being sentenced in France. Those in the ministry had been watching events unfold in France with apparent horror. Crisp wrote to Lord Jenkin with an apology: he, too, was concerned that important files no longer existed. The destruction, he said, should never have happened. 'There are many of us who think that one of the reasons you can't get all of these documents was they cleaned them up because there was a panic going around the world in the middle 80s that these issues would reach court,' Lord Owen later said. Lords Jenkin and Morris were equally incensed by what appeared to be a systematic destruction of important evidence. They urgently raised the issue in Parliament, demanding a promise that all surviving documents would be preserved.

The government showed no signs of relenting on a public inquiry: it was unfortunate that a previous administration had destroyed papers, but it had been done in error and there was little more to learn. It did, however, offer one concession, agreeing in 2003 to give ex-gratia payments to people infected with hepatitis C by NHS treatment before September 1991. The Skipton Fund would pay a lump sum of £20,000 to each person and a further £25,000 to those whose hepatitis C had progressed. It was a far cry from the £522 million compensation deal the Haemophilia Society had requested. Up to 80 percent of people with hepatitis C develop a chronic infection, which can lead to liver cirrhosis and cancer within twenty years.

People had already started to have liver problems and the list of those awaiting transplants was growing. Added to that, the first hepatitis C treatment, Interferon, had punishing side effects that could last years, including fatigue, muscle pain, fever, depression, anxiety and excessive irritability.

Without a public inquiry, people with hemophilia had a real fear that history could repeat itself; fears that came close to being realized with vCJD. In the early years of the vCJD outbreak, British people were banned from donating plasma at home and abroad. But this swift response was not applied to hemophilia treatment. Using Professor Edward Tuddenham's early research, the factor VIII protein had been genetically sequenced and used to make a synthetic treatment, called recombinant Factor VIII, which was approved for use in 1992. But it wasn't immediately available to all British patients because of how expensive it was. It cost around 10 cents per unit to make, but the manufacturers charged around $1 per unit. 'The pharma companies as usual had a cash cow and were very happy to maximize their income,' says Professor Tuddenham. Depending on where they lived, some patients could access synthetic Factor VIII, while others were still reliant on the version made with human plasma. The new treatment wouldn't work for everyone, because some had inhibitors that prevented their bodies from accepting it. But people with hemophilia wanted the choice. Instead, they felt the government in Westminster continued to gamble with their lives.

Peter Longstaff fought the government for access to recombinant Factor VIII. After a five-year battle that included an unsuccessful judicial review and a hazardous treatment strike from Peter, the government agreed in 2003 to give more than four thousand patients the right to access synthetic Factor VIII. For them, it had been painfully reminiscent of the AIDS crisis. In 2004, the government wrote to more than eight hundred people with hemophilia to inform them they had been treated with Factor VIII containing plasma from a donor who later developed vCJD. Thankfully, no one developed symptoms.

The fight had taken its toll on Peter, who passed away in April 2005 after a painful and debilitating fight against hepatitis C and

AIDS-related illness. His widow, Carol, vowed to continue the fight. 'For some of us, it has literally taken our whole lives,' she says.

In a statement to a local newspaper following Peter's death, the Department of Health doubled down. 'The government of the day acted in good faith, relying on the technology available then. There is no evidence of any wrongful practice and therefore the Department of Health does not feel a public inquiry would provide any real benefit to those affected.'

Clair wanted to move to London for a fresh start. In the years after Bryan's death, she questioned why she was still in Warwickshire, having only returned there because her husband had wanted to be near his family in his final years. She found solace at work, where she could focus on preserving Shakespeare's folios, but her empty house was a constant reminder of what she had lost. Not only her husband, but also contentment with herself and her world. Inside, she was anguished about her health and what the future would look like.

Wanting an escape, Clair spent more and more time in London, where she met people who could relate to her experiences of the past fifteen years. Her colleagues in Stratford-upon-Avon were supportive after she was widowed, sending her letters of condolence and praising her courage in the face of Bryan's death from cancer. In London there were people with whom she could be more honest. On one of these trips, she saw an advert for a job supporting people with HIV. She wanted to leap on the opportunity, but there was an obstacle.

Before Bryan died, as he became increasingly unwell, Clair had struggled to keep them afloat financially. She was working and caring for Bryan, who had lost his job because of his non-Hodgkin's lymphoma. Basics like heating had become too costly so, in desperation, she had gone to the Macfarlane Trust, the charity that had received ex-gratia payments from the government to assist those infected with HIV. Survivors had to apply to the Trust for each payment in a process that many describe as degrading. When Clair asked for regular support to replace Bryan's income and help with their spiraling bills, she felt like a character in a Dickens novel, begging bowl in hand.

John Williams, administrator of the Macfarlane Trust, put forward a strange offer. 'We can take the mortgage off you and make an equity loan,' he said. The Macfarlane Trust could support people with grants, but Williams explained he would only give them money in exchange for a share of their house.

Clair and Bryan had felt cornered: the building society might withdraw their mortgage altogether if it discovered Bryan was dying from AIDS. With no other choice, they agreed to sign away a portion of their home in order to keep a roof over their heads. After nine frugal months, the Macfarlane Trust paid them a first installment.

Now that Clair wanted to move to London, it became clear the Macfarlane Trust was going to get in her way. To the trustees, her home was an investment, and if Clair sold up she would have to pay back both the loan and a proportionate amount of the additional value the house had gained since Bryan's death. 'They would have made about £40,000 worth of profit and I was not going to let them have it, not off the back of my husband,' says Clair.

The full extent of the Macfarlane Trust's abusive treatment of Clair only emerged years later when she filed a subject access request asking for the communication it held about her. In a letter, Williams had written to trustees: 'I am afraid the lady wants to eat her cake and still have it. She conveniently forgets the rent-free living she has enjoyed for seven years.' Rent-free living in the home she had *owned* with Bryan before he became severely ill. Seeing that letter, Clair realized how much contempt those at the Macfarlane Trust had for her, a grieving widow. In another document, Williams said he had offered the loan to Clair and Bryan because both of them were HIV positive, so the trustees would soon recoup their investment. 'They were expecting us to die,' says Clair. 'They did not expect that thirty years later I would still be alive.'

As Clair fought to regain control of her life, she was treated dismally by those who worked for the Macfarlane Trust. On one occasion, Williams shouted at her, 'You would be thrown out by your ears if it wasn't for this Trust.' Clair was disgusted by the way the government had washed its hands of them with meager ex-gratia money to the Macfarlane Trust, which was in turn retraumatizing them every time they asked for help.

Seven years after Bryan's death, the Macfarlane Trust agreed to transfer its stake to a new property. Clair could move to London. But a precedent had been set: whenever she wanted to move, she had to ask the Macfarlane Trust. She couldn't break free from the organization that had treated her as nothing more than an ungrateful nuisance.

Shortly before the millennium, Clair gave up her career at the Shakespeare Birthplace Trust and moved to north London to help other people with HIV and AIDS. Here was a community that had reframed being HIV positive to focus on the 'positive.' They offered one another counseling, ran support groups, disseminated the latest research and had specialist hospice care; well-funded services that weren't available in the rest of the country. As she became more integrated and received welcome support, she began to realize just how isolated she had been. She worked with many of the leading HIV organizations, including the Elton John AIDS Foundation and Positively Women.

After a few years in London Clair regained her confidence and decided to return to her career. She had come to understand Bryan's philosophy in the years before he died, of seizing every day while you still had the time. She accepted a place at the Royal College of Art for a master's degree in conservation that was based in part at the Victoria and Albert Museum. She would finally realize her teenage dream of going to art school.

Having seen Bryan's deterioration while taking AZT, Clair had refused HIV medication for herself. She didn't want her identity to be subsumed by being a patient, and didn't want to put her life in the hands of pharma companies. Instead, she found alternative ways to look after herself, keeping fit with yoga and herbal teas, only occasionally treating herself to a pint of Guinness. But the thought of HIV was never far from her mind. When her tutor offered her a research trip to Austin, Texas, she had to turn it down without explanation because the US still restricted people who were HIV positive from entering the country (the rule was in place for twenty-two years and only lifted in 2010). She wasn't ready to tell people at university her HIV status.

While Clair was focusing on her studies, her health started to work against her. As had already happened to thousands of others, her T-cell count dropped. At first she ignored the symptoms, putting them down to tiredness and continuing to push herself each day. But she soon felt so unwell that daily life became difficult. Having always been petite, she shrank to six stone. Out of necessity, she told her tutor and course director the truth: she had HIV. But in reality, it was progressing to AIDS. They said they had thought she had anorexia, because of how thin she was. Clair convinced them to give her a year off to recover. The time would prove pivotal.

Reluctant to submit herself to the potentially degrading treatment Bryan had experienced, Clair put off going to the hospital for as long as she could. By the time she relented, she was desperately ill. Her consultant at the Royal Free told her she was within days of death. Clair had become so diminished, physically and emotionally, that all she could muster was a shrug of her shoulders. She was admitted to hospital with PCP, an AIDS-defining illness she knew had killed millions of patients in the last two decades. She also had Cytomegalovirus, or CMV, not in the eyes, which often caused blindness in people with AIDS, but in the brain. Her greatest fear had come to pass: she was in hospital far from home, weak and frighteningly alone. With her family back in Warwickshire, she had no one to offer her comfort when she needed it. Even though the Royal Free's AIDS ward had been open for nearly twenty years, Clair was wary of the staff. She balked when a nurse assumed she had acquired HIV from drug use. And she told the consultant she only wanted to have medication at the last possible moment. Clair feared she would become one of the more than two million people per year who were dying from AIDS-related illness.

When the time came that Clair couldn't survive any longer without medication, her doctor gave her antiretrovirals. Gradually, she became stronger. Having recovered sufficiently to leave hospital, she went straight back to the Royal College of Art, determined to finish her course. She wanted life to continue.

Whenever Clair, timorous but defiant, took the rare leap of telling someone she had HIV she could almost see their brains tick into gear and the nasty questions begin: How did she *get* HIV? She must be a drug user; the way she is behaving must be related to her drug use. Clair didn't want to have to preface her diagnosis with the fact she was the widow of a hemophiliac; no one should be discriminated against because they were HIV positive. It might have been 2004, but society still harbored the same prejudices from the 1980s. And Clair herself harbored the memories. She couldn't escape the terror of that era: in her mind she was still a timid twenty-three-year-old living with the stigma of the early years of the AIDS epidemic.

Clair succeeded in getting a number of extensions, but she pushed her recovery too hastily and became ill again. While she was back in hospital, a letter arrived from the Royal College of Art. She had missed too many deadlines, it said, and the university was terminating her place. Her last ember was now extinguished. She had been expelled from her course; her childhood dream snatched away from her.

As if to kick her while she was down, another message landed with her in the hospital on the anniversary of Bryan's death. This was an update from the Macfarlane Trust about the ongoing fight over her house and the profit it was trying to extract from her. She was just one of hundreds of people asking for assistance, it said, many of whom 'have dependent families, which you do not.' Only because the opportunity to do so had been cruelly taken from her, she thought.

When Clair eventually left the hospital, she went to the UK Coalition of People Living With HIV and AIDS in south London, seeking support. She told a charity worker how she had lost her place on the master's course while she was in hospital with AIDS. They said the decision amounted to discrimination and promised to help her challenge it. The compassion this stranger showed her provided the lift she needed. At an appeal meeting, Professor Sir Christopher Frayling, the rector of the Royal College of Art, said he was shocked by the decision of his colleagues. Clair felt a rare dose of warmth and understanding.

'I should not have been given deadline after deadline, but given the opportunity to go away and get better,' she said.

Afterwards, Frayling sent Clair a letter of apology and promised to change the university's HIV policy. He praised her courage and said she could have her place back when she was better. Caught off guard by this uncommon act of humanity, Clair felt relief at having been heard. She knew she could keep going.

In 2005 someone hacked into the Macfarlane Trust's computer system and leaked internal emails that showed just how derogatory its employees had been about beneficiaries. For years, HIV survivors felt like they had been mistreated by the Trust – and here was the proof. One trustee had called them 'the great unwashed.' Writing to a colleague about Birchgrove co-founder Haydn Lewis, chairman Peter Stevens had said: 'It is irritating that somebody so thick can come up with such meddlesome suggestions.' In another email about a group of recipients he saw regularly, he wrote, 'What a monumental waste of time not just this afternoon but all the previous hours spent nurturing that lot of moaners.' (Stevens later apologized, saying his language had been 'totally inappropriate' and 'disgraceful.')

The leak gave survivors motivation to start a new campaign group for people with HIV and hepatitis C, called Tainted Blood. Former Treloar's pupils Richard Warwick, Gary Webster, and Ade Goodyear all joined. Founding member Andrew March was an experienced researcher and he set about compiling into a manifesto all the evidence of wrongdoing that survivors had so far collected. The result was a seventy-page 'Accusations Document,' which listed the people and organizations they held responsible for their infections and the deaths of their friends.

The manifesto opened with eight allegations, each paragraph beginning 'We accuse' – a nod to Émile Zola's *J'Accuse . . . !*, an open letter about the unlawful jailing of Alfred Dreyfus. Tainted Blood accused the UK government of gross maladministration for failing to achieve self-sufficiency; ignoring warnings about AIDS and hepatitis; failing to protect them; and unlawful and immoral behaviour in the HIV litigation when it made people sign Dr Rejman's hepatitis waiver despite knowing thousands had been infected. They accused hemophilia doctors of conducting unethical research on them without their consent; of deliberately using children at Treloar's for hepatitis trials; and withholding test results. The final accusation: 'We accuse the government and the Department of Health of a COVER-UP regarding the contaminated blood catastrophe – in ATTEMPTING TO VANISH crucial evidence, and in allowing the shredding of documents.' Over the following pages, Tainted Blood outlined the evidence in detail, before concluding:

> We are fighting for closure, not only for the survivors but for those who have been left behind. We all deserve answers as to why this has happened and we need to be able to live, not just exist. The people we entrusted our lives to have wronged us, but they have also grossly underestimated the will and strength of the survivors of this tragedy. . . . Against overwhelming evidence, no fault has ever been admitted by either the government or the pharmaceutical companies who supplied the contaminated blood products. We start the process towards the end here.

12. Breakthrough

Snow was piled high on the streets of Manchester at the beginning of 2010. After consecutive days of snowfall, it had become the coldest January in the UK since 1987. Newspapers called it the 'big freeze' as temperatures plummeted to minus 17.6°C in parts of the city, wreaking havoc on the roads.

Andy Burnham was in the garden with his son, kicking a football through snow clouds. It was a Monday morning but, given the weather, schools were closed and children were at home. Burnham had a few minutes to spare before leaving for his constituency office in Leigh. He was seven months into his new job as secretary of state for health and was due to meet people who had contracted chronic viruses from infected Factor VIII on the insistence of his good friend Paul Goggins, the Labour MP for another Manchester constituency, Wythenshawe and Sale East. Goggins believed the contaminated blood scandal could prove to be a cover-up as grave as the Hillsborough disaster – in which ninety-seven football fans had been killed during a crush at a poorly policed football stadium in Sheffield – only with thousands of victims.

'Just sit down, talk to them,' said Goggins. 'Do what you did with the Hillsborough families.'

Before joining the Department of Health in 2009, Burnham had been instrumental in getting the government to set up the Hillsborough Independent Panel, which led to over twenty-five thousand documents being brought to light that revealed how the police had covered up the fatal lack of control. The panel concluded forty-one victims could have survived, and that the police had amended 116 statements to remove unfavorable comments. Prime Minister David Cameron consequently apologized to the Hillsborough families for the 'double injustice.'

It had taken Burnham months to set the date with Goggins. Infected blood was low on his list, falling behind the demands of a swine-flu pandemic and an NHS crisis after more than four hundred deaths at Stafford Hospital because of poor care and patient neglect. Additionally, a briefing from his civil service colleagues at the Department of Health had convinced him that people with hemophilia had been 'inadvertently infected' and that 'there was now little more to be learnt.'

Two years earlier, in 2007, Lord Peter Archer had opened an inquiry into contaminated blood products at the request of Lord Morris. Because the inquiry wasn't established by a government minister, Lord Archer didn't have the power to compel witnesses to give evidence. With that in mind, the Department of Health and the health secretary had refused to participate. Still, Lord Archer concluded after two years of investigation that the infection with HIV and hepatitis C of thousands of people by blood products was 'a horrific human tragedy.' He was dismayed at how long it had taken the government and scientific agencies to respond to the dangers of AIDS. If Britain had stopped importing Factor VIII earlier, the 'scale of the catastrophe would have been significantly reduced,' he said. Lord Archer added that the paternalistic relationship between doctors and patients in the 1980s – with doctors making decisions on behalf of patients without obtaining their consent – had unfortunate consequences. But the ultimate burden of responsibility rested with the pharmaceutical companies.

'Long after alarms had been sounded about the risks of obtaining paid-for blood donations from communities with an increased incidence of relevant infections, such as prison inmates, this practice continued,' he said. 'It is difficult to avoid the conclusion that commercial interests took precedence over public health concerns.'

Lord Archer recommended the UK government provide compensation that was 'at least the equivalent' to that paid in Ireland – where each victim had received on average £150,000. He also said it should set up a patient advisory panel to give people with hemophilia more say over their treatment, as had been established in the US. 'Commercial interests should never again override the interests of public health,' he said.

The government's mistakes had, at least in part, been exposed, but it refused to give up its steadfast position of the last twenty years. When the Labour government responded to Lord Archer's findings on May 20, 2009, the prime minister, Gordon Brown, didn't issue a formal apology. Nor did Health Secretary Alan Johnson address the findings in Parliament. Instead, the Department of Health issued a written statement from Public Health Minister Dawn Primarolo. The government would double the annual payments for people with HIV who were still alive to £12,800 per year, and would review the annual £5,000 for people with hepatitis C in five years' time. The money would still be funneled through the Macfarlane and Skipton Trusts, as the previous £150 million had been. Lord Archer's other recommendations were ignored; 'Steps to safeguard blood products against HIV and hepatitis C have been in place since 1985,' said Primarolo. The Department of Health believed the matter had been dealt with – and it told Burnham as much when he became health secretary a couple of months after Lord Archer released his report.

A fortnight into Burnham's tenure, the Manor House Group had held a significant protest outside his constituency office. Defying his staff's advice to avoid going in that day, he entered through the back door. One of the protestors was David Tonkin, chair of the Manor House Group. Campaigning had become a full-time job for David, who had a small office under the stairs at home and would often be on the phone until the early hours of the morning. He handed Burnham a letter that outlined how he and thousands of others had been infected with hepatitis C by blood products. In response, the Department of Health sent Tonkin a defensive letter signed by Burnham, which said:

> There is no evidence that individuals were knowingly infected with contaminated blood and blood products. Although there was recognition at the time among the medical community that there was some degree of risk, it was not possible to test donors for these infections. The overwhelming consensus among the experts was that the risks were outweighed by the benefit that these new treatments brought.

Burnham's office was subsequently bombarded with letters from campaigners – all of whom received similar replies.

When the time came for Burnham to meet the constituents who had been infected and affected by contaminated blood along with Goggins and another MP, Brian Iddon, the Department of Health yet again briefed him that the matter was closed. He didn't want to disbelieve his colleagues, but he was willing to listen.

One constituent, Fred Bates, explained how he had received a diagnosis for hepatitis C in 1993 after he read a leaflet about the condition and asked his doctor outright if he was positive. By 2010, Fred had cirrhosis of the liver and continuously felt cold. But what stood out to Burnham was how Fred discovered he had hepatitis B. In 1994 he and his wife were talking to his solicitor, who casually mentioned he had tested positive for hepatitis B back in 1977. He had never been told he had the virus.

Goggins was in contact with other campaigners, including Manor House co-founder Peter Mossman and his friend Carol Grayson, who had both shared a wealth of documents that showed the government had known about the dangers of hepatitis but hadn't warned patients. Among these was a 1981 letter from the Department of Health to the Treasury which said that, because of insufficient Factor VIII supplies from Blood Products Laboratory, it was having to supplement 'with expensive and, because of the hepatitis risk, less safe imported commercial blood products at a cost of £10 million annually.' Patients like Fred had been put directly in harm's way and then deliberately kept in the dark.

Burnham realized the Department of Health had given him a certain version of events, but something was very badly wrong. If he was understanding correctly, it appeared his colleagues had been lying to him and a cover-up had been underway for decades.

After the meeting, Burnham asked his colleagues in the civil service to reopen the issue. The Department of Health conducted a review of the Macfarlane and Skipton support schemes, which led to some more funding, but it wasn't enough. Burnham was now committed to getting to the truth. A few months later, in April 2010, a separate judicial review into the government's decision not to compensate victims found its approach 'has been, and remains, infected by error.' But in May Labour lost the general election and Burnham was relegated to fighting from the opposition benches.

Back in 2008, with the Archer Inquiry underway in London, Scotland's deputy first minister Nicola Sturgeon announced her government's own inquiry into how blood products and transfusions had come to infect seventy-eight Scottish people with HIV and nearly three thousand with hepatitis C. Like Lord Archer, Lord George Penrose couldn't compel members of the Department of Health to give evidence to his inquiry, even though he was looking at England alongside Scotland. Survivors and bereaved family members held on to the hope that his report could bring them the truth.

By 2015, after six years and £12 million, Lord Penrose had finished his report. He was seriously ill in hospital, so it fell to the inquiry's secretary to present his findings. On a cool, bright late-March day in Edinburgh, Maria McCann addressed hundreds of victims and family members in the auditorium of the National Museum of Scotland. Lord Penrose's report ran to eighteen hundred pages, but the crux was that very little could or should have been done differently. Lord Penrose had one clear recommendation: the Scottish government should offer a hepatitis C test to anyone who had a blood transfusion before September 1991. Parallel to the scandal of Factor VIII, up to 26,800 people in the UK were estimated to have been infected with hepatitis C from blood transfusions before screening began in 1991. But the national testing was restricted to Scotland, so thousands of people in the UK remain unaware. From 2019 to 2023, 110 people learned they had been living with hepatitis C as a result of blood transfusions they'd had more than three decades earlier.

When McCann conveyed Lord Penrose's sympathy for the clinical staff who had suffered throughout the infected blood disaster, the room erupted. Believing his support misplaced, people stood up and shouted 'whitewash,' pointing angrily at McCann. Others threw the report to the ground and left the auditorium in protest. Some wept at the verdict. Insults from survivors echoed across the news: travesty, obscene, waste of time. One campaigner called the report a '£12 million door stop.' Another said they wanted those responsible to be charged with murder. Again, their hopes of justice had been dashed.

But there was one unprecedented outcome of the Penrose Report. Down in Westminster, Prime Minister Cameron stood at the Despatch Box in the House of Commons and apologized to the victims of contaminated blood.

'It is difficult to imagine the feelings of unfairness that people must feel at being infected with hepatitis C or HIV as a result of totally unrelated treatment within the NHS,' he said. 'I would like to say sorry on behalf of the government for something that should not have happened.'

He offered £25 million to improve the way support money reached survivors and their widows, and promised proper compensation to recognize the damage done to people's lives. But the compensation, which could exceed a billion pounds, never materialized.

'They have just been biding their time, waiting for as many people to die as possible before ultimately they will do something when there's half a dozen of us left,' says former Treloar's pupil Richard Warwick. 'In the eyes of the government, we were expendable. An inconvenient afterthought that should have gone away a long time ago. And they just wanted rid of us.'

The legacy of the Penrose Report was captured in stark footage. Outside the museum, a group of campaigners who had traveled from England started ripping up its pages. Then, on the pavement in Edinburgh, they set fire to it sheet by sheet.

As the embers of the Penrose Report smoldered on Jason Evans's computer screen, something shifted in his mind. Jason was a twenty-six-year-old hip-hop DJ from Coventry, who had been following the contaminated blood campaign from afar. He had booked the day off from his nine-to-five marketing job knowing the Penrose Report was due to be released, and was following updates on Facebook. The day had mostly been spent waiting for what he hoped would be answers that explained his life to date. But when news started to filter through about Lord Penrose's conclusions, it became clear the report was a disaster. Jason heard the shouts of 'whitewash' and saw the flaming papers. As Lord Penrose's findings literally turned to ash, there was one phrase that stuck in his mind: 'little could or should have been done differently.' In his dad's case alone, he knew that wasn't true. There were multiple times when things could have been done differently, things that might have saved his dad's life. Anger built inside him. Looking at the screen, he made a promise to himself: he would do something to avenge his dad.

Jason had one memory of his father, Jonathan, from his fourth birthday. It was approaching the end of summer in 1993 and his mum had taken him to his grandparents' house to visit his dad. Jason remembers clutching his Game Boy; his dad was in bed. Jonathan was too weak to get up and play with him, but that felt normal for Jason, whose dad had been ill for so much of his short life. Six weeks later, on October 8, 1993, Jonathan had died from AIDS-related illness, aged thirty-one. Jason's next memory was from his father's funeral. Too young to comprehend that he would never see his dad again, he remembered the enveloping sadness in the church, a sea of crying adults, his grandma looking down at him through tears. Someone later told him he had placed a rose on his dad's coffin and said, 'Bye bye, Daddy, I'll miss you.' From that day, he would always think of his dad whenever he heard 'In the Air Tonight' by Phil Collins, which had played at the funeral.

After his death, Jonathan became a mystery to his son. Jason's mum would cry every time she tried to talk about her deceased husband, so for years Jason knew very little about his father. He didn't know that his mum had given birth to him surrounded by medical staff wearing protective equipment that made them look like they were going into space. Nor did he know that on his birth certificate, next to the place where a midwife had written his birth weight, there was a stamp that said BIOHAZARD. On the day he was born, Jason had an HIV test. But he didn't know any of that when, at primary school, he was using the water fountain and two girls approached him from behind.

'Don't use that, that's the AIDS boy,' one of the girls said to the other. 'There's going to be AIDS on the fountain.'

That evening, as Jason recounted the story to his mum, she looked away before explaining that AIDS was an illness and his dad had died from it. That was it; she didn't elaborate. She contacted the school and asked them to make sure Jason wasn't exposed to more hurtful comments. But children were soon telling him his dad must have been gay. They lived in a small village where anonymity was impossible. Learning more about AIDS as he went through primary school, Jason started to come up with theories of how his dad had contracted the illness. Perhaps his dad had been secretly gay? Or maybe he was an intravenous drug user? His mum's reticence made him feel like there was a family conspiracy to keep him in the dark.

Needing answers, Jason braced himself to ask his mum about his dad again. What was the secret she had been keeping from him? This time she told him his dad used to take a medicine called Factor VIII, which contained AIDS. And then she started to cry. Trying to get answers from his mum was futile. The subject was too triggering for her. If he really wanted to know what had happened to his dad, he would have to find out for himself.

The opportunity came in his first computer lesson at secondary school when the teacher said they would be trying out a new thing called Google, on which they could search for anything they wanted. Jason opened Google and typed 'AIDS,' then 'blood.' In the results, he read about how AIDS had been transmitted to people with hemophilia. His father must have had hemophilia – and he wasn't the only person who had died in this tragic accident. But the knowledge did little to help Jason in the face of continuous nasty jokes about AIDS. As he went through secondary school, the feeling that he was an outlier threw Jason off the rails. 'The system' had killed his dad and he didn't want to be a part of it. He bunked off school and skipped multiple GCSE exams. While his friends followed traditional paths – taking gap years and going to university – Jason became engrossed in his main passion: hip-hop music. He became a DJ and performed to audiences across Europe. All the while, he tried to ignore the permanent lump that had developed in his throat. He worried it could be throat cancer, but tests showed it was globus pharyngeus – a physical symptom of anxiety. At night, he was tormented by panic attacks.

When Jason was eighteen, his grandfather gave him a small collection of his dad's medical records. He read how Jonathan had asked to return to cryo because of the dangers of AIDS. But after one round of cryo, Jonathan's doctor had encouraged him to continue with Factor VIII, saying what he had heard in the press was mere sensationalism. Then, Jonathan had been told he was positive for HTLV-III around six months after the hospital had known. That was the extent of Jason's knowledge when the Penrose Report came out.

Having made the promise to himself to avenge his dad, Jason started to investigate how blood products had become contaminated. He read about the Freedom of Information Act, which gave UK citizens the right to access public records. He filed his first FOI request to the Oxford Health NHS Foundation Trust, where his dad had been treated, and asked to know all of the brands of Factor VIII it had used in the 1980s. To his surprise, the Trust responded with a spreadsheet containing a list of manufacturers and batch numbers. Jason wasn't sure what to do with it, but he had discovered that he could get information simply by asking for it. He sent request after request to the Department of Health and the Cabinet Office. Within two years, he had filed a thousand of them.

The sheer quantity of information was overwhelming. When the documents shared with the Penrose Inquiry became available through the National Archives, Jason downloaded all of them onto his computer – amounting to tens of thousands of pages. He quickly figured out what to look for and started piecing together evidence of wrongdoing and negligence. Deep in those pages was the story of how his dad ended up dying at thirty-one. He became obsessive, reading documents late into the night. After finishing work, he would have dinner then continue his research, often taking his laptop to bed. His girlfriend broke up with him and his music career took a back seat, but he didn't care: he had a chance to have a real impact in the world and understand what had happened to his dad.

Realizing there was more material to be found at the National Archives themselves in Kew, he started driving a hundred miles from Coventry to south London most Saturdays. He would spend the day sifting through files from decades past. Forbidden from bringing food or drink into the reading rooms, he wouldn't eat or drink anything for eight hours. On leaving the archives for the drive home he always had a pounding headache.

Jason's first major breakthrough came when he discovered a government memo from 1987 outlining how the Department of Health's knowledge of AIDS had developed from 1982 to 1984. The typewritten document showed the government had said there was 'no conclusive evidence' AIDS was transmitted through blood 'to reduce public anxiety.' But behind closed doors, it had in fact 'assumed in its policy decisions that AIDS <u>was</u> transmitted by an infective agent.' The worst part for Jason was that the government had accepted there was conclusive proof AIDS was caused by a blood-borne virus in April 1984, when Dr Gallo's team discovered HTLV-III. 'However by then public interest had waned,' said the memo, so the government hadn't publicly acknowledged that until December 1984. In those eight months, Jason's dad had wanted to switch to cryo, but his doctor had told him the press reports weren't to be trusted. In November 1984, Jonathan tested positive for HTLV-III.

Jason believed he had new evidence on his hands – and he contacted a journalist at the *Daily Express* with his discovery. That week, his research was printed in a national newspaper.

Another document he found was from the Treasury in 1991, around the time of the HIV litigation, which contained a rough calculation of how much money would be saved on people with hemophilia over the next two years as they died from AIDS: '147 will die, wives will claim [housing benefits] for 18 months,' said the memo. In that time, Jason's dad had passed away and his mum had become a widow; they had been little more than a number.

The first time Jason met other campaigners was at a protest in Westminster in April 2016, which he had helped to organize. In all the years of campaigning, it was one of the first protests to bring the groups together under one banner. The boys from Treloar's were there, as well as Frankie. One person who caught Jason's eye was Tony Farrugia, who had painted himself bright red in honor of his father and two uncles who had died from HIV and hepatitis C. Jason had printed off a selection of around ten key documents and put them into brown paper envelopes.

'Please read this,' he said as he handed them to journalists and MPs.

Inside was the letter John Major had sent in 1987 warning the government against a 'sympathetic response' when it made the first payments to the Macfarlane Trust because it could lead to a lawsuit, and the 1985 memo that showed the FDA's Dr Meyer had asked the pharmaceutical companies to 'quietly' stop using unheated Factor VIII. Later that day, MP Dr Philippa Whitford read both documents aloud in the House of Commons. Jason was amazed at his achievement: something he had printed off at home was being read inside Parliament. He still felt like a kid who liked to DJ with his friends, but here he was holding power to account.

Jason met more campaigners, some of whom had known his dad. Through them, he learned disquieting details about his father's life, such as how his dad would have been expecting a painful death after seeing his friends pass away before him. He also discovered his dad had been adopted at birth. Meeting his father's biological sister for the first time, she told him she and Jonathan had another brother who had also died from AIDS-related illness and hepatitis C. The two estranged brothers had passed away within a couple of years of each other.

The weight of unearthed history was taking its toll. Jason wasn't the type to talk about how he was feeling; he had hardly told his mum about his campaign work. In need of support, he asked the Macfarlane Trust for a counseling grant. Facing some resistance, he had to push for it and tell them it might save his life. When he eventually spoke to a counselor, they helped him understand why he had become so obsessive about investigating the blood scandal: poring over the history had the same effect as listening to a piece of music that reminded him of his dad. His research had given him a new connection to his father: a closeness he had been lacking. It made sense. Every hour he spent reading documents was stretching out the limited time they had together.

In November 2016 Jason went to London to watch a House of Commons debate about contaminated blood. As he sat in the public gallery, looking at the chamber where so many evasions had taken place, he heard a statement from a government minister that he knew was false. 'It is difficult to see what more information could be made available through a public inquiry given that action was taken as soon as possible to introduce testing and safety measures for blood and blood products as these became available, with the introduction of heated products,' said Nicola Blackwood, parliamentary undersecretary of state for public health and innovation.

Jason knew he had exhumed enough evidence to challenge the government. He had been sharing documents with BBC's investigative documentary program *Panorama*, which was making an hour-long special about contaminated blood. But Jason knew public attention was just one weapon in the campaigners' arsenal. What he really wanted was the government's attention – and a recourse to justice. For that, he needed a lawyer.

When Des Collins agreed to attend an event Andy Burnham was holding in Westminster for justice activists at the start of 2017, he had been toying with the idea of retiring. He had a reputation for being a fierce litigator, winning fights for ordinary people against corporations and public bodies. But for those who bumped into him on the streets of Watford, where his firm, Collins Solicitors, was based, he had a far more unassuming air, speaking with halting care and an easy laugh. He had the approachable look of an old-fashioned private detective, with a silver moustache and watery blue eyes. Des was sixty-eight and wasn't looking for new cases, but he and his colleague Dani Holliday had gone along to support two clients whose child had died in a flood.

Des's type of legal work involved risk – he could easily work on a case for ten years before the chance of getting paid came close – but he found it gratifying to know he was helping fight corporate wrongdoing and negligence. He earned his reputation with a toxic-waste case in his hometown of Corby. In the years after Corby's steelworks had closed down, babies had been born with limb defects at a rate three times higher than in the surrounding area and ten times higher than expected in a town of sixty thousand people. With Des's help, the parents of eighteen children brought a multimillion-pound legal case against Corby Borough Council. In a landmark victory, he proved the council had put people at risk by not disposing of toxic material properly. Internationally, it was the first time a case like that had been fought – let alone won. The press described it as 'the worst child poisoning case since thalidomide' and said it echoed Erin Brockovich. Lauding their victory, Collins Solicitors' public relations team emailed Brockovich, whose work investigating the contamination of drinking water in Hinkley, California, had ended with a $333 million settlement and a film starring Julia Roberts. Brockovich replied with congratulations, and for months afterwards Collins Solicitors had a cardboard cutout of her in their office.

In the House of Commons for Burnham's Justice Summit, Des listened as half a dozen groups told the lawyers and politicians in the room how their cases of injustice had never progressed. One of the speakers was a young man in his twenties called Jason Evans who said his dad had died from AIDS-related illness after a medical treatment infected him with HIV. And he had evidence it could have been prevented. Des looked at Dani.

'You're too young to know about this,' he said under his breath. 'But I thought this was all settled back with the HIV settlement. I can't believe this is still going on.'

After the talks, Dani gave her business card to Jason and his friend Max, who had been infected with HIV and hepatitis C himself.

'If you want to have a chat sometime, give us a ring,' she said.

Jason wasn't going to wait around. He had contacted over a hundred solicitors, but they had all refused to take him on. Within a week of meeting Des and Dani, he called Collins.

Des arranged for Dani and four of his colleagues to join them for a meeting with Jason and Max. In the event they had a case, he wanted to be able to make the call there and then.

Jason and Max didn't look like the bookish, activist types; they just seemed like normal blokes, which made Des even more surprised when, every time he asked a question, Jason had the answer.

'What's your evidence for that?' Des would ask, and Jason would slide a document across the table.

Jason had brought with him a selection of around twenty key documents that he believed proved wrongdoing by the Department of Health. He showed Des how doctors and politicians had known about the risk of hepatitis and HIV in Factor VIII long before patients developed illnesses. Des couldn't believe what he was hearing. He had one thought: this was dynamite. They spoke for two hours, with Jason laying out the potted history of contaminated blood. As the meeting drew to a close, Des had a suggestion.

'Why don't we write to the Department of Health and tell them we're going to bring legal action?' he said.

'Yeah, that sounds OK to me,' said Jason, holding in somersaults of excitement. Finally, he thought, someone wanted to act.

Des suggested they sue the Department of Health for misfeasance in public office, which meant it had knowingly and willingly caused loss or harm to a third party. Although the case had been closed in 1991 and people with hemophilia had waived the right to bring further legal action, Des knew that could be overruled if they proved the government was guilty of misfeasance. The case would be complicated, but for Des it boiled down to a simple set of facts: something was wrong, the department hadn't told people, and those people had then died.

Collins Solicitors was lucky to have enough resources to throw at the case. Major law firms had rejected it, which Des thought was because of the risk of taking on a difficult case without the guarantee of earning money. That was one of the reasons he liked running his own firm: he could unilaterally decide to do something while shaving first thing, develop the idea in the shower and implement it by 10:30 a.m. Once he had the approval of his colleagues and wife, of course. Des knew he would be taking a massive risk by agreeing to represent Jason and Max. Suing the Department of Health was an initial step, but even in that first meeting, Des had a bigger goal in mind. If they hit hard enough and quickly enough, they might be able to force the government at long last to announce a public inquiry into infected blood. With little more than Jason's two-hour rundown, Des came to believe a public inquiry would end up reporting 'this was badly handled by the government, that it was a cover-up and that these people should have been compensated.' He believed true compensation could be anywhere from hundreds of thousands of pounds per person to several million.

Within a few days, Collins Solicitors had roughly a hundred new clients, all of whom were either survivors of contaminated blood or bereaved relatives. Within a couple of weeks, that number had hit five hundred. In May 2017 the BBC aired its *Panorama* episode about the infected blood scandal and Jason's mum told him how proud she was of him. With awareness at a high, Des, Jason and Max went public with the news: they were suing the Department of Health for misfeasance in public office.

On July 4, the front page of the *Daily Mail* read: 'NHS Tainted Blood Shame.' Jason had fed journalists documents that showed patients were given Factor VIII contaminated with deadly hepatitis for at least five years after officials knew about the dangers. He gave the paper notes from an international meeting in Glasgow held in September 1980 at which virologist Dr John Craske had warned hematologists to expect problems in their patients within a decade. Dr Craske had said: 'There is a high risk from the use of Factor VIII or IX concentrate that the patients will contract non-A, non-B hepatitis, and a 20–30 percent chance of resultant chronic hepatitis.' Within nine months, minutes showed, doctors and scientific advisers had known up to fifty cases of non-A, non-B hepatitis were being reported each year. Rather than warning patients or changing treatment, they decided to use patients for a study into hepatitis. This same attitude had then continued as AIDS emerged.

Jason had put contaminated blood back onto the front page of a national newspaper. On the day that article ran, Des went to the High Court to lodge the civil action against the Department of Health.

Andy Burnham was preparing to leave Parliament in April 2017 and take up his new position as mayor of Greater Manchester. Before doing so, he had one last opportunity to address the House of

Commons – and he wanted to use it to raise the issue of infected blood. He had faced resistance within the civil service to reopening the matter ever since his meeting with Goggins and campaigners back in January 2010, and had come to believe this was because the establishment was resistant to addressing historical injustices. He took to the Despatch Box to make a final plea to his colleagues.

'Knowing what I know, and what I believe to be true, I would not be able to live with myself if I left here without putting it on the official record,' he began. 'I will be honest: this is a speech made with a sense of guilt in that all of us here are collectively culpable of failing to act on evidence that is there before us if only we cared to look. And, by extension, failing thousands of our fellow citizens who are the victims of perhaps the greatest untold injustice in the history of this country.'

Burnham wanted to pull on the heartstrings of his fellow MPs, but he didn't want to just reiterate what so many before him had already said in Parliament. He wanted to compel his colleagues to act. Following Cameron's apology, there had been an expectation among survivors and politicians that the government might offer proper compensation.

'However, following those expectations victims now feel that they have been led up to the top of the hill only to be let down once again,' he said.

The more Burnham had thought about the contaminated blood scandal, the more parallels he could see with Hillsborough. 'Both relate to the 1980s and both resulted from appalling negligence by public bodies,' he said. But, more importantly, the two scandals involved an 'orchestrated campaign to prevent the truth being told.'

Here Burnham reached the crux of the problem. Once the truth was revealed the government would have no choice but to offer full compensation to the victims of contaminated blood, just as it had done with the families of those crushed at Hillsborough Stadium. Survivors had been silenced by the stigma of their illnesses. They were dispersed across the country, too, which had made it harder to campaign collectively. And, of course, many of them had already died. On their behalf, Burnham wanted to convince Parliament to give them the two things they had so longed for but never had: the truth and justice.

'This scandal amounts to a criminal cover-up on an industrial scale,' he said. His evidence? He knew hundreds of victims could show crucial pages were missing from their medical notes. He told the story of three individuals. There was an eight-year-old child who was infected with hepatitis C after being treated with twelve infusions of contaminated blood products for a swollen knee. His medical records contained details of everything from his knee problem to his test for HIV – but the batch numbers for the products that infected him were missing. The next was a child whose doctor had tested them for hepatitis C without their parents' consent.

'In my view, it is a criminal act to test a child without a parent's knowledge,' Burnham said.

Third was the story of Ken Bullock, a high-ranking civil engineer with hemophillia who had been infected with hepatitis C. His medical notes contained his initial infection in 1983, but from the end of that year, all mention of blood products in his notes had ceased. Doctors instead put his liver damage down to alcoholism. When Ken needed a liver transplant in 1998 it was refused to him because of the assertions that he was an alcoholic. He only ever drank an occasional glass of wine – and the last was on his wife's sixtieth birthday in 1995. Without the transplant, he died.

As a final conclusion, Burnham said he had two letters that proved the knowledge of real risk to patients' lives – and what the establishment wanted to cover up. He had the letter Dr Joseph Garrott Allen had sent from Stanford University to Britain's Blood Products Laboratory in 1975 saying that American plasma was being procured '100 per cent from Skid Row derelicts.' The second was the 1983 'cheaper than chimps' letter in which doctors said they would test the 'infectivity' of Factor VIII on patients.

'We soon start to see that there was something here that needed to be hidden,' said Burnham.

With that, he listed the wrongdoing he had seen evidence of: people were treated as guinea pigs; they were given inappropriate treatment; tests were conducted without consent; those test results were often withheld for years – and in some cases decades – even when positive; medical records had been falsified.

'Just as the evidence of amended police statements provided the thread that we eventually pulled to unravel the Hillsborough cover-up, so I believe the evidence that I have just provided must now become the trigger for a wider inquiry into establishing the truth about contaminated blood,' said Burnham. 'My suspicion is that there are documents held at a national level, either by the government or by regulatory or professional bodies, that point to a more systematic effort to suppress the truth.'

Momentum was building. There was more public awareness after the *Panorama* documentary, the media was paying attention and Burnham had roused his parlimentary colleagues with his final speech. Then the final piece of the puzzle slotted into place. In June 2017 Prime Minister Theresa May called a snap general election, which the Conservatives narrowly won. With her party lacking an overall majority, May formed a coalition with Northern Ireland's Democratic Unionist Party, which had supported a cross-party call for a Hillsborough-style inquiry into the contaminated blood scandal.

A month into the new Parliament, on July 11, May made an announcement that thousands of survivors had waited more than thirty years to hear: there would be a full public inquiry into infected blood. It would be funded by the government and would have statutory powers. The NHS had failed patients and the government had denied them answers for too long. She promised those wrongs would now be addressed.

13.   Inquiry

A couple of hundred meters north of the Thames, down a narrow lane that opens into a peaceful square, there is a tired grey office block that reflects the austerity of postwar London. Fleetbank House stands at the crossroads of truth and justice, sandwiched between Fleet Street, the historical home of British journalism, and the Royal Courts of Justice, the country's most important courthouse. Despite its humble appearance, Fleetbank House was about to become a home away from home for thousands of people. The core participants of the Infected Blood Inquiry would travel to London for weeks at a time from the end of April 2019 until February 2023 to hear the reality of their lives laid bare.

Within Fleetbank House's stone walls, people who had been infected with and bereaved by HIV, hepatitis C and other blood-borne viruses would find a fragile sense of community. Outside, they could seek solace in the leafy Salisbury Square. There would be days when the courtyard reverberated with anger; on others, it provided a quiet space for tears. People would break for cigarettes between hearings. The press would broadcast the latest evidence from politicians. Lawyers would debrief with their clients. And survivors would stand proudly together, shoulder to shoulder. Passersby could identify some of them by their uniform, a black-, red- and yellow-striped tie, or breast pin with the same colors. The yellow was for hepatitis; red for HIV; and black for the 2,900 or more people who had died after treatment with infected blood products and transfusions (by 2019, at least 1,170 people with bleeding disorders had died after contracting HIV and hepatitis C from plasma products, and 1,675 from blood transfusions).

On a warm spring morning at the end of April 2019, Sir Brian Langstaff arrived at Fleetbank House for the opening day of hearings at the Infected Blood Inquiry. He had been a judge in Britain long enough to know today wasn't about him; it was about the thousands of participants who had waited thirty-five years for answers. Sir Brian commanded a reassuring presence despite his small stature and self-effacing manner. He would become known for his forensic questioning style. Sir Brian understood the weight of responsibility he had taken on in chairing the inquiry: after decades of obfuscation he finally had the power to compel witnesses to give evidence. He wanted to convey as much to the 2,007 core participants who were either infected with HIV and hepatitis, or affected by a loved one being so. Stepping up to the plinth, Sir Brian began his opening address by thanking campaigners for their passionate resilience; if not for them, this moment would never have come. He had already spent a year reading evidence and going through the detailed histories people had put together, which he knew had stirred up painful memories.

'Some are harrowing, some incredibly moving, and some chillingly factual,' he said. 'There may be moments in the testimonies that you are about to hear, which may bring you close to tears, or they may excite indignation in any reasonable person. That is only human and I do not ask you to be anything else.' Sir Brian acknowledged that there would be times ahead when evidence would be 'unpalatable,' when people would want to blame witnesses for their infections, or when speakers would be evasive. No matter how high tensions ran, he asked people to treat one another considerately.

The inquiry's hearings would end up stretching across three and a half years, during which time Sir Brian would come to feel like a protective guardian for those who had been ostracized and ignored for so long. He understood this was their last chance for justice, and to know the truth.

'Finally, I am here to listen,' Sir Brian drew to a close. 'I know enough to realize that I have much more to learn.'

Derek Martindale made the courageous step of being the first witness on the stand. Wearing a suit and tie, his son accompanying him for support, he told Sir Brian how he had been diagnosed with HIV aged twenty-three on Friday, September 13, 1985. His brother Richard tested positive, too, after they had both been treated with contaminated Factor VIII. Derek struggled to support his brother, having himself been robbed of his future in those four words that had echoed across Britain's hospitals – 'a year to live.' They were both warned not to tell anyone, including family members, about their diagnoses.

'Richard knew he was dying; he knew he had AIDS,' said Derek, his son placing a reassuring hand on his back as his voice broke. 'He just wanted to talk about that, talk about his fears, how scared he was. But I couldn't. It was too close to home for me and I wasn't there for him. It was the biggest regret of my life, because he's gone and I can't do anything to make amends for that.' Richard died in 1990, shortly before his twenty-fourth birthday. Those who had come to watch – including Richard Warwick, Jason Evans, Frankie and Joe – gave Derek a standing ovation.

Throughout the opening week of the inquiry, one survivor after another told heartbreaking accounts of lethal infections, confronting their mortality, the difficulty of forming relationships with HIV, broken homes, and the battle for some kind of government support. They spoke about being tested without their consent and results being withheld for years. There were also those who had contracted hepatitis C from blood transfusions years ago but had only recently discovered they had the virus, because public awareness was still so low.

On the third day of hearings, it was Clair's turn to take the stand. She looked calm and self-possessed, with a long grey dress and her hair pulled back into a plait. Over the years, she had felt silenced as a woman with HIV: her story didn't fit with the accepted narratives. This was her chance to put her experience on the record – to tell an authority that was finally willing to listen. Clair retained her composure as she recalled how her husband, Bryan, had tested positive for HIV, and how she herself had contracted it a few years later as they tried for a baby. She maintained the same composure as she described Bryan's 'horrendous and painful' death from AIDS-related illness. But when she revealed the treatment she had received from the Macfarlane Trust, she finally foundered. Pain took over as she relived how worthless it had made her feel. People in the room gasped as she described how the Trust's stake had increased in value until someone there told her she was 'in hock to the MFT to the tune of over £168,000.' She described how, in 2017 after the government closed down the Macfarlane Trust, the stake in her home had been transferred without her knowledge to the Terrence Higgins Trust. She had remained shackled.

For Clair more than most, that week marked a new chapter in her life, because a few days before she gave evidence she had regained control of her house. The Terrence Higgins Trust had canceled her 'debt.' No longer could the organizations that had been designed to help people infected with HIV continue to profit from her and her dead husband. Leaving the witness stand, she felt like she had shed a skin.

Clair didn't have long to reflect after stepping into Salisbury Square, because she needed to get on the road. She was running late for a hospital appointment. She had made the daunting decision to come out publicly with her HIV status in that week, first by giving evidence without anonymity and then through an interview with me for the *Telegraph*. We climbed into the back of the photographer's car so we could speak on the way to Chelsea and Westminster Hospital.

'We've had it so embedded in us that we are toxic, we're poisoned and everybody will hate us,' said Clair in the car. 'Even though I know that's not true, it was how I felt right up until today.'

In many ways, her mind had ossified as a twenty-three-year-old's, conditioned as she was to be silent about HIV. Her generation had been some of the first to contract the virus. They had faced fear, ignorance and sudden death. Clair had carried the mental scars from 1985 right through to 2019; they had deepened in the face of further injustice and cover-up.

Clair had a full afternoon of appointments ahead of her at the hospital. She was in good physical health now, doing yoga every day and keeping her virus levels undetectable with antiretroviral therapy. But she still feared what age would bring. HIV exacerbated the signs of aging, while the treatment came with a higher risk of type two diabetes and cardiovascular disease. Clair lived some three hours from Chelsea but opted to receive her care there because of the hospital's brilliant reputation for treating patients with HIV, and her fear of encountering stigma in rural England. As we entered Chelsea and Westminster Hospital, she turned to me and said, 'This is my life.' Endless afternoons in hospital waiting rooms. Today was different, though. Her face wore a smile as she intermittently browsed a property website on her phone. For the first time in decades she was free to dream again – she could move house if she wanted to without having to battle the Trust.

Through the years of campaigning and long weeks at the inquiry, survivors found solidarity in unlikely places. For Clair, it was in friendship with Frankie. The two thought of themselves as very different people, who might never have been friends if it weren't for their similar experiences. But they had a common cause: to ensure women were not forgotten in this struggle (of seventy-one partners who had been infected in the UK, they were among those who were still alive). At the inquiry, they were often seen together, supporting one another when they were upset or incensed. Eventually, they decided to launch a campaign group of two called Positive Women via Factor 8.

On Frankie's day to give evidence, she was shaking with nerves. She had worn a pair of high heels, refusing to look like, or be known as, a victim. Trembling violently, she wondered as she approached the stand if she had made the right decision. Just about staying upright, she reached the witness box and sat on her hands, trying to still them. She was hot. Her voice shook. Within a couple of minutes, she was in tears.

'I've got no chance if I'm crying already, have I?' she said, twiddling her mum's rings and thinking of her parents.

Frankie had kept her life story hidden for thirty-six years, unable to shake the persistent guilt and shame that clung to her. After her dad died and she tested positive for HIV, she had distanced herself from her family. They knew Joe was HIV positive, but nothing more. They didn't know about her own diagnosis, or about her two terminations. A fragment of the truth would only lead to more questions. Living a double life, she had never shared her past with anyone, never written it down and never confronted it. With the secrecy, her personality had mutated, becoming jagged and insular. She became a skilled liar, locking away her past so effectively that even her family was unaware. As a result, she sometimes lashed out, once becoming violent towards a relative. She wouldn't advise anyone to hide their trauma in the way she had, but she couldn't see any other way.

A couple of years before the inquiry was announced, Frankie had finally told her mum and siblings the truth about her HIV diagnosis. Her brothers found it difficult. For years, they had behaved as though they were walking on eggshells around her, scared of her snapping if they said the wrong thing. She had refused to join them on holidays and take part in normal family life. Now at least they understood why she had been so cold and sullen.

Graciously, her mum took the news in stride, telling Frankie they would get on as they had always done. She had died knowing the truth, but they had lost so much time without being close or honest with one another.

'I just do not know how you did that,' one of her brothers confessed at her mother's wake. 'And I can't even compute how you did it on your own.'

'I can't either,' said Frankie. But she had no choice.

As Frankie neared the end of her evidence, she said her physical health had improved and her HIV was undetectable, but she still suffered from intermittent pain and was working on her mental health. 'I just want to say to everyone in this room, I know we have all been infected, I know we have all had crappy lives,' she said. 'I have probably been guilty of lashing out and appearing discompassionate. That's what has been shown to me. . . . My PTSD counseling is bringing my compassion forward. That's where I want to be.'

Sir Brian listened quietly as witnesses spoke, writing notes with a fountain pen. Every now and then, he interjected with a question. He always spoke with unwavering care and precision, whether he was addressing a traumatized widow or a defiant politician. At the end of Frankie's evidence, he showed her the empathy she had desperately craved.

'Can I be very clear: in this room you are not being judged for what you did, but valued for what you are,' said Sir Brian. 'I wouldn't myself use words like "angry" or "bitter" to describe what you have said. I think rather the words that come to my mind are "fierce" and "passionate" about what has happened to you and what should happen in the future.'

Watching his ex-wife, Joe relived some of the worst days of his life. He had taken the stand himself that morning, but hearing Frankie give evidence he realized she had been traumatized by the experience in a way he couldn't begin to understand. He almost wished they had never got married. If Frankie had walked away from him as a teenager, she could have saved herself. Despite knowing there was a mountain of evidence against those he held responsible for destroying their lives, he couldn't help but blame himself.

On a Friday afternoon in late June 2021, Jenni Richards, lead counsel for the inquiry, was rounding off a week of punishing evidence about the on-site hemophilia center at Treloar's. With her signature black suit and long silver chain necklace, Richards grilled former ministers about their mistakes and gently coaxed survivors when they were overcome with emotion. But there were days like this when the documents themselves told the harrowing story.

'Lord Mayor Treloar College is a unique establishment since there are more than fifty boys suffering from various coagulation defects in residence at the College for approximately 264 days each year,' said Richards, reading from a funding application from the early 1970s. 'It is the only establishment in the United Kingdom which can provide the opportunity and the facilities for extensive clinical trials of various kinds of treatment which cannot, at present, be conducted anywhere else.'

Richards was outlining evidence her team had gathered on the trials conducted on children at Treloar's. From the end of the 1960s, when the school had first taken on pupils with hemophilia, the center had received additional funding from the National Fund for Research into Crippling Diseases. The research began with Dr S. G. Rainsford, a former surgeon rear admiral in the Royal Navy, who had started treating boys at the school in 1969 and had set up a laboratory to study their bleeding patterns. This had continued through the 1970s and into the 1980s under Dr Tony Aronstam. After the introduction of Factor VIII, this research had expanded to include the effectiveness of prophylaxis and the safety of different brands. Some patients were treated with a placebo for extended periods of time as a control, while others were restricted to cryo. Then there were those who were treated solely with imported American Factor VIII – despite the known risks. Pharmaceutical companies had paid the school to conduct research trials, 'generously' contributing to the work that formed the basis of Dr Aronstam's book.

'In terms of the question of the significance of this research activity, there may be three issues which arise,' said Richards. Firstly, did doctors follow ethical guidelines and get consent from patients or their parents? Secondly, was research that exposed patients to viruses or resulted in them receiving a less safe version of treatment unethical? And finally, did the focus on research at Treloar's mean doctors lost sight of how to treat patients properly? In other words, asked Richards, had the doctors seen 'pupils as objects for research and study foremost, rather than as individual patients'?

One of the more controversial pieces of research conducted by British hemophilia doctors in the mid-1970s was the 'hepatitis study' coordinated by Dr Craske at the Public Health Laboratory Service. For this, doctors had monitored which brands of Factor VIII were most likely to transmit hepatitis, the effects on patients and the emergence of the more virulent non-A, non-B hepatitis. Treloar's formed a key part of the study. Research fellow Dr Peter Kirk, who worked with Dr Rainsford for a year, monitored forty-five boys for hepatitis from September 1975, each of whom was treated with either cryo, commercial imported Factor VIII or NHS-made Factor VIII. The doctors drew up a template for getting parental permission, but the inquiry had found limited evidence of parents actually receiving consent forms. Former pupil Nicholas Sainsbury said he had found a letter in his medical records saying he had been selected to be treated solely with Kryobulin, which was made in Europe with American plasma. The letter intended for his parents didn't say the change was for research, but so it would be 'easier to trace the source should he contract hepatitis.' When Nicholas asked his parents years later if they had received such a letter, they said no, they had never been contacted about his treatment when he was at the school. Even if they had got this particular letter, it didn't include a request for consent to their twelve-year-old taking part in a hepatitis study. 'There was nothing consensual,' said Nicholas, who died in 2023. 'They called us ticking time bombs . . . we were given a treatment that was supposed to enhance our lives. It was killing us.'

Richards and the inquiry's legal team discovered a pattern: although the Treloar's hemophilia center had a policy of asking parents to consent to their children taking part in studies or having a treatment change, there was little evidence in practice to show doctors had actually done so. A mother whose son died with HIV and hepatitis C after attending Treloar's said she wasn't asked or informed when he was moved from cryo to Factor VIII. Former pupils said they were never asked for consent. Had parents been informed of the risks of Factor VIII and given a choice in their children's treatment, they could have requested doctors stick to cryo, thereby drastically reducing the risk of infection with HIV and hepatitis C. John Peach, whose two sons died five months apart, said he had no idea Dr Aronstam had been testing his children for signs of AIDS from as early as January 1983. No idea until it was too late and his sons were already ill.

Following the Nazi war-crime trials at the end of the Second World War, the Nuremberg Code established a set of ten standards for doctors to follow when conducting experiments with human subjects. The principal rule stated: 'The voluntary consent of the human subject is absolutely essential.' That means people should be free to choose whether they participate in research, and be given sufficient information about the study to be able to make an informed decision, including knowing the hazards and possible side effects. 'The experiment should be so conducted as to avoid all unnecessary physical and mental suffering and injury,' said the code.

Before the inquiry began, former Treloar's pupil and tailor Gary Webster had requested his medical records on the advice of his lawyer, Des Collins. He was initially told they had been destroyed, but a member of staff at the Treloar's hemophilia center then discovered them at the back of a cupboard along with the records of some other former pupils. Gary found a general consent form from when he joined the school, containing scant detail, which his mum had signed. Personally, he remembered taking part in one trial as a teenager, when he was paid £35. But in his notes there was evidence he had been involved in more than ten research projects. As he listened to Richards talk about research at Treloar's, he heard another detail that astounded him: in 1976 there had been a trial involving three boys from the junior school at Holybourne. Back then, Gary was ten years old and in his first year. Sitting in the inquiry's hearing room, he realized he must have been one of the three guinea pigs, because there had only been three boys in the lower school then. Gary had been made a subject of research less than a year after he joined – and his parents hadn't been told. In sending him to Treloar's, they had unwittingly handed over his life to the school. The utopian vision he and his fellow ex-pupils used to have of the school now felt completely absurd.

Six months into Dr Kirk's hepatitis study, in April 1976, three pupils had contracted hepatitis, one of whom experienced tiredness, anorexia and nausea for a whole term. Within eighteen months, all of those treated with Factor VIII had abnormal liver enzyme readings. By December 1977 two boys on Baxter's Hemofil had chronic hepatitis, and the results showed there was a higher chance of contracting the disease from Factor VIII than from cryo. But Dr Kirk's research didn't stop there. Despite clear evidence of a higher risk with some products, he suggested a follow-up study: treat one group of children with commercial Factor VIII and the other with British Factor VIII. The safer cryo wouldn't be included. When Dr Aronstam joined Treloar's, fifteen of the forty-five boys in the hepatitis study had signs of chronic liver damage. Convinced by Dr Craske of the important role he could play in progressing their scientific understanding, Dr Aronstam had agreed to pick up from Dr Kirk and continue to monitor the boys. Although he expressed reservations about the research at times, he didn't introduce any major changes at the center, such as informing parents about his work.

Nationally, Dr Craske concluded there was a 'very high' risk of patients contracting hepatitis from Baxter's Hemofil. As a result, he broadened his study to look at the risk of non-A, non-B hepatitis from different brands of Factor VIII. Dr William Maycock, director of Blood Products Laboratory, had tried to warn Dr Craske against the research in 1978: if patients who contracted chronic hepatitis found out about the 'close investigation' of them, they could conclude 'they had been negligently treated and that a claim for compensation might be in order.' Regardless, Dr Craske went ahead. And he had the support of the Department of Health. By 1980 half of Britain's hemophilia patients were showing signs of chronic hepatitis. 'It seems likely that some patients will develop severe chronic liver disease over the next ten years,' Dr Craske wrote, estimating it would affect around a third of patients. They were all deliberately left in ignorance for a decade.

Had doctors addressed hepatitis as a serious risk – either of their own accord or at the behest of patients – they might have curtailed prophylactic treatment to minimize the exposure each patient had to viruses. They could have sought out safer versions of Factor VIII – made with voluntary European or heat-treated plasma – or chosen to go back to cryo. These steps could have protected people against AIDS before it emerged. But the country went in the opposite direction. A 1976 internal memo from the Austrian company Immuno, which made Kryobulin, illustrated Britain's priorities. Immuno had two versions of Factor VIII, one made with paid-for American plasma and the other with safer, volunteer-given European plasma. 'The British market will accept a higher risk of hepatitis for a lower-priced product,' said the memo. 'In the long-term Kryobulin [made with European plasma] will disappear from the British market.' Put simply, Britain was willing to buy a more dangerous product because it was cheaper.

Other research took place across Britain without patients' knowledge. For Clair, the most disturbing was the 'heterosexual study' of thirty-seven wives whose partners had tested positive for HIV following treatment with Factor VIII. Hearing about this, she realized exactly why her doctor had wanted her to come back to hospital every month for tests when she and Bryan were trying to conceive. 'We'll monitor you,' they had said. As with any new virus, doctors needed to research the transmission of HIV in order to learn how it spread, but decades later patients were angry about the apparent lack of care they had been given, and how little they were told.

Throughout the Treloar's week at the inquiry, the rooms of Fleetbank House and the courtyard outside vibrated with fury. Surviving pupils' worst suspicions had been confirmed: as children they had been seen as captive guinea pigs to be used in medical trials, often without their parents' knowledge. 'They were using dangerous products known to be infected,' says Richard Warwick. 'It was awful.' The usually mellow Richard couldn't help but raise his voice in anger. As he listened to the evidence, he had to pinch himself to believe it was true. Treloar's had been a research facility with a school attached. Pupils there received more treatment with Factor VIII than elsewhere across Britain. At Treloar's, prophylaxis was given every other day, in comparison to twice a week at other hemophilia centers. When AIDS became a threat in 1982, the trials and prophylaxis continued. That year, Ade Goodyear was one of fifty boys involved in a study of Factor VIII from Speywood, which distributed American Factor VIII. Many of these children developed adverse, and later fatal, side effects.

Former headmaster Alec Macpherson unsettled ex-pupils further by confirming the school's apparent complacency. Macpherson said he had known doctors were undertaking research, but he had avoided probing too much, because he trusted them. When the risk of AIDS emerged, he thought the doctors had reacted promptly. But over the course of his day on the stand, the evidence Richards showed demonstrated otherwise.

'With the benefit of hindsight, do you think that the school should have had greater oversight into the activities of the hemophilia center?' she asked.

'I always thought they were doing the best they could, and that they were honest,' said Macpherson. 'If they didn't immediately take action when they knew that infected blood was being used, I'm very surprised, and I think that was remiss and that was a mistake, which I would say was culpable. I think that's what you've been implying to a certain extent here. . . . If that was true, then that's disgraceful. But as for us in the school, we didn't know about it, and we didn't have any authority or reason to interfere. No reason whatsoever. I mean, let's face it, doctors are gods, aren't they?'

Gary was furious as he listened to Macpherson. Treloar's should have looked after them as children in its care, but it had let them down in the most brutal way imaginable. A few months after hearing this evidence, in October 2021, Gary sued Treloar's for negligence and breach of statutory duty in its care of 122 boys with hemophilia. Twenty-one other survivors soon joined the claim, including Richard and Ade. The school insisted liability lay with the NHS. As a child, Gary had been made a research subject without his parents' knowledge. As an adult, his liver was shot because of hepatitis C. He couldn't work because of the damage done – and he wanted the school to be held responsible.

Former head of Bradford's hemophilia center Professor Liakat Parapia was certain he had fallen into a corrupt system as a young consultant. In the 1970s and '80s, each hemophilia center director was in charge of buying their own supplies of Factor VIII, which meant they could be influenced by companies into buying more of their products. Alpha, Armour, Baxter, Bayer and Immuno had offered Professor Parapia support for his center that he couldn't get through the NHS, such as training for his nurses and doctors. Center directors could go to the companies and say, 'I really need a physiotherapist,' and they would fund the position for a year. They also sponsored residential weekends for patients through the Haemophilia Society and home-treatment kits. 'It was almost like a conspiracy,' says Professor Parapia. 'We all fell for the marketing from the pharma companies because we needed the support and scientific information they were giving. The pharma companies were brainwashing us.' Having limited funds for his NHS hemophilia center, Parapia accepted research materials and financial support for his staff, but insisted on always paying his own expenses.

'Put crudely, what were the companies getting out of it?' Richards asked Dr Winter, who had run the hemophilia center at Thanet General Hospital.

'They got a sort of closer relationship and understanding of the way in which hemophilia centers worked,' said Dr Winter. 'They wanted our business, of course, and they said to themselves this would be a way of making it more likely that they would get our business.'

Like many others, Parapia had been wooed by the promise of better products from pharma companies – their treatments contained more of the factor VIII protein, which made them more soluble and effective. They also came with an applicator and distilled water, so were easier to administer than the NHS version. But they had a far greater risk of containing viruses. 'The safety measures were not totally explained to us,' says Professor Parapia. 'It's a personal tragedy for me because I was responsible for starting to use commercial products in Bradford. I feel terribly guilty. If I had carried on using cryo, there would have been a far lower number of hepatitis and HIV cases.'

As Parapia had realized imported Factor VIII carried a greater risk of hepatitis and then AIDS, Professor Arthur Bloom and the Department of Health had said there wouldn't be enough British-made Factor VIII to provide for all patients. 'The companies promoted prophylactic and home treatment, which meant the amount needed was ten times more,' he says. 'That was one of their marketing ploys.' He had tried to use a reasonable mix of British and American Factor VIII depending on the availability. But there were other hospitals where doctors prioritized imported Factor VIII, because of their close relationships with the manufacturers.

In Newcastle, Dr Peter Jones, who had complained to the Press Council about Sue Douglas's 'Killer Blood' article, had such a preference for commercial Factor VIII imported from the US that in August 1983 a colleague had admonished him for having an 'embarrassingly large supply' of unused British Factor VIII in his fridges. By then, doctors were well aware of the warnings that American Factor VIII could contain AIDS. But those who preferred the imported product argued it was easier to use, more soluble, caused fewer allergic reactions and had 'a more attractive presentation.' Dr Jones said he chose commercial products because he knew there was a shortfall in the version made by the NHS. Three-quarters of Dr Jones's patients contracted HIV, according to author Virginia Berridge.

During the inquiry, Sir Brian drew a stark comparison between Alder Hey Children's Hospital in Liverpool and Sheffield Children's Hospital. Alder Hey had continued to treat children with imported Factor VIII after advice in the summer of 1983 to restrict them to the British version. As a result, 90 percent of its patients were infected with HIV. Sheffield had used only cryo – or NHS Factor VIII when cryo wasn't available – and just one of its patients contracted the virus.

'They may be separated only by a few miles in the Pennines, but they're worlds apart,' said Sir Brian. 'The result couldn't be more different.'

Among those who contracted HIV at Alder Hey were two of Sue Hallwood's sons, Stephen and Brian, both of whom were treated with commercial Factor VIII in 1985, well after the dangers were known. After testing positive for HIV when he was five, Stephen died in 1989 aged nine. Brian passed away less than five years later, aged sixteen. Sue's third son, Thomas, was infected with hepatitis C. An expert report into Stephen's death found his doctor at Alder Hey, Dr John Martin, had been negligent in not treating him with cryo in 1983 and 1984, and for giving him unheated commercial Factor VIII in 1985. 'I hate him; I hate that man,' Sue erupted while giving evidence. She described the hospital as a 'conveyor belt' of child deaths.

Day after day, doctors were at the end of the poison line – the final people with the power to make decisions that might have prevented infections. They could have stuck to cryo when they realized how rife hepatitis was; refused to use imported Factor VIII; petitioned the British government to prioritize self-sufficiency; avoided prophylaxis to reduce the amount that patients infused; given them an informed choice about their treatment; reacted more quickly to the first signs of AIDS; moved to heat-treated Factor VIII as soon as it was available. The benefits and convenience of the miracle treatment seemed so great it blinded doctors to its dangers. Some denied the risk of AIDS for longer than others, and there were those who conducted unethical research and allowed commercial relationships to influence their treatment. Most significantly, doctors had failed 'to apprise their patients – or when they were children, their parents – of the true state of affairs at the time,' said Steven Snowden, barrister for Collins Solicitors. 'Or own up quickly afterwards.'

By the time of the inquiry, many of the doctors whom survivors most wanted to hear from had passed away, taking the full story to their graves, including Bloom, Aronstam and Rizza. Of those still alive, Dr Jones said he was too frail to give evidence, as did Dr Craske, who had led the hepatitis study. Professor Tuddenham was willing to answer all of Sir Brian's technical questions about how much doctors had known about the risk of viruses. He said he greatly regretted how their efforts to improve hemophilia care had resulted in disaster. 'I hope we learn from it and guard against any similar catastrophic consequences,' he said.

Parapia said he ultimately wished the Department of Health had been more strict in its regulation of blood products. In Scotland, where the blood transfusion service became self-sufficient in the early 1980s, the HIV infection rate was far lower: only sixty people contracted it from blood products there, which was around 5 percent of their hemophilia population. Those with hemophilia B – a less common form caused by deficiency in clotting factor IX – were also less at risk of blood-borne viruses because Britain could more comfortably meet the Factor IX demand with plasma given by volunteer donors. The proportion of people with severe hemophilia A who contracted HIV was ten times higher than in those with severe hemophilia B.

At the end of his time on the witness stand, Parapia said something core participants needed to hear from a doctor: 'I'm sorry.' The next day, his apology was on the front page of the *Yorkshire Post* and his inbox was filled with thank-you notes from survivors. They were grateful to him for admitting mistakes that had led to needless infections and deaths.

In the decades leading up to the inquiry, former health secretary Ken Clarke, now sitting in the Lords, had become a sort of bogeyman for survivors, who had come to believe that the buck stopped with him. His face had been pasted onto their placards along with the slogan 'blood on his hands.' Contaminated Factor VIII had been imported into the UK and prescribed to patients on his watch. He had gone on television to encourage people to keep infusing as he played down the risks. Ahead of his evidence in July 2021, Birchgrove member Alan Burgess wanted to hear Lord Clarke say, 'I was in charge; it was down to me. We did fuck up, I admit that. I'm going to hold my hands up now.'

Lord Clarke had a self-confessed garrulous manner, which had only become more entrenched as he entered his eighties. He spoke with the confidence of an upper-class man who had spent half a century in Parliament, maintaining unshakeable certitude even in the face of intense criticism. For decades, he had been unconvinced of the merits of holding a public inquiry into infected blood. The events were in the past – a distant past of which he could conveniently remember very little – and the government had done all it could at the time and thereafter. But, having been compelled to give evidence, Clarke arrived at Fleetbank House in late July 2021 for three days on the stand. They would be among the inquiry's busiest days, the hearing room filled with participants sitting in socially distanced clusters, along with another five hundred people watching from home. The boys from Treloar's were there, along with Jason, Joe and Clair.

Dashing the hopes of survivors, Lord Clarke quickly made it clear that he wouldn't be giving the answers they wanted. Instead, he was belligerent: blood products had been a small part of his role; he had never heard of cryo; he thought Factor VIII was a pill; the Department of Health had reacted appropriately and warned the public of the dangers of AIDS in a timely manner.

'If things were done by the department that either should not have been done or could have been done better,' said Richards, 'does the minister of state not bear some responsibility for the actions –'

'Well, we're a team, yes,' said Lord Clarke, cutting her off. 'I'm not trying to escape by saying, "It wasn't me, guv." I don't think the department did anything wrong. I've never heard anybody suggest anything that, in the real world, a minister or a civil servant might have done that would have prevented it. I've already said, had we taken the step we now know would have saved lives [withdrawing American Factor VIII and banning further imports], we would have been treated with outrage by the Haemophilia Society and most hemophiliacs by denying them their Factor VIII.'

Lord Clarke's manner was bullish, interrupting Richards and firing questions back at her. Eventually, Sir Brian intervened after he had retorted, 'What's the relevance of all this?'

'I think the relevance, ultimately, Lord Clarke, is for me to determine,' said the chairman. 'If I think that the questions are unhelpful, then I will indicate that.'

But Lord Clarke wouldn't relent. In fact, he believed he had been unfairly singled out.

'I was not directly responsible for any of this,' he said in exasperation. 'I only play such a prominent part in evidence because I nowadays have the misfortune to be slightly better known than any of the others. I'm the nearest to a B-list celebrity you've got.' The only other public figure in Lord Clarke's eyes was his fellow peer, former health secretary Norman Fowler. For his part, Lord Fowler told Sir Brian the government had been slow to change its view that there was 'no conclusive proof' AIDS could be transmitted through blood products, and that early compensation for victims had been 'doomed to failure' because of Thatcher's resistance to paying victims.

Eventually, Lord Clarke did concede on something. 'Obviously, we'd have behaved totally differently in 1980 if anybody had told us, "You do realize 2,800 people are going to die because they're being given this product,"' he said. 'Of course the behavior of everybody in the department would have been dramatically different. That's the wisdom of hindsight.'

Before Sir Brian dismissed those who had come to watch Lord Clarke, he pointedly thanked them for having shown patience and courtesy to every witness so far, no matter how much they may have disagreed with them. But that patience had worn thin by the time Lord Clarke left Fleetbank House after his third day on the stand. Clive Smith, chair of the Haemophilia Society, spoke for many when he described Clarke's behavior as a 'shocking slap in the face,' which was reflective of the government's 'shameful indifference' towards them.

One of Lord Clarke's main defenses was that he hadn't been made aware of the finer points of decision making: that had been the responsibility of civil servants. As an example, he was surprised when Richards showed him that by now well-known warning letter Dr Galbraith had sent in May 1983 imploring the Department of Health to ban imports of American blood products.

'Suppose that this document, which rather shocked you when you looked at it now, had come to you – do you think you would have said, "What's the alternative?"' said Richards. 'You'd have asked questions, perhaps, wouldn't you?'

'Had I seen that, yes,' said Clarke.

No politician appeared to have seen the letter. Lord John Patten, parliamentary undersecretary of state for health from 1983 to 1985, said he had lacked the full picture in those crucial months when the dangers of AIDS emerged. He believed he should unequivocally have been shown Dr Galbraith's letter. Had he seen it, he said, 'I probably would have pressed the panic button.'

The Department of Health was fatally slow in responding to the AIDS crisis in the spring and summer of 1983. Rather than listening to the country's leading epidemiologist, Dr Galbraith, or international organizations like the Council of Europe, it relied on the advice of Professor Bloom and the pharmaceutical companies, neither of whom had expertise in epidemics.

Professor Richard Tedder, the virologist behind the early HTLV–III tests, told the inquiry he had also tried to sound the alarm in May 1983 in a meeting with Dr Diana Walford, the government's senior principal medical officer. But, like Dr Galbraith, he had been brushed off. Dr Walford had told him to 'go away and stop rocking the boat,' he wrote in a note at the time. For her part, Dr Walford couldn't remember the meeting with Tedder. 'It sounds most unlike me,' she said. 'I don't know what I can have said that could have possibly given him the feeling that I was asking him to go away.' Lord Simon Glenarthur, a parliamentary undersecretary who worked closely with Dr Walford and Lord Clarke and who had responsibility for blood products, defended the Department of Health, saying they had taken AIDS 'extremely seriously and diligently,' even if their actions might look 'slow and perhaps even too bureaucratic' with hindsight.

But this evidence appeared to confirm what survivors had always suspected. An echo chamber in the Department of Health had allowed government ministers and civil servants to downplay the risk of AIDS from 1982 to 1985. In wanting to stave off panic and protect the public purse, the government had presided over a string of mistakes that allowed dangerous Factor VIII to continue to be imported into Britain and injected into patients. The government never achieved self-sufficiency, despite the risk of hepatitis and then AIDS, because of underinvestment in Blood Products Laboratory. It was then slow to respond to the emerging AIDS epidemic and, having recognized the dangers of non-A, non-B hepatitis, failed to act upon them appropriately. The government had given doctors and manufacturers too long a leash over the safety of its citizens and delayed the switch to heat-treated Factor VIII. Then, after the scale of the disaster emerged, it attempted to bury those choices.

Some politicians struck a more conciliatory tone than Lord Clarke had. John Major, Thatcher's Chancellor of the Exchequer and her successor as prime minister from November 1990 until 1997, initially offended onlookers when he testified, 'What had happened was incredibly bad luck' – the hearing room erupted in a unified gasp – 'awful, and it was not something that anybody was unsympathetic to.' His use of the phrase 'bad luck' implied the infections had happened by chance. For survivors and family members, it felt like another denial of the government's failures. At the end of the day, Major said he was sorry if he had upset people. He told Sir Brian he had not been informed when the government of Japan apologized to its citizens with hemophilia, nor had he taken the time to find out. To his knowledge, his government had never considered a similar investigation in Britain, even as the inquiry into BSE was underway.

'In your experience, how good are governments at acknowledging that things have gone wrong?' asked Richards.

'Oh, I don't think they're very good at all,' said Major.

On the stand forty-five years after he was health minister, Lord Owen said, 'We should be humble enough to admit as politicians that this inquiry is not taking place because of a conscious decision to do so. Successive governments, Labour, Conservative and the Liberal-Conservative coalition, all refused it. It was eventually done because there was a parliamentary majority that was going to vote it through and the government had no option. So we have, all of us politicians, failed to face up to the fundamental thing: when things go wrong, be prepared to have a post-mortem.'

The fortnight in mid-July 2022 threatened to bring the hottest temperatures on record to Britain. As the country prepared for the heat wave, railway lines were painted white to prevent them from buckling and people were told to stay at home to avoid severe sunstroke. On the 18th and 19th, the heat was like nothing the country had experienced. The fire service faced its busiest day since the Second World War, with parched ground igniting across the capital. Forty-one properties would be destroyed before cooler winds arrived later in the week. At the inquiry, Sir Brian had recently heard two days of evidence from Sir Robert Francis, a judge who had been asked to conduct a parallel review into how the government might compensate survivors and their families. Sir Robert recommended that an immediate payment should be made, given how long people had waited. It was a 'matter of justice,' he said.

On the morning of Friday July 15, before the intense heat arrived in London, Sir Brian said he had taken the time to reflect on Sir Robert's report and would be opening a ten-day consultation for core participants to send him their thoughts on immediate, partial compensation. He had set a clock ticking for the government.

With the inquiry abuzz over this development, it was Andy Burnham's turn to be sworn in. Now the mayor of Greater Manchester, he was also campaigning for a Hillsborough Law that would bring an

end to 'the depressingly familiar pattern of cover-ups and conceal-
ment' by creating a legal duty for officials to be candid in the wake of
national tragedies. Burnham had reviewed reams of documents in
preparation for his evidence, including letters he sent to constituents
when he was health secretary. Letters he could now see were riddled
with inadvertent lies. Like the one he sent to David Tonkin after the
Manor House Group protested outside his office, which contained a
false statement: 'There is no evidence that individuals were knowingly infected.' Reading those words again, more than a decade after
they were written, Burnham saw them in a fresh light. 'I would say
that is evidence of the cover-up going right to the top, when you're
giving a secretary of state a letter to sign that includes sentences that
are not truthful,' he says. Then there were the briefings created by
civil servants, which he believed were falsified.

'As a ministerial team, in my view, we were given a number of
inaccurate lines by departmental officials in this particular period –
lines that I now know to be false,' Burnham told Sir Brian.

The reason the government had lied for so long, he now believed,
was because it had wanted to avoid having to pay exorbitant compensation if it was found to be at fault. 'Embedded deep within the civil
service psyche, the response to this particular issue was primarily
driven by fear of financial exposure,' said Burnham. 'That explains to
me why the UK government has comprehensively failed the victims
of infected blood over five decades.'

For the first time in over three years, the inquiry hearing room
erupted in applause in the middle of evidence. He knew there would
be people in the Department of Health who would be cursing him.
'But if you don't confront people with what you believe to be the truth,
no matter how hard it is, then how does the system learn?' he says. After
six and a half hours, Burnham reached a rousing conclusion. 'I think
the Department of Health and the bodies for which it is responsible
have been grossly negligent of the safety of the hemophilia community in this country,' he said. He outlined the evidence he had seen
substantiating this claim: the failure of successive governments to
become self-sufficient; medical trials being conducted without proper
consent and safeguards; the scraps of financial support that had

compounded rather than alleviated people's distress; and the subsequent cover-up. 'When you add it all together, I personally can come to no other conclusion. I appreciate the inquiry may take a different view, but I think there is a clear case to me that there is a massive legal liability here for being grossly negligent.'

With this indictment of the government's failures, Burnham said he believed there was a 'rock-solid legal case' for significant compensation and scope for criminal investigation. 'I would say there is even the possibility that the Crown Prosecution Service should be asked to consider charges of corporate manslaughter,' he said. 'I don't say that lightly.'

Towards the end of the blistering fortnight, Jeremy Hunt took the stand. Hunt was the epitome of the establishment politician – foreign secretary at the time of giving evidence and later Chancellor of the Exchequer – but he was prepared to be similarly explosive. Throughout his six years as health secretary from 2012 to 2018, Hunt had held firm that this was a historic injustice, having first come alive to it in 2007, when his constituent Mike Dorricott told him how he had been infected with hepatitis C from Factor VIII during routine dental surgery as a child. It had taken Dorricott fourteen years to discover he had the virus, which had attacked his liver so aggressively he needed two transplants. Dorricott passed away in 2015, just as the Penrose Report was published. The failure to deliver justice before he died had weighed on Hunt's conscience ever since.

Hunt had his own assessment of why the government had for so long covered up the infected blood disaster. 'I am afraid that institutions and the state close ranks around a lie sometimes – and I think that's what happened in this case,' he said. The civil service had perpetuated the lie that infected blood had been an 'unavoidable problem' before tests for HIV and hepatitis C became available. Ministers like him had been fed what appeared to be a conclusive history of the scandal, he said, when they should in fact have been told the Department of Health's narrative was highly contentious.

'The totality of this was a failure by the British state. I don't think there's any other way to describe it,' said Hunt. 'Although in some ways you could look at this as a huge failing of our democracy that it's taken so long to resolve this issue, in another way, the families and campaigners, including Mike, were entirely responsible for justice being done in the end.'

Two days after Hunt gave his evidence, something finally shifted. The inquiry was winding down before the summer break and Sir Brian had one last announcement to make. 'I have decided to recommend that interim payments of no less than £100,000 are made to all infected people and to all bereaved partners,' he said.

By October the government had made the payments. Survivors had waited nearly forty years for this recognition.

In April 2023, Sir Brian said other bereaved relatives, including parents who had lost children and children whose parents had died, would also receive £100,000. He urged the government to pay full compensation to everyone who had been infected and affected by blood and blood products contaminated with HIV, hepatitis C, hepatitis B and vCJD. The final sum could far exceed a billion pounds, with people expected to receive anything from a few hundred thousand pounds to several million. In July 2023, Sir Brian took the unprecedented step of reopening the inquiry hearings to address the government's lack of response to his recommendation for compensation.

'My conclusion is that wrongs were done at individual, collective and systemic levels,' said Sir Brian. 'The infections themselves and their consequences merit compensation, but so, too, do the wrongs done by authority, whose response served to compound people's suffering.'

For survivors it felt like a Pyrrhic and bitter victory. Thousands of people had already been killed, including more than five hundred who had died since the inquiry began.

Sitting in the small workshop in the bungalow that he shared with his wife, Tina, in the countryside near Scarborough, Richard ruminated about moving house. After thirty years in their modest home, which had one bedroom and a postage-stamp lawn, he could now afford a new place to live. They had bought the bungalow in 1991 after he received £23,500 from the settlement of the HIV litigation. In a way, he considered himself lucky. He had friends who were living in council housing because of their infections from Factor VIII; who had never found a life partner to accept them with their HIV positive statuses; who had passed away before they had a chance to attempt either.

Now in his late fifties, Richard was thinking about using the £100,000 to move closer to his parents. Save for the six years he spent at Treloar's, he had never strayed far from them. He and Tina lived in a small village in Yorkshire, fifteen miles from his parents. But even that was becoming a stretch now that both his parents were approaching their eighties. Tina's knees were starting to give up and he wasn't getting any healthier, having recently had a heart attack and surgery to have four stents inserted. One thing was easier, at least: society had evolved and the stigma had receded. If he did move, he could worry less about the barriers he had once faced.

Divided across four decades of harm, Richard worked out that the interim payment amounted to a paltry £2,500 per year. It would bring some comfort, at least in the short term, helping people clear debts and pay off their mortgages. But Richard was seeking justice from the inquiry, not money. 'Over the years we've been pushed aside, dismissed, made to feel like moaners. We haven't had the recognition that we've all craved,' he says. He wanted a sincere apology from the parties who harmed them.

Wrapping up the inquiry, the lawyers who represented the survivors were forceful about the mistakes that had been made. Clair, Joe and Frankie's lawyer, Sam Stein, said the use of imported blood products after 1982 was 'morally, ethically and criminally wrong' and that the trials conducted on hemophilia patients had breached the Nuremberg Code.

'This was a brutal, unacceptable, unforgivable and unnecessary travesty visited upon patients in the grossest breach of medical trust imaginable, with truly devastating consequences,' said barrister Steven Snowden, speaking on behalf of the 1,074 clients Des Collins represented. 'Why, in the United Kingdom in the twenty-first century, did it have to come to this? Why has the truth had to be squeezed out of government by campaigners?'

On February 3, 2023, lead counsel Richards stood in front of Sir Brian for the final address of the Infected Blood Inquiry. She outlined how unprecedented it had been: tens of thousands of people infected by blood products and transfusions in a disaster that stretched across five decades and the four nations of the UK. The inquiry had collected over five thousand statements, disclosed more than a hundred thousand documents and spent upwards of £100 million by March 2022 (costing an average of £30 million a year).

'This is not simply an inquiry into matters of history,' said Richards. 'This is an inquiry into the here and now. It is an inquiry with ongoing relevance and resonance to decision making by the government and the NHS today.' Only recently, England's patient safety commissioner, Dr Henrietta Hughes, had released a report on her first hundred days in the position, which outlined concerning findings: the NHS was focused on financial control and productivity rather than safety. The culture was getting worse, and unless there was a change, Dr Hughes warned, there would be a repeat of 'other health scandals, severe harm and death.' 'This is a sentence which I think will resonate with all of you,' said Richards, quoting the report: '"Medicine is industrialized when it needs to be humanized."'

Richards outlined the issues she thought Sir Brian might want to consider as he drew his conclusions. The first was the state's obligation to protect life under the European Convention on Human Rights, and its moral duty to shield its citizens from harm. Second, many witnesses had implored the inquiry not to let hindsight cloud its view. 'Something may be done in accordance with the standards and norms of the time and yet be wrong,' said Richards. She suggested Sir Brian could consider this when assessing the 'dearth of guidance from the chief medical officer or General Medical Council' and the 'culture of paternalism' in medicine at the time which had led to doctors keeping patients in the dark. Politicians and civil servants had a duty to act with integrity and honesty; doctors to 'do no harm.'

Before concluding, Richards left Sir Brian with two key quotes. The first was Thatcher's claim, which had been repeated ad nauseam: 'All patients received the best treatment available in light of the medical knowledge at the time.' And the later claim from the Department of Health as it rejected the need for an inquiry: 'The government does not accept that any wrongful practices were employed.'

★

With everything now laid out before the inquiry, those who had spent their lifetimes fighting for justice were left with a bittersweet feeling. Jason Evans knew there would be no celebratory moment when Sir Brian released his final report. Those infected and affected by contaminated blood products and transfusions would never stand together outside the Royal Courts of Justice and cheer victoriously. There was no such thing as winning, he thought. It was too late; the majority of people who had been infected with HIV and hepatitis C had already died.

Even though there was no victory, Jason wanted to honor the memory of those who had passed. 'For me, that's what this is about – it's about respecting and honoring my dad,' he says.

Through the eight years he had been investigating the death of Jonathan Evans, he had forged a connection with his late father. When the inquiry ended, he knew he would have to relinquish this strange new father–son relationship.

14. Living

On a Friday afternoon in autumn 2021, Clair was in the garden tending to three new trees. The colors were radiant and burning, and the birds were singing. She had found a corner of peace in her verdant garden, which had a wrought-iron archway amid scatters of wildflowers. She could sit on the bench at the far end with the birdsong around her and watch her dog bound towards her. Out there, Clair tried to escape. Her house was empty of the family she had dreamt of having by the time she reached sixty. She wanted to be thinking about children going to university, grandchildren, retirement, but those things would never exist for her. Instead, she was still fighting. The question remained of who was ultimately to blame for her husband Bryan's death. And she would come back to the same answer: the American manufacturers of Factor VIII.

'My husband, Bryan, a hemophiliac, was so low down in the pharmaceutical companies' eyes that he just didn't matter,' she says. 'He died never knowing. Perhaps that was the best thing for him, as he went to Iceland and enjoyed that last adventure – that he didn't spend his time campaigning.'

Eighteen months later, walking down the aisles of his local supermarket, Jason saw one of those regular reminders of his dad. In late January 2023, he and his wife, Prisca, had a baby daughter. There was no 'biohazard' on her birth certificate, she didn't need an HIV test and the midwives who delivered her were dressed in ordinary scrubs. The process of becoming a father had stirred up a lot of memories for Jason. Looking at nappy-rash creams in the supermarket, he rejected the most popular brand: Bepanthen. Staring at him from the front of its box was a circular logo with a cross in the middle that said BAYER. *They killed my dad*, he thought. He refused to buy their products, just as he had banned makeup from Revlon in his house. No matter how much he tried to move forward, there would always be triggers. But he pushed on, like he always did.

'The villains in this story are clearly the pharma companies,' says Des Collins. 'I don't say that because they're easy to hit. They produced this material. They have also produced a lot of lifesaving material. But in this particular case I don't believe they can rely on that fact as an excuse for killing people.' Sir Brian's inquiry was focused on the UK – on how the government and doctors had acted – and he didn't have powers to compel international witnesses, so he only heard from two representatives from pharma companies. Christopher Bishop was the UK marketing manager for Armour for more than twenty years until 1993. During his seven hours of evidence, Bishop admitted that Armour had known Factor VIII could transmit hepatitis B when it first launched its version in 1976. Within five years, the company became aware that it also contained non-A, non-B hepatitis, which could lead to severe and chronic liver damage. Despite warnings about traces of AIDS in its defective heat-treated Factor VIII, Bishop insisted Armour's plasma collection had been 'beyond reproach' and, in a move that infuriated those watching, that he didn't think there was anything Armour could have done differently.

'I'm very proud of the fact that we did everything in the right way,' he said.

'Were any lessons learnt by Armour from what had happened?' Richards tried again.

'Not that I –' he faltered. 'No. No specific lessons.' Instead, he said, 'The whole thing, the development of AIDS and hepatitis B, has been a terrible tragedy.'

The American companies who made Factor VIII had avoided repercussions in the UK, but Des thought they should be in the frame. Michael Baum said there was still a chance of them facing justice in countries where they had so far avoided it. He believed the documents he had used for lawsuits in the US proved fraud and could pave the way for further legal action – if only someone was willing to put the time and money into fighting it. But pinning a case to a single company would be difficult. 'Pharma companies are very quick to go on the attack if there's any suggestion they are involved,' says Des. 'They'll say, "We're a completely different company to the one which had involvement in the import of contaminated material into England."' Today, none of the four companies exists in its original form. Those who made Factor VIII in the US back then – Alpha, Armour, Baxter and Bayer – and their European counterparts, such as Behringwerke and Immuno, have been sold, merged, spun out or rebranded, obfuscating the line of responsibility.

After the fallout from Factor VIII infecting people with HIV, Green Cross sold Alpha to a Spanish pharma company called Grifols in 2003 for $100 million, accelerating its expansion in the US. Grifols later bought Bayer's plasma business, too, which had been made up of two laboratories, Cutter and Miles, making it the third largest producer of plasma products in the world.

Armour was owned by Revlon Healthcare. In 1985 the company split, selling its makeup brand to Pantry Pride and its healthcare division to French company Rhône-Poulenc Rorer. Through a number of deals, assets from Armour ended up with Sanofi and CSL Behring, which also bought Behringwerke. Today, the brand Armour is better known in the US for its canned meats, in particular jumbo hot dogs.

Baxter initially expanded its blood products and plasma business, buying Austrian company Immuno for $715 million in 1996, before splitting off the division to make a separate company called Baxalta, which was worth $1.6 billion in sales. In 2016 Baxalta agreed to a $32 billion merger with Shire, both of which Japanese pharma giant Takeda bought three years later.

This constant flow of capital allowed the companies who made Factor VIII in the 1970s and '80s to slowly syphon off responsibility, just as they had syphoned off human plasma for decades.

Baxter and Bayer are still well-known pharmaceutical giants, worth $23 billion and $62 billion, respectively, but neither is in the plasma business any longer. Four companies dominate the fractionation industry today, collecting more than 80 percent of plasma in the US. Australian company CSL Plasma, which is owned by CSL

Behring, is responsible for almost 30 percent of the US market. Grifols now owns 20 percent of America's plasma centers, while another 16 percent is held by Takeda. The industry is prospering; in 2022 it was worth nearly $40 billion and was expected to almost double in value in the next five years.

As they did in the 1980s, the majority of the world's countries still rely on imported plasma. Only a third of them make their own plasma products, and more than half are entirely reliant on imports. The main supplier of the world's plasma today? The US, because it allows companies to pay donors, despite the WHO advising against it.

Most people will receive plasma products at some point in their lives. Some pregnant women are given immunoglobulin, like Lorraine Mull, while people who have suffered major blood loss, serious injury or burns can be treated with albumin. Rare immune conditions and liver failure can also require plasma products. The growth of the industry is due in part to an aging population and a rising prevalence of hemophilia. Although there is now widely available recombinant Factor VIII, a significant proportion of patients are still treated with Factor VIII made with human plasma, because they can develop inhibitors that stop the synthetic version from working.

There is a vast amount of money to be made in the plasma game. Wolfgang Marguerre started his business career at Baxter's Travenol Laboratories in Europe in the 1970s before joining Revlon Healthcare as head of its plasma division in 1978. As the AIDS crisis was emerging in 1983, Marguerre left Revlon Healthcare to co-found Octapharma in Switzerland. He is now worth $5.6 billion personally, and his company has more than 180 plasma donation centers in the US, around 15 percent of the market. 'Octa' is a subtle nod to Factor VIII. 'They gave the most lavish parties of all,' remembers Professor Tuddenham.

Octapharma's website reveals how the industry works today: 'New donors can earn over $800 during the first 35 days!' CSL Plasma, meanwhile, offers $100 for first donations, $125 on the second and $115 for the third. After giving eight times, the reward drops. Companies are known to pay between $20 and $50 per donation. In the US, people can give plasma twice a week just two days apart; whereas in other countries donations are limited to twice a month.

That means in America an individual can give plasma 104 times a year and earn $2,080 to $5,200 depending on the center, compared with twenty-four times a year in the UK, where donors aren't paid. 'The United States has the least restrictive regulations in the world,' says Analidis Ochoa, a researcher at the University of Michigan. She has seen billboards advertising for people to 'give plasma, make $900 a month.' Incentives for first-time donors encourage them to return eight times within the first month, not waiting to see how giving regularly affects their bodies in the long term. 'The intention is to recruit long-term donors,' Ochoa says.

In destitute districts of American cities, queues form in strip malls each morning as people arrive for their ninety minutes spent giving around a pint of plasma. Inside, they answer some questions about themselves, including whether they have HIV, if they have had a tattoo or piercing in the last four months, and if they do drugs. After a quick health and blood-pressure check, they move to a bed to be hooked up to the plasmapheresis machine, which separates plasma from blood cells, returning the latter to the body. Prepaid credit cards are then loaded with their earnings. This is the dark side of the American dream: poor people willing to sell their plasma just to get by. The resultant products are treated for viruses now, but there has been little research into the long-term health impacts of regular plasma donation. Companies say the short-term side effects can include dizziness, fatigue and bruising or inflammation at the puncture site; long term, it can lead to reduced levels of immunoglobulin, or antibodies, making donors vulnerable to infections.

There are more than a thousand plasma collection centers in the US, a number that has boomed in the last fifteen years, ever since the 2008 financial crash. Most are concentrated in high-poverty areas, such as cities that have been hit by unemployment, factory closures and the aftershocks of the Covid-19 pandemic. There are also more centers near state-funded universities and along the border with Mexico, according to Ochoa. In 2021, US Customs and Border Protection closed the immigration loophole that allowed people from Mexico to travel across the border to donate plasma, following an investigation by ProPublica. But a year later, a judge in Washington,

DC, overturned the decision, saying officials had 'failed to consider' how much plasma companies relied on those donors. As much as 10 percent of the plasma collected in the US came from people crossing the border. It is illegal to pay for plasma in Mexico.

The ethical quandary of Richard Titmuss's 'gift relationship' has not gone away. The Plasma Protein Therapeutics Association, which represents manufacturers, says that without the US supply there would be a global shortage of plasma treatments and people would die. There is some truth in the supply argument, given how much of the world relies on American plasma. But it is also true that the US system is unethical and exploitative, leeching off impoverished people. It is too easy to point the finger at the US plasma industry, since countries that forbid paying for plasma donations at home, including the UK, continue to import treatments made with paid-for American plasma. If each country invested in self-sufficiency, as the WHO recommends, then the world might be less reliant on the American plasma trade. The current system, with countries placing trust in the profit-driven industry, increases the risk of history repeating itself.

The HIV and hepatitis C disasters didn't pass without statutory consequence. In the US, as part of the Ricky Ray Act and legal settlement, the government and pharmaceutical companies agreed to implement measures to safeguard the blood supply. The government tightened its regulation of blood products, while the companies agreed to lower the limit of their pool sizes from one hundred thousand donations to sixty thousand following pressure from Congress. Patients became involved in the Advisory Committee on Blood and Tissue Safety and Availability, which now had to prioritize safety over cost. Dana Kuhn was the first consumer to be appointed, followed by Corey Dubin. Without their efforts, blood safety measures might not have come to fruition and the industry may never have regained the trust of hemophilia patients. At their insistence, companies have introduced more rigorous questioning of donors before they give plasma and a host of viral screening tests. Only recently was the total ban on gay men donating lifted in the US and UK.

Britain has introduced stricter regulations on the pharma industry, limiting how companies can spend money and increasing transparency.

In 2012, the Association of the British Pharmaceutical Industry updated its code of practice to say companies had to disclose all money they had paid to healthcare professionals, as well as grants and donations given to organizations. 'I'm glad that has been reined back,' says Professor Tuddenham. 'It was an abuse of process.' In 2016 pharma companies gave American doctors and hospitals more than $8 billion, compared with £116 million given to British health workers that year.

As the Covid-19 pandemic showed, there will always be new pathogens that aren't immediately treatable. Already, there are diseases that are resistant to heat and chemical pasteurization, including vCJD and hepatitis E. Other blood-borne diseases have also raised concerns among researchers, including babesiosis, which is transmitted by the ticks that carry Lyme disease and is the most frequently reported parasitic infection transmitted through blood and blood products. Symptoms can be flu-like, including a fever, body aches and nausea, and it can be life-threatening in elderly people and those with a weak immune system. There is currently no FDA-approved test that could be used for screening donors. After someone in Brazil contracted Zika virus from a platelet transfusion, the FDA introduced screening for it, which was lifted in 2021.

The hope is that the plasma industry would react more quickly next time, with technological advancements helping researchers detect and identify viruses and other pathogens, and the new regulations preventing financial concerns from overriding patient safety. But some of those who lived through the HIV and hepatitis C epidemics are skeptical. Journalist Donna Shaw says, 'It absolutely could happen again. We're all going to have to have constant vigilance, because when you forget these things happened, you're opening the door for it to happen again.' Whistleblower Dr Kay Noel doesn't have a lot of faith in her former industry. 'Do I think the corporate world will be faster to respond to the next risk that arises?' she says. 'I'm too cynical to believe that.'

The infected blood disaster has painful similarities with other pharmaceutical scandals in the past seventy years. From the mid-1950s, thalidomide was sold as an over-the-counter treatment for morning sickness. As reports emerged of babies with birth defects, the drug continued to be sold. It wasn't until the end of 1961, after more than ten thousand babies had been affected – around half of whom died within a few months of birth – that thalidomide was finally withdrawn. Even then, it remained in people's medicine cabinets for months until the UK government issued a warning about the dangers to pregnant women in May 1962. As a result of that scandal, governments changed how they licensed pharmaceuticals, making sure they had been tested on humans, controlling which could be bought without a prescription and introducing ways to report side effects. Within a decade, British families had received compensation.

More recently, parallels can be drawn between the infected blood scandal and the opioid crisis. Companies including Purdue Pharma, McKesson Corporation and Cardinal Health aggressively marketed addictive opioid painkillers, causing a spike in dependency and overdoses. But in spite of well over two hundred thousand deaths, the companies mostly walked away with fines. The opioid crisis wasn't anywhere near as sharp in the UK, in part because of stricter rules on how aggressively companies can market their products to doctors and centralized purchasing. 'It's very similar because it's profits over patients,' says Gerald Posner, author of *Pharma: Greed, Lies, and the Poisoning of America*. 'When they eventually have to pay a fine for having done something terrible, it reduces the amount of their profit, but it never eliminates it. For them, it's the price of doing business.' Leadership is purged, regulations are tightened and patients die. But for the most part, pharma companies bounce back from scandal.

Wrongdoing doesn't equate to intent – and most people affected by contaminated Factor VIII draw a clear line between their experiences and any medical conspiracy. Des Collins put four companies in the frame for the infected blood scandal, but he was clear not to criticize big pharma in general. He praised the work of Pfizer, Moderna, AstraZeneca and others in rolling out Covid-19 vaccinations. He was glad to have his vaccine and the boosters, especially when he contracted Covid himself. 'But,' he says, 'that doesn't give them carte blanche to kill people.' For all the fears about the Covid-19 vaccine, many of those infected with viruses by Factor VIII were able to trust the science when it came to being vaccinated in the pandemic. Richard, Gary and Joe all had the Covid-19 vaccine. But some have held onto an unresolvable fear about when to have treatment and when to say no. In Louisiana, Karen Cross supported her daughter Jennifer's decision not to be vaccinated.

People with hemophilia face an impossible choice: trust the pharmaceutical companies who gave them HIV and hepatitis C or refuse the treatment they need in order to stay alive. Joe and Clair, like many others, avoided HIV treatments for as long as they could after experiencing the damage wrought by Factor VIII. But the antiretroviral therapies produced by the same industry allowed their health to recover and virus levels to become undetectable, meaning they couldn't pass it on to someone else. We will never know how many died because of reluctance to trust these innovations.

Today there is also pre-exposure prophylaxis (PrEP), which can prevent people from contracting HIV in the first place. In 2021, 1.6 million people around the world took PrEP. The NHS, meanwhile, said it expects to eradicate hepatitis C from England by 2025. The marathon effort to create an effective HIV vaccine continues.

Once a week, Professor Tuddenham takes the train from Rye, on England's south coast, to Hampstead, in north London, where he has his office at the Royal Free's hemophilia center. Now in his late seventies, he is an Emeritus Professor at University College London and still researching hemophilia treatment. After an effective treatment became available for AIDS, he returned to hospital work, treating patients alongside his research. On one of these days at the Royal Free in late July 2022, Tuddenham was celebrating a breakthrough. Research he was involved in had been splashed all over the news: a trial of gene therapy for hemophilia B had successfully stopped bleeding in nine out of ten patients.

Gene therapy could fix the defect that prevents the body from being able to make vital clotting factors. One injection of FLT180a – a virus that instructs the body to manufacture missing clotting factor – was enough to take a patient's levels of factor IX from 1 percent to normal, preventing the need for weekly infusions. There had been side effects, with one patient developing a blood clot after receiving a high dose, but the results were an epoch-shifting step forward. Tuddenham scrolled through emails of congratulation from colleagues in the UK and abroad. Among them was a kind message from a patient who had been involved in an earlier, unsuccessful stage of the trial.

Tuddenham had found patients were keen to be involved in research, despite their history, because they wanted to help further scientific development. If anything made recruitment difficult, it was how many competing pieces of research there were, not hesitancy about the dangers. Ethical procedures were now followed more rigorously and doctors were no longer seen as gods – they were fallible human beings whose statements could be questioned. Within medical culture, patients were now part of the process, being given the facts so they could make an informed decision. And perhaps more than anything, the advent of the internet has provided people with access to more knowledge about their health than ever before. No longer would a doctor be able to keep patients in the dark in the way Frankie, Joe, Clair and Bryan had been.

In late 2022, the FDA approved the first gene-therapy treatment for hemophilia B from CSL Behring, which had bought Tuddenham and his team's early research. One dose could prevent bleeding for eight years or more – and it cost $3.5 million per patient. CSL Behring defended the high cost, saying it would save hospitals money in the long term, given regular injections of Factor IX could cost upwards of $700,000 per year. 'Even now their take on things always ends up at the bottom line,' says Professor Tuddenham. The European Medicines Agency approved the first gene therapy for hemophilia A in 2022 based on his research, but it currently doesn't last as long as the treatment for hemophilia B.

As he walks through the corridors of the Royal Free wearing a cream suit jacket and a protective face mask, Tuddenham cannot help but see the scars of the hemophilia AIDS crisis. Having started in a caravan in the hospital's car park, the hemophilia center had moved into a hospital with a grant from a man whose son had the bleeding disorder. When the disaster hit, that man's son was one of those who contracted HIV and died. A few meters from the entrance to the hemophilia center was the ward which had become an emergency AIDS unit, where many of Tuddenham's patients passed away.

Forty years on, as he enters the hemophilia center, he thinks of the young boys who never made it to adulthood, of the patients who suffered avoidable deaths. 'As a Christian, I look to meet them again,' he says.

In houses the world over, fragments of the infected blood disaster are preserved. Unworn baseball caps, neglected cuddly toys, childhood posters, handwritten diaries, tapes containing voices that vanished, wedding rings hidden away. All that remains of those who died are pictures of smiling faces in happier times; memories in grieving minds. Survivors and the bereaved exist in a place that's full of lost things. Children who never became adults. Adults who never had children. People who never found partners. Grandparents who never were.

Lawyer Des Collins's unwavering old-school composure cracks as he recalls one of the worst stories he has heard from a client: a funeral director who told a family to put their loved one's dead body in a black bag and place it in the garden until the day of the funeral to prevent the spread of AIDS. 'It's just inhuman,' he says. Tom Mull's PTSD is triggered whenever he talks about the hemophilia cases, reopening old wounds. 'Closure is such an overused and misleading aspiration, an unattainable goal, and I thought it was actually an emotional albatross,' he says. Having shared the full story, he reflects, 'I now think it does exist and that I am somehow at least partially "closed," and it feels so good, so unburdening.'

Amid the bloodshed, life continues. When Gary Cross developed cancer in the years after the US legal fight ended, he discovered a new fortitude in himself. Lying in bed, feeling mortally unwell, he said to himself, 'Brad, I'm coming.' By thinking about his son, he realized he wasn't scared of death. After a series of operations, he pulled through. 'Brad made us stronger,' says Karen, sitting next to her husband in their Baton Rouge home, their daughter, Jennifer, in the other room. Memories of Brad surround them, a framed watercolor of him bundled up in the snow, another with his arms wrapped around his sister. Stored away, they have a collection of unused Factor VIII bottles and newspaper clippings about their fight for justice.

Many of those who made it to the Infected Blood Inquiry were plagued by survivors' guilt. Every hour, Ade Goodyear would remember the classmates he lost. A song could cause time to unravel. Whenever the film *Gremlins* was shown on the television, he was back in the cinema as a child alongside nine friends, seven of whom are now dead. There was a continuum of guilt. But having promised his late classmates and brothers that he would keep their memories alive, Ade was determined to keep talking, to keep living. Richard Warwick feared the emptiness that would come when he no longer had a reason to travel to London to campaign with the other surviving Treloar's boys. His sister had chosen not to start a family with her husband because she felt too guilty that he and Tina couldn't have children. Their family line was coming to an end. But he would always have a support network. Ade says, 'We're a unique set of people in history.'

Frankie felt like a husk of the person she was meant to be, but eventually, after her mum passed away, she decided she needed to try to heal. Her mum's last words to her had been, 'take care of yourself,' and she wanted to do just that. During the pandemic, she moved to the southwest of England to live on the coast with her new partner. Down there, she did her best to shut away her life's trauma and enjoy spending time with her partner's grandchild. But every time she went to London there was a painful reminder of all that had been taken from her – of the forty years that Factor VIII had disfigured.

Frankie's ex-husband Joe had a new partner who was widowed when her husband, a former Treloar's pupil, developed AIDS-related illness and passed away. There was a strange symmetry to Joe being with her; she could understand him in a way others couldn't. At the end of each day at the inquiry, Joe would remove his red AIDS ribbon and hide it in his pocket, fearing how people on the outside would react if they knew. HIV and hepatitis C would always be there in the back of his mind. He tried to turn away from the past, but as he had dinner with his solicitor he couldn't help but think how the lawyer was exactly the same age his and Frankie's child would now have been. The shadows of a lifetime lost.

As the trial investigating the death of Ken Dixon had drawn to a close in New Orleans back in March 1999, each lawyer had a couple of hours in which to deliver their closing arguments to the jury. For those representing Alpha, Armour, Baxter and Bayer, this was the opportunity to defend their clients – to prove they couldn't have reacted any differently to the dangers of hepatitis and AIDS. To make the case for their 'wonder treatment' Factor VIII, which had transformed the lives of people with hemophilia.

Terry Tottenham, the lawyer representing Bayer, had an idea to capture the jury's imagination as he made his final argument. While the jurors were out of the courtroom on their lunch break, he opened a box containing dozens of small glass vials, each about the size of a salt shaker. Inside, there was white powder. The lids were made from a soft metal, which could be punctured to inject the sterile distilled water so the mixture could then be extracted with a syringe for infusion. A white sticker across the front had a clinical, sterile appearance that said: ANTIHEMOPHILIC FACTOR KOATE. Tottenham approached the ledge in front of the witness box and started lining up vials along the top, one next to another. When he had created enough of a base he began a second row, placing more vials on top of the first ones. His plan was to make a tower with the bottles.

Something about the triangular construction looked strangely beautiful – the sleek glass bottles symmetrically balanced, with the backdrop of the courtroom behind them.

Tom looked at Lorraine, whose eyes reflected his thoughts. 'He's gonna knock that over,' he said.

After lunch, the jury came back and Tottenham stood up to address them. To his mind there was only one responsible party in this whole tragedy: AIDS. The virus had stolen into the blood supply without anyone knowing and infected people before they had a chance to stop it. Before the companies could have changed their manufacturing process to make it safer. He gestured towards the tower of Factor VIII bottles: this was truly a miraculous treatment for people with hemophilia. Hepatitis was an unavoidable by-product, not a warning of what was to come.

At some point in his rousing speech, Tottenham accidentally bumped the railing. The bottles shook. Then they started to tumble down in a cascade of glass and metal. As they hit the floor they exploded, sending a cloud of white powder into the air. Panicked, the members of the jury instinctively covered their faces and ran from the courtroom. Judge Tobias scarpered, too. The trial paused for the rest of the day so that cleaners wearing hazmat suits could make sure it was completely safe before everyone reentered.

In that moment, Tom was conflicted. Watching the jury flee, he knew his side would win the case. In their terrified faces he saw they understood just how lethal Factor VIII had been and the risks the companies had taken. Risks that killed thousands of people, many of whom were children. Every single bottle of Factor VIII manufactured in America in 1983 had been contaminated with HIV and hepatitis. But the people who had known the dangers had continued to pump it out regardless. 'A medically necessary product, sourced by cheap labor, manufactured with an economy of scale, a permanent captive audience, governmental acquiescence and cooperation,' says Tom. Those who needed its life-changing properties were caught in a deadly confluence of opportunity and greed. It was sick, he thought; the whole system was sick. But at least people would now know the truth.

Acknowledgments

The many people who shared the intimate and traumatic details of their lives for this book should never have had to do so. A cruel combination of stigma and outright suppression meant they were largely ignored or dismissed for decades. The infected blood scandal has ultimately come to light as a result of survivors' tireless investigation, as well as the work of family members, lawyers, journalists and politicians – some of whom appear in *Blood Farm*, but many more of whom do not, given the sheer scale of this global disaster. The evidence that forms the bedrock of this book has been unearthed by hundreds of people, each of whom have worked determinedly and doggedly to expose the truth. I am one writer, but the voices in this book are many.

I am grateful to everyone who trusted me with their individual stories and for their dedication to getting the facts right. My hope is to have done them justice. Recollections of events from forty years ago can be hazy, but I have tried to verify as much as I can by cross-checking personal accounts with official documents, witness statements, medical records and other people who were present at the time. Any mistakes are my own. Some names have been changed to protect anonymity.

I want to acknowledge the team at the Infected Blood Inquiry, who have spent five years meticulously combing through half a century's worth of evidence. The full record of their work can be found at www.infectedbloodinquiry.org.uk. Thank you to Tom and Lorraine Mull for sharing all of the documents from their court cases in the US, with the technical assistance of Andy White, and to Jason Evans and Donna Shaw for being so generous with their own forensic research. Donna's book coauthored with Eric Weinberg, *Blood on Their Hands*, as well as Douglas Starr's *Blood: An Epic History of Medicine and Commerce*, are both vital resources, particularly in the US and international context, for explaining how Factor VIII became a deadly poison. Gary Cross's memoir, *Vial 023: A Father's Pursuit of Justice*, moved me to tears more than once, while Marcus Plowright's ITV documentary *In Cold Blood* is a clear telling of how Britain failed its hemophilia population.

The amazing editorial team behind this book have lived and breathed it like I have. Thank you to my editor Greg Clowes, Liz Gassman in the US, and my agent Nick Walters, all of whom understood that this story needed to be told and committed to helping me do so with the utmost care. Thanks also to the indefatigable teams behind them at Viking, Diversion Books and David Luxton Associates – especially my copyeditor Trevor Horwood; the legal team, Martin Soames and Lucy Middleton; and rights and contracts director Rebecca Winfield.

The genesis of this book was two features I wrote for the *Telegraph* in the opening week of the Infected Blood Inquiry in 2019. Two years later, my incredible colleagues Sarah Peters and Theodora Louloudis wholeheartedly agreed we should investigate further for the second series of our podcast *Bed of Lies*. I'm indebted to Theo for giving us the support and freedom to report on this story with the time it needed. Sarah has been the best producer I could have asked for, patiently sharing her knowledge with me and answering my calls anytime day or night.

Thank you to everyone who read chapters in draft form, especially my two writing groups for their encouragement during the pandemic and beyond. I am grateful to my family – Mum, Dad, Callie, Fergus and Granny – and to all the friends who let me write this book from their sofas and gardens in Europe and America. Without the escape from my desk and a chance to debrief over cups of tea it would have been much more difficult to make *Blood Farm* what it has become. I hope the stories shared in this book go some way towards preventing history from repeating itself.

Responses from the Pharmaceutical Companies

The author approached the pharmaceutical companies involved in the production of Factor VIII for comment. They responded as follows.

Bayer

Bayer has been cooperating fully with the Infected Blood Inquiry in the UK, examining the circumstances in which men, women and children treated by the National Health Service, in particular in the 1970s and '80s, were given infected blood and infected blood products. Bayer understands the importance of the inquiry's work to those infected and affected by this tragedy and expresses deep sympathy for people living with hemophilia who contracted HIV or hepatitis C infection through use of blood therapies in the 1970s and '80s and for the family members of those that were infected.

Bayer is truly sorry that this tragic situation occurred and that therapies that were developed by us, and that were prescribed by doctors to save and improve lives, in fact ended up causing so much suffering to so many.

As the full findings of the Infected Blood Inquiry are still to be published, it would be inappropriate for Bayer to comment further.

Baxter

Baxter did not respond to our request for comment, but provided the following statement for *Bed of Lies* in November 2021:

Patient safety and quality are of the utmost importance to Baxter and are critical in pursuing our mission to save and sustain lives. The business involved in the situation you describe was spun-off from Baxter in 2015, along with all associated records and data. While we have cooperated with the Infected Blood Inquiry to the fullest extent possible, Takeda currently owns this business and would be the appropriate party to respond to your inquiry.

Takeda

Takeda is aware of the Infected Blood Inquiry, and is fully engaging with any requests made to Takeda by the inquiry. We have great sympathy with anyone impacted by this issue, and their families. It is not appropriate to comment further given the independent inquiry is ongoing.

CSL Behring

We are deeply saddened that in the late 1970s through to the early 1990s many people contracted devastating diseases from new and emerging pathogens through contaminated blood and plasma-derived products. Plasma-derived therapies undergo rigorous safety controls and inspections throughout every step of the manufacturing process from the collection of plasma to the final packaging of the finished product, ensuring plasma-derived therapies are of the highest quality and safety.

Grifols

We provided testimony to the Infected Blood Inquiry indicating that during the relevant time frame, 1970 to 1993, Grifols did not manufacture or distribute any pooled plasma-protein therapeutics in the UK. The first distribution of Grifols products in the UK was in 1997; all of which products were virally inactivated and have not been implicated in the transmission of any viral agents.

Sanofi

Did not respond to request for comment.

Notes

Prologue: The Farm

It is here that Isaac Franklin . . . www.crt.state.la.us/Assets/OCD/archaeology
/discoverarchaeology/virtual-books/PDFs/Angola_Pop.pdf.

Tom Mull had driven up from New Orleans, et seq. Author interviews with Tom Mull, July 12,
2021, October 26, 2021 and April 4, 2023.

Chapter 1: Schoolboy Games

Ten-year-old Richard Warwick . . . et seq. Author interviews with Richard Warwick, July 11
and August 12, 2022, April 4, 2023.

But the largest group was Richard's . . . Infected Blood Inquiry, Presentation about Treloar's,
June 21, 2021.

Within a year, he had raised enough money . . . www.treloar.org.uk/about-us/our-history/.

Although Treloar's was for children with physical disabilities . . . Author interview with Amanda
Beesley, July 7, 2022.

If a child was in a wheelchair . . . Author interviews with Richard Warwick, and Ade
Goodyear, June 24 and August 9, 2021.

a fibrin clot . . . www.hog.org/handbook/article/1/3/how-blood-works-in-a-person-with
-hemophilia.

Haemophilia A is caused by . . . www.hemophilia.org/bleeding-disorders-a-z/types
/hemophilia-a.

von Willebrand disease . . . www.hemophilia.org/bleeding-disorders-a-z/types/von
-willebrand-disease.

more than eight thousand people . . . UKHCDO annual report 2020, www.ukhcdo.org
/wp-content/uploads/2021/03/UKHCDO-Annual-Report-2020-2019-20-Data
_FINAL.pdf.

Queen Victoria was a carrier . . . et seq. www.hemophilia.org/bleeding-disorders-a-z
/overview/history.

a breakthrough in 1964 . . . C. K. Kasper, 'Judith Graham Pool and the Discovery of
Cryoprecipitate,' *Haemophilia*, vol. 18 (2012), 833–36.

In each treatment, children . . . Author interview with Professor Liakat Parapia, April 24,
2023.

In the late 1960s . . . et seq. Eric Weinberg and Donna Shaw, *Blood on Their Hands: How
Greedy Companies, Inept Bureaucracy and Bad Science Killed Thousands of Hemophiliacs*
(Rutgers University Press, 2017), and Douglas Starr, *Blood: An Epic History of Medicine
and Commerce* (Sphere Books, 2000).

Gary found Factor VIII life-changing . . . et seq. Author interview with Gary Webster, July
14, 2022, and Infected Blood Inquiry, June 21, 2021.

After the war, his family . . . et seq. Author interview with Professor Edward Tuddenham, August 6, 2021 and July 26, 2022; Infected Blood Inquiry, Professor Edward Tuddenham, oral evidence, October 22, 2020.

the median age of death was around sixty . . . C. Mejia-Carvajal, E. E. Czapek and L. A. Valentino, 'Life Expectancy in Hemophilia Outcome', *Journal of Thrombosis and Haemostasis*, vol. 4, no. 3 (March 2006); Infected Blood Inquiry, Expert report to the Infected Blood Inquiry: Fractionation; Alfred H. Katz, Social Adaptation in Chronic Illness: A Study of Hemophilia,' *American Journal of Public Health*, vol. 53, no. 10 (October 1963).

Haemophilia care was unique in medicine . . . Author interview with Professor Jean-Pierre Allain, July 21, 2022.

They worked long hours . . . 'Frances Rotblat Obituary,' *The Times*, June 12, 2021.

After an initial grant . . . Author interview with Professor Edward Tuddenham, May 28, 2023.

Clair was seventeen when . . . et seq. Bed of Lies, Telegraph podcast Infected Blood Inquiry, Clair, oral evidence, May 2, 2019, and Clair, written evidence, WITN1589001.

Three years older than her . . . Cara McGoogan, 'The Tainted Blood Scandal Left Me Widowed, Childless and with HIV,' *Telegraph*, May 5, 2019.

They all had haemophilia . . . Author interview with Richard Warwick, July 11, 2022.

Chapter 2: Outbreak

Ade turned and made his way . . . et seq. Author interviews with Ade Goodyear, June 24 and August 9, 2021, July 12 and August 24, 2022, and Infected Blood Inquiry, Adrian Goodyear, written evidence, WITN1243.

Adults always remarked . . . Author interview with Amanda Beesley, July 7, 2022.

the British Navy, which had a history . . . Richard E. Hawkins et al., 'Risk of Viral Hepatitis among Military Personnel Assigned to US Navy Ships,' *Journal of Infectious Diseases*, vol. 165, no. 4 (April 1992), 716–19.

Over successive years . . . Infected Blood Inquiry, Adrian Goodyear, oral evidence, June 5, 2019.

Dr Aronstam was responsible for . . . et seq. A. Aronstam, *Haemophilic Bleeding: Early Management at Home* (Baillière Tindall, 1985).

Dr Aronstam had an open-door policy . . . et seq. Infected Blood Inquiry, Presentation about Treloar's, June 25, 2021, and Adrian Goodyear, oral evidence, June 5, 2019.

Macpherson didn't question . . . Author interview with Amanda Beesley, July 7, 2022.

Richard's treatment would remain the same . . . et seq. Richard Warwick's medical records, shared with the author, and Infected Blood Inquiry, Richard Warwick, oral evidence, June 20, 2019.

Gary's friend Stephen, along with . . . et seq. Author interview with Gary Webster, July 14, 2022, and Infected Blood Inquiry, Gary Webster, June 21, 2021.

Ade's bout of hepatitis . . . Infected Blood Inquiry, Adrian Goodyear, oral evidence, June 5, 2019.

Compared to the revolutionary upsides . . . Author interview with Professor Edward Tuddenham, August 6, 2021.

The head told the children . . . Infected Blood Inquiry, Alec Macpherson, oral evidence, and presentation about Treloar's, June 24, 2021.

'We have found from observations . . .' Infected Blood Inquiry, Letter from J. Craske to Dr A. Aronstam, May 10, 1979, HHFT0000916_00.

'As far as your suggestion . . .' Infected Blood Inquiry, Letter from A. Aronstam to Dr J. Craske, May 14, 1979, HHFT0000916_002.

'I am increasingly wary . . .' Infected Blood Inquiry, Presentation about Treloar's, June 23, 2021.

'Don't worry, boys . . .' et seq. Infected Blood Inquiry, Adrian Goodyear, written evidence, WITN1243.

Ade's friends at Treloar's . . . et seq. Author interviews with Ade Goodyear, June 24 and August 9, 2021, July 12 and August 24, 2022, and Infected Blood Inquiry, Adrian Goodyear, oral evidence, June 5, 2019.

Some of the more exciting items . . . Infected Blood Inquiry, Presentation about Treloar's, June 21, 2021.

He was prescribed phenytoin . . . Richard Warwick's medical records, shared with the author.

Among them was Gary . . . Author interview with Gary Webster, July 14, 2022.

Joe lived to the extreme . . . et seq. Author interviews with Joe, July 27, 2021 and July 7, 2022, author interviews with Frankie, July 20, 2021 and July 12, 2022, and Infected Blood Inquiry, Frankie, oral evidence, October 31, 2019.

'I came to office with . . .' www.margaretthatcher.org/document/105617.

Chapter 3: Do No Harm

Kevin Slater developed . . . et seq. Infected Blood Inquiry, Presentation on First Cardiff AIDS Patient, February 2, 2021, and Lynda Maule, written evidence, WITN3517001.

The first sign . . . et seq. www.cdc.gov/mmwr/preview/mmwrhtml/00001126.htm.

gay-related immune deficiency . . . www.cdc.gov/mmwr/preview/mmwrhtml/su6004a11 .htm, and 'Clue Found on Homosexuals' Precancer Syndrome,' *New York Times*, June 18, 1982.

Early research had shown . . . Lauren Martin, 'How Does a Person's T Cell Count Indicate AIDS?,' *Medical News Today*, April 29, 2021.

UK Haemophilia Centre Directors Organization . . . Infected Blood Inquiry, Professor Edward Tuddenham, oral evidence, October 22, 2020.

Dr Tuddenham and the others . . . Minutes of the 13th meeting of the UK Haemophilia Centre Directors, September 13, 1982, courtesy of Tainted Blood.

Cases of AIDS in America had doubled . . . www.cdc.gov/mmwr/preview/mmwrhtml /00001163.htm.

'We are becoming aware that . . .' Dr Jane F. Desforges, 'AIDS and Preventative Treatment in Hemophilia,' *New England Journal of Medicine*, vol. 308, no. 2 (1983).

Christine Doyle wrote . . . Christine Doyle, 'Mystery Disease Threat,' *Observer*, January 16, 1983.

Less than two weeks later . . . et seq. Penrose Inquiry, Notes of meeting with Immuno at London Airport, January 24, 1983.

There was mounting evidence . . . et seq. Virginia Berridge, *AIDS in the UK: The Making of Policy, 1981–1994* (Oxford University Press, 2002).

'The recognition of disease . . .' 'Acquired Immune Deficiency in Haemophilia,' *The Lancet*, April 2, 1983.

There were other doctors . . . Infected Blood Inquiry, Professor Christine Lee, oral evidence, October 21, 2020.

'barrage of viruses' . . . Penrose Inquiry, Notes of meeting with Immuno at London Airport, January 24, 1983.

Tuddenham and Kernoff mulled . . . *et seq.* Author interview with Professor Edward Tuddenham, August 6, 2021, and Infected Blood Inquiry, Professor Edward Tuddenham, oral evidence, October 22, 2020.

'If we didn't move to concentrates . . .' Author interview with Professor Liakat Parapia, July 21, 2021.

In Cardiff, he called his patients 'my boys' . . . Infected Blood Inquiry, Janet Smith, written evidence, WITN1523001.

'Blood products or blood . . .' www.cdc.gov/mmwr/preview/mmwrhtml/00001257.htm.

'As you can imagine . . .' *et seq.* Infected Blood Inquiry, Professor Bloom and Cardiff Haemophilia Centre presentation, September 30, 2020.

These groups all had vested interests . . . National AIDS Memorial HIV Story Project video, www.youtube.com/watch?v=G4mFmwmCXSw.

'the evidence suggests . . .' *et seq.* Infected Blood Inquiry, Professor Bloom and Cardiff Haemophilia Centre presentation, September 30, 2020.

A new episode . . . *et seq. Horizon,* 'Killer in the Village', BBC TV, April 25, 1983, www.bbc.co.uk/iplayer/episode/p01z2lbp/horizon-19821983-killer-in-the-village, and author interview with Richard Warwick.

three new AIDS cases . . . National Research Council, *AIDS: The Second Decade* (National Academies Press, 1990), and www.cdc.gov/mmwr/volumes/70/wr/mm7022a1.htm.

'This young man . . .' Infected Blood Inquiry, Richard Warwick, oral evidence, June 20, 2019.

'Acquired Immunodeficiency Syndrome new.' *et seq* . . . Infected Blood Inquiry, Presentation on First Cardiff AIDS Patient, February 2, 2021.

Sue Douglas landed her job . . . *et seq.* Author interview with Sue Douglas, July 22, 2022.

fear over the 'gay plague' . . . *Aids: The Unheard Tapes,* BBC TV, 2022, www.bbc.co.uk/programmes/m0018t1c.

the true number was thought . . . 'US Blood Products Face Ban in AIDS Scare,' *Guardian,* May 2, 1983.

He had resigned from . . . 'Obituary, Stewart Steven,' *Guardian,* January 20, 2002.

Back in Treloar's at break time . . . *et seq.* Author interviews with Ade Goodyear, June 24 and August 9, 2021, July 12 and August 24, 2022; and Infected Blood Inquiry Presentation about Treloar's, June 21, 2021, and Adrian Goodyear, oral evidence, June 5, 2019.

'BLOOD imported by the NHS . . .' Susan Douglas, 'Exclusive: Virus Imported from U.S – Hospitals Using Killer Blood – Spread of the Gay Plague,' *Mail on Sunday,* May 1, 1983.

Sue Douglas was back . . . *et seq.* Author interview with Sue Douglas, July 22, 2022.

'As an experienced doctor . . .' *et seq.* Infected Blood Inquiry, Susan Douglas, oral evidence, September 15, 2022.

Dr Aronstam was on the front line . . . *et seq.* 'Warning Against AIDS "Panic,"' *Guardian,* May 4, 1983.

In the hemophilia center at Treloar's . . . Infected Blood Inquiry, Alec Macpherson, oral evidence, and presentation about Treloar's.

When Gary and Stephen arrived . . . *et seq.* Author interview with Gary Webster, July 14, 2022, and Infected Blood Inquiry, Gary Webster, June 21, 2021.

Reports from America of AIDS . . . et seq. Infected Blood Inquiry, Letter from Revd Alan J. Tanner, May 4, 1983.

He attended a meeting . . . et seq. Infected Blood Inquiry, Presentation on First Cardiff AIDS Patient, February 2, 2021.

Dr Galbraith was the UK's . . . 'Dr Spence Galbraith Obituary,' *British Medical Journal*, vol. 338 (2009).

'The mortality rate of AIDS . . .' Infected Blood Inquiry, Letter from N. Galbraith to Dr I. Field, May 9, 1983.

'We have absolutely no doubt . . .' *In Cold Blood*, ITV, September 27, 2020.

'very real threat' . . . et seq. Author interview with Sue Douglas, July 22, 2022, and Infected Blood Inquiry, Susan Douglas, oral evidence, September 15, 2022.

researchers at the Pasteur Institute . . . 'Luc Montagnier, Nobel-Winning Co-Discoverer of H.I.V., Dies at 89,' *New York Times*, February 10, 2022, and Françoise Barré-Sinoussi et al., 'Isolation of a T-lymphotropic Retrovirus from a Patient at Risk for AIDS,' *Science*, vol. 220 (1983), 868–71.

The New York Times *ran . . .* 'Health Chief Calls, AIDS Battle "No. 1 Priority"' *New York Times*, May 25, 1983.

Chapter 4: Missed Warnings

In the weeks before Clair's . . . et seq. Bed of Lies, *Telegraph* podcast; and Infected Blood Inquiry, Clair, oral evidence, May 2, 2019, and Clair, written evidence, WITN1589001.

They could now seize the future . . . Cara McGoogan, '"What were we to them – expendable?" The Story Behind the Biggest Treatment Scandal in NHS History,' *Telegraph*, October 8, 2021.

The weather grew warmer . . . et seq. Infected Blood Inquiry, Presentation note on Treloar's, June 2021, INQY0000281.

'neurotic about getting too associated' . . . Justin Parkinson, 'AIDS Campaign: Thatcher "Fought Against Risky Sex Warnings,"' BBC News, February 8, 2021.

Scientific experts in the Department of Health . . . Infected Blood Inquiry, Dr Diana Walford, oral evidence, July 20, 2021.

370 recorded AIDS deaths in the UK . . . Hilary E. Tillett, N. S. Galbraith, et al., 'Routine Surveillance Data on AIDS and HIV Infections in the UK: A Description of the Data Available and Their Use for Short -Term Planning,' *Epidemiology and Infection*, vol. 100 (1988), 157–69.

Into this hesitant and distracted . . . Infected Blood Inquiry, Bloom and Cardiff Haemophilia Centre presentation, September 30, 2020.

the 'line to take' was . . . et seq. Infected Blood Inquiry, Dr Diana Walford, oral evidence, July 20, 2021.

Years later, Norman Fowler, Ken Clarke . . . Infected Blood Inquiry, Lord Simon Glenarthur, oral evidence, July 22, 2021.

'false conclusions' . . . et seq. Infected Blood Inquiry, Bloom and Cardiff Haemophilia Centre presentation, September 30, 2020.

'little evidence . . .' Infected Blood Inquiry, Presentation on Armour and Bayer, September 29, 2021.

'health hazards' of Factor VIII . . . Infected Blood Inquiry, Lord Simon Glenarthur, oral evidence, July 22, 2021.

'confidential, largely because . . .' Infected Blood Inquiry, Sir Joseph Smith, written evidence, WITN5281001, and Bloom and Cardiff Haemophilia Centre presentation (continued), September 30, 2020.

As health minister, Clarke . . . Berridge, *AIDS in the UK.*

Thatcher later asked Fowler . . . Parkinson, 'Aids Campaign.'

the government decided to provide . . . Infected Blood Inquiry, Lord Kenneth Clarke, oral evidence, July 27, 2021.

'There is no conclusive proof . . .' Infected Blood Inquiry, Dr Diana Walford, oral evidence, July 21, 2021.

'It has been suggested that AIDS . . .' Infected Blood Inquiry, Lord Simon Glenarthur, oral evidence, July 23, 2021.

In the middle of June 1983 . . . et seq. Infected Blood Inquiry, Presentation on First Cardiff AIDS Patient, February 2, 2021.

'We have not laid down . . .' et seq. Infected Blood Inquiry, Bloom and Cardiff Haemophilia Centre presentation, September 30, 2020.

At Treloar's, Dr Aronstam tried . . . et seq. Infected Blood Inquiry, Presentation note on Treloar's, June 2021, INQY0000281, and Alec Macpherson, oral evidence, and presentation about Treloar's, June 24, 2021.

Doctors Tuddenham and Kernoff . . . Infected Blood Inquiry, Presentation on Armour and Bayer, September 29, 2021.

For every 250,000 units . . . Inter-Pharma memo, January 27, 1981, courtesy of Jason Evans.

In July 1983 the Haemophilia Society . . . Infected Blood Inquiry, Bloom and Cardiff Haemophilia Centre presentation, September 30, 2020.

Kevin's diagnosis was recorded . . . et seq. Infected Blood Inquiry, Presentation on First Cardiff AIDS Patient, February 2, 2021.

In his letter to Dr Aronstam . . . Infected Blood Inquiry, Presentation note on Treloar's, June 2021, INQY0000281; author interview with Tony Farrugia, April 4, 2023.

Dr Tuddenham traveled to Stockholm . . . et seq. Author interview with Professor Edward Tuddenham, August 6, 2021.

For Dr Peter Foster . . . Infected Blood Inquiry, Dr Peter Foster, oral evidence, March 24, 2022.

He also mentioned a version . . . Infected Blood Inquiry, Professor Edward Tuddenham, oral evidence, October 22, 2020.

Back at the Royal Free . . . Infected Blood Inquiry, Professor Christine Lee, oral evidence, October 21, 2020.

When Ade returned to school . . . et seq. Author interview with Ade Goodyear, August 24, 2022, Infected Blood Inquiry, Adrian Goodyear, oral evidence, June 5, 2019, and Adrian Goodyear, written evidence, WITN1243.

Sue and her editors believed . . . Susan Douglas, 'The Scandal of [Hemophiliac's] Death,' *Mail on Sunday*, October 2, 1983, and author interview with Sue Douglas, July 22, 2022.

'Susan Douglas uses . . .' Infected Blood Inquiry, Letter from Peter Jones to The Press Council re complaint about *Mail*'s article entitled 'Hospitals Using Killer Blood,' October 5, 1983, PJON0000001_126.

Andrew Veitch reported . . . et seq. Department of Health photocopy of Andrew Veitch, 'US Blood Causes AIDS,' *Guardian*, November 1, 1983.

Dr Walford could see no justification . . . Infected Blood Inquiry, Dr Diana Walford, written evidence, WITN4461001.

'I would like to put on record . . .' et seq. Infected Blood Inquiry, Lord Simon Glenarthur, oral evidence, July 23, 2021.

In a debate in the House of Commons . . . House of Commons Hansard Debates for November 14, 1983, vol. 48, https://hansard.parliament.uk/Commons/1983-11-14/debates /2a367b68-2c97-42cd-9bcd-1a6b8155f1f0/BloodProducts(Imports).

'no conclusive proof . . .' Jim Reed, 'Blood Inquiry: Former Health Minister Defends Blood Products Advice on Aids,' BBC News, July 28, 2021.

Kevin's case of AIDS was 'confirmed' . . . Infected Blood Inquiry, Presentation on First Cardiff AIDS Patient, February 2, 2021.

On April 23, 1984 . . . Penrose Inquiry Final Report – Chapter 29.

Their findings ran in Science . . . Robert C. Gallo et. al., 'Frequent Detection and Isolation of Cytophathic Retroviruses (HTLV-III) from Patients with AIDS and at Risk for AIDS,' *Science*, vol. 224, no. 4648 (May 4, 1984), 500–3.

'public interest had waned . . . Department of Health memo, 'Use of Factor VIII by Haemophiliacs,' October 20, 1987, courtesy of Jason Evans.

'At what point did we . . .' Author interview with Professor Edward Tuddenham, August 6, 2021.

Ade had been having a difficult . . . et seq. Author interviews with Ade Goodyear, June 24 and August 9, 2021, July 12 and August 24, 2022, Infected Blood Inquiry, Adrian Goodyear, oral evidence, June 5, 2019, and Adrian Goodyear, written evidence, WITN1243.

he continued to prescribe . . . Infected Blood Inquiry, Presentation note on Treloar's, June 2021, INQY0000281.

Professor Montagnier in Paris . . . et. seq. Penrose Inquiry, Final Report – Chapter 29.

Tedder invited hemophilia doctors . . . Infected Blood Inquiry, Professor Richard Tedder, oral evidence, October 13, 2022.

His results revealed the true scale . . . et seq. Berridge, *AIDS in the UK*, and Penrose Inquiry Final Report – Chapter 29.

Bloom brought the hemophilia . . . et seq. Infected Blood Inquiry, Minutes of a Haemophilia Reference Centre Directors Meeting re blood donor testing and screening for HTLV-III antibodies, December 10, 1984.

set of recommendations . . . Infected Blood Inquiry, UKHCDO Report Suggesting Unheated Concentrate Almost Certain to be Contaminated, December 14, 1984.

But the British government was skeptical . . . In Cold Blood, ITV, 27 September 2020.

Dr Mark Winter was director . . . et seq. Infected Blood Inquiry, Dr Mark Winter, oral evidence, October 1, 2020, and Penrose Inquiry, Dr Mark Winter submission, PEN0150292.

The Lancet *published an editorial . . .* Justice Horace Krever, Commission of Inquiry on the Blood System in Canada (hereafter Krever Report), Part IV: 'International Responses to the Risk of HIV in the Blood Supply.'

doctors were told to stop using . . . Infected Blood Inquiry, Archer Inquiry Transcript, June 12, 2008.

'a proper protection against AIDS . . .' In Cold Blood, ITV, September 27, 2020.

'I am sure you have been . . .' et seq. Infected Blood Inquiry, Bloom and Cardiff Haemophilia Centre presentation, September 30, 2020.

Dr Aronstam blamed the government . . . 'Specialist Hits at UK Inaction on AIDS Blood,' *Sunday Times*, October 8, 1989.

At the beginning of 1985 . . . www.collinslaw.co.uk/contaminated--blood-timeline.

Britain's Blood Products Laboratory . . . *et seq.* Berridge, *AIDS in the UK*.

some hospitals in England and Wales . . . *et seq. In Cold Blood*, ITV, September 27, 2020.

Kevin's health was deteriorating . . . *et seq.* Infected Blood Inquiry, Presentation on First Cardiff AIDS Patient, February 2, 2021.

On June 23, 1985 . . . *et seq.* Infected Blood Inquiry, Lynda Maule, written evidence, WITN3517001.

Chapter 5: Lethal Injections

At the beginning of March 1985 . . . *et seq. Bed of Lies, Telegraph* podcast, and Infected Blood Inquiry, Clair, oral evidence, May 2, 2019, and Clair, written evidence, WITN1589001.

around three hundred and fifty people . . . Institute of Mathematics, 'Urban Maths: World AIDS Day 2018,' https://ima.org.uk/10941/urban-maths-world-aids-day-2018/.

After Hudson's death . . . Ella Braidwood, ' "Gay Plague": The Vile, Horrific and Inhuman Way the Media Reported the AIDS Crisis,' *Pink News*, November 30, 2018.

Late one morning in May . . . *et seq.* Author interviews with Ade Goodyear, June 24 and August 9, 2021 and August 24, 2022, Infected Blood Inquiry, Adrian Goodyear, oral evidence, June 5 2019, and Adrian Goodyear, written evidence, WITN1243.

Dr Tuddenham knew tragedy . . . *et seq.* Author interviews with Professor Edward Tuddenham, August 6, 2021 and July 26, 2022.

Between 1970 and 1991 around 1,250 people . . . Infected Blood Inquiry, Expert Report to the Infected Blood Inquiry: Statistics.

'This looks like HTLV-III . . .' et seq. Author interviews with Joe, July 27, 2021 and July 7, 2022; author interviews with Frankie, July 20, 2021 and July 12, 2022, Infected Blood Inquiry, Mr AN, oral evidence, October 16, 2019, Frankie, oral evidence, October 16, 2019.

Bryan became obsessed with . . . *et seq. Bed of Lies, Telegraph* podcast and Infected Blood Inquiry, Clair, oral evidence, May 2, 2019, and written evidence, WITN159001.

It made Ade feel isolated . . . Infected Blood Inquiry, Adrian Goodyear, oral evidence, June 5, 2019.

Amanda Beesley was a member . . . Author interview with Amanda Beesley, July 7, 2022.

Staff felt ill-equipped . . . Infected Blood Inquiry, Presentation note on Treloar's, June 2021, INQY0000281.

Those who had avoided . . . *et seq.* Infected Blood Inquiry, Adrian Goodyear, written evidence, WITN1243, and Adrian Goodyear, oral evidence, June 5, 2019.

The infamous 'Monolith' advert . . . Health Departments of the United Kingdom, *AIDS: Monolith*, 1987, player.bfi.org.uk/free/film/watch-aids-monolith-1987-online.

In April 1987 Princess Diana . . . Rob Miller, 'I Met Princess Diana on One of Her AIDS Ward Visits – She Changed Everything,' *Metro*, August 31, 2022.

In the quiet of their dorm . . . *et seq.* Author interviews with Ade Goodyear, July 12, 2021 and August 24, 2022, and Infected Blood Inquiry, Adrian Goodyear, written evidence, WITN1243.

'uncomplainingly given up . . .' Aronstam, *Haemophilic Bleeding*.

'There are gloomier predictions . . .' et seq. Infected Blood Inquiry, Presentation about Treloar's, June 25, 2021.

couldn't escape the guilt . . . BBC TV South, November 1987, www.youtube.com/watch?v=1q6Y4PeNWeQ.

Colin Smith was . . . Infected Blood Inquiry, Janet Smith, written evidence, WITN1523001.

The pattern was repeated . . . World Federation of Hemophilia, 'Report on the Annual Global Survey 2020,' www1.wfh.org/publications/files/pdf-2045.pdf.

Richard Warwick had left . . . *et seq.* Author interviews with Richard Warwick, June 24, 2021 and April 4, 2023, and Infected Blood Inquiry, Richard Warwick, oral evidence, June 20, 2019.

cause patients to develop epilepsy . . . C. Kellinghaus et. al., 'Frequency of Seizures and Epilepsy in Neurological HIV-Infected Patients,' *Seizure*, vol. 17 (2008), 27–33.

Bryan was planning . . . *et seq.* Bed of Lies, *Telegraph* podcast, and Infected Blood Inquiry, Clair, oral evidence, May 2, 2019.

Bryan was being treated . . . 'The Story Behind the First AIDS Drug,' *Time*, March 19, 2017.

Chapter 6: Evasion

David Owen had been dreading . . . Infected Blood Inquiry, Lord David Owen's evidence to the Archer Inquiry.

On December 1, 1975, an investigative documentary . . . World In Action: Blood Money, ITV, 1 and December 8, 1975.

'It in no way requires . . .' cited in Weinberg and Shaw, *Blood on Their Hands*.

The World Health Organization advised . . . World Health Organization, 'Utilization and Supply of Human Blood and Blood Products,' May 28, 1975.

And a number of British doctors . . . In Cold Blood, ITV, September 27, 2020.

Solicitor Graham Ross . . . *et seq.* Author interview with Graham Ross, October 14, 2022, and Infected Blood Inquiry, Archer Inquiry Transcript, June 12, 2008.

Most came after a public outburst . . . *et seq.* Berridge, *AIDS in the UK*.

'the final outcome would be . . .' Letter from Graham Ross to David Watters, December 4, 1986, courtesy of Tainted Blood.

By June 1989 the lawyers . . . Author interview with Des Collins and Dani Holliday, April 12, 2023.

Dr Aronstam decided in early 1990 . . . Minutes of the nineteenth meeting of the AIDS group of Haemophilia Centre Directors, February 12, 1990, courtesy of Jason Evans.

Ade had a bleed in his elbow . . . *et seq.* Author interview with Ade Goodyear, 2023.

'gross maladministration' . . . *et seq.* Infected Blood Inquiry, Lord David Owen, oral evidence, September 22, 2020.

Only one memo . . . 'HIV Blood Disaster Papers "Were Pulped,"' *Telegraph*, July 12, 2007.

'Does it not follow . . .' Letter from David Owen to Sir Michael Buckley, March 22, 2002, courtesy of Carol Grayson.

'I feel personally responsible . . .' House of Commons Hansard Debates for November 23, 1989, vol. 272, publications.parliament.uk/pa/cm198990/cmhansrd/1989-11-23 /Debate-5.html.

'sympathetic response' might 'give rise . . .' Infected Blood Inquiry, Sir John Major, oral evidence, June 27, 2022.

the amount available per person . . . www.collinslaw.co.uk/contaminated--blood-timeline; Department of Health, 'Infected blood: reform of financial and other support,' https:// assets.publishing.service.gov.uk/government/uploads/system/uploads/attachment _data/file/494004/Infected_blood_cons_doc.pdf.

The case Graham Ross was building . . . et seq. Author interview with Graham Ross, October 14, 2022, and Infected Blood Inquiry, Archer Inquiry Transcript, June 12, 2008.

'Grave errors of judgement . . .' et seq. Clare Dyer, 'Justice Versus Equity for Haemophiliacs with AIDS,' *British Medical Journal*, vol. 301 (1990), 776.

One morning at the end of June 1990 . . . et seq. www.taintedblood.info/timeline/.

Thatcher thought the particulars . . . Author interview with Des Collins and Dani Holliday, April 12, 2023.

'no one's fault. . .' et seq. Dyer, 'Justice Versus Equity.'

'The Forgotten Victims . . .' Margarette Driscoll and John Davison, 'Haemophiliacs Demand End to Official Secrecy,' *Sunday Times*, August 5, 1990.

'I don't believe that the Health Service . . .' In Cold Blood, ITV, September 27, 2020.

By November 1990 over two hundred people . . . Celia Hall, 'Of the Infected Haemophiliacs 208 Have Already Developed AIDS and 130 Have Died', *Independent*, November 9, 1990.

'I will however make clear . . .' Cara McGoogan, 'Government "Pressured Infected Blood Scandal Victims to Accept Payout,"' *Telegraph*, May 18, 2022.

Pharmacist Brian Brierley . . . Infected Blood Inquiry, Sean Brierley, written evidence, WITN1104001.

Alcohol had become an anaesthetic . . . et seq. Author interviews with Joe, July 27, 2021 and July 7, 2022, author interviews with Frankie, July 20, 2021 and July 12, 2022, and Infected Blood Inquiry, Joe, written evidence, WITN1387001.

Nearly every person with hemophilia . . . Infected Blood Inquiry, Expert report to the Infected Blood Inquiry: Statistics.

The idea had come . . . et seq. Infected Blood Inquiry, Dr Andrzej Rejman, oral evidence, May 11, 2022.

Lawyers can ask witnesses . . . Author interview with Des Collins and Dani Holliday, April 12, 2023.

civil servant J. C. Dobson said . . . Paul Gallagher, 'Tainted Blood Scandal: Health Officials Thought Victims Would Win Court Case, Secret Memo Reveals,' *i News*, February 4, 2022.

Chapter 7: Survival

A similar tragedy to that . . . Krever Report, Part IV.

'deception over the quality of a product . . .' Starr, *Blood*.

Allain maintained . . . et seq. Author interview with Professor Jean-Pierre Allain, July 21, 2022.

The president of the hemophilia association encouraged . . . Starr, *Blood*.

They collected samples . . . Steve Connor, '"I am a scapegoat, I am innocent": Steve Connor Talks to the Cambridge Professor Facing Two Years in a French Jail for His Part in the Aids-in-Blood Case,' *Independent*, October 24, 1992.

Allain wasn't too . . . et seq. Author interview with Professor Jean-Pierre Allain, July 21, 2022.

The tensions worsened in late 1984 . . . Eric Favereau, 'Sang contaminé: Garretta et son magot insaisissables depuis dix-huit ans,' *Libération*, February 7, 2018.

Allain had watched . . . et seq. Author interview with Professor Jean-Pierre Allain, July 21, 2022, Starr, *Blood*, and Krever Report, Part IV.

'*must be used until . . .*' Sharon Waxman, 'Transfusion of Death,' *Washington Post*, May 29, 1993.

Allain told Anne-Marie . . . et seq. Author interview with Professor Jean-Pierre Allain, July 21, 2022.

At the end of 1991 . . . Krever Report, Part IV.

Although he believed . . . Author interview with Professor Jean-Pierre Allain, July 21, 2022.

Former Treloar's pupil Stephen . . . et seq. Author interview with Gary Webster, July 14, 2022.

The trial of the French doctors . . . Krever Report, Part IV.

Allain started to lose faith . . . Author interview with Professor Jean-Pierre Allain, July 21, 2022.

sometimes shouting 'Assassins! . . .' Starr, *Blood*.

Allain was compared to Josef Mengele . . . Ibid.

'*I don't have to come anymore, . . .*' *et seq.* Author interview with Professor Jean-Pierre Allain, July 21, 2022.

'*The deliberate nature of the actions . . .*' *et seq.* Krever Report, Part IV.

Dr Roux . . . Dr Netter . . . Diana Brahams, 'Trial and Tribulations of J-P Allain,' *The Lancet*, July 24, 1993.

Allain lodged an appeal . . . Author interview with Professor Jean-Pierre Allain, July 21, 2022.

'*My conscience is completely clear . . .*' Sharon Waxman, 'French Officials Sentenced in AIDS Case,' *Washington Post*, October 24, 1992.

In one protest in March 1992 . . . Waxman, 'Transfusion of Death.'

It was with great sadness . . . Dr Ian Peake, 'Professor Arthur Bloom: A Tribute,' published online, since removed.

Dr Tuddenham believed . . . et seq. Author interviews with Professor Edward Tuddenham, August 6, 2021 and July 26, 2022.

'*He and Dr Peter Jones . . .*' Author interview with Professor Likat Parapia, July 21, 2021 and April 24, 2023.

Ade lost friend after friend . . . et seq. Author interviews with Ade Goodyear, June 24 and August 9, 2021, July 12 and August 24, 2022, and Infected Blood Inquiry, Adrian Goodyear, written evidence, WITN1243.

Librarian Suresh Vaghela . . . Infected Blood Inquiry, Suresh Vaghela, written evidence, WITN1577001.

sixty-five pairs of brothers . . . House of Commons Hansard Debates for June 27, 1991, vol. 193, https://hansard.parliament.uk/Commons/1991-06-27/debates/ea7e5b6f-d609 -4cf1-a5e9-35f4a354dbe5/BloodTransfusions(Hiv).

John Peach lost his two sons . . . Infected Blood Inquiry, John Peach, written evidence, WITN3896001.

six families in which three brothers . . . Author interview with Tony Farrugia, April 4, 2023, and Infected Blood Inquiry, A. V. Farrugia, written evidence, WITN1218001.

Lee Turton in Cornwall . . . Infected Blood Inquiry, Denise Turton, written evidence, WITN157500.

Lauren Palmer became an orphan . . . Lauren Palmer, 'My Parents Died in the Infected Blood Scandal, but I Won't Get a Penny in Compensation,' *Telegraph*, August 8, 2022.

Gary Cornes was the first . . . et seq. Infected Blood Inquiry, John Cornes, oral evidence, June 11, 2019.

Gary Webster went on a mission . . . Author interview with Gary Webster, July 14, 2022.

Meanwhile, Joe and Frankie . . . et seq. Author interviews with Joe, July 27, 2021 and July 7, 2022, and Frankie, July 20, 2021 and July 12, 2022.

Chapter 8: Mother's Curse

Karen Cross refused . . . et seq. Author interview with Gary and Karen Cross, November 1, 2022, and Gary Cross, *Vial 023: A Father's Pursuit of Justice* (Kudu Publishing, 2012).

The legal practice Mull & Mull . . . et seq. Author interviews with Tom and Lorraine Mull, July 12, 2021, October 29, 2022 and April 5, 2023.

One boy in particular . . . https://ryanwhite.hrsa.gov/about/ryan-white and https://ryanwhite.hrsa.gov/livinghistory/.

On May 21, 1991 . . . Court Listener, *Cross v. Cutter Biological,* www.courtlistener.com /opinion/1720316/cross-v-cutter-biological-div-of-miles-inc/.

the number of those infected . . . Institute of Medicine, *HIV and the Blood Supply: An Analysis of Crisis Decisionmaking* (National Academies Press, 1995).

Corey, a radio host in Los Angeles . . . 'Corey S. Dubin: 1955–2017,' *Santa Barbara Independent,* February 2, 2017.

Dana contracted HIV . . . Author interview with Dana Kuhn, November 18, 2023.

Tom and Lorraine made . . . Author interviews with Tom and Lorraine Mull, July 12, 2021, October 29, 2022 and April 5, 2023, and Cross, *Vial 023.*

Dr Thomas Drees had been the president . . . et seq. Dr Thomas Drees trial testimony, *Gary Cross et al. v. Cutter Biological et al.,* October 12, 1993, trial transcript courtesy of Tom and Lorraine Mull.

thousands of prisoners of war were experimented on . . . Justin McCurry, 'Japanese Veteran Admits Vivisection Tests on PoWs,' *Guardian,* November 27, 2006.

Dr Drees believed . . . et seq. Dr Thomas Drees depositions, May 23 and August 29, 1990, April 11 and November 20, 1991, courtesy of Tom and Lorraine Mull.

That month, the CDC also advised . . . www.cdc.gov/mmwr/preview/mmwrhtml /00001183.htm.

'How many people have to die? . . .' Randy Shilts, *And the Band Played On* (Souvenir Press, 2011).

He believed they had been reckless . . . et seq. Dr Don Francis deposition, August 3, 1993, courtesy of Tom and Lorraine Mull.

He wrote a letter to all parties . . . et seq. Dr Don Francis memo, January 6, 1983, courtesy of Tom and Lorraine Mull.

eight cases had so far . . . Court Listener, *Cross v. Cutter Biological.*

Most patients were never told . . . Congressional Record, vol. 140, no. 36 (March 25, 1994), www.govinfo.gov/content/pkg/CREC-1994-03-25/html/CREC-1994-03-25-pt1 -PgH104.htm.

Dr Francis now told the lawyers . . . et seq. Dr Don Francis deposition, August 3, 1993, courtesy of Tom and Lorraine Mull.

Dr Francis maintained this view . . . Global Health Chronicles, 'The Early Years of AIDS: CDC's Response to a Historic Epidemic,' www.globalhealthchronicles.org/items /show/6874, and CPAC, 'Pillars of Democracy: Tainted Blood – Dr Don Francis,' www.youtube.com/watch?v=yTV333zzV1Y.

The film was rough and gritty . . . et seq. Author interviews with Tom and Lorraine Mull, July 12, 2021, and Michael Baum, August 12, 2021.

Another whistleblower from Alpha . . . Author interview with Dr Jeanne Kay Noel, September 2, 2021.

fourteen workers in one . . . J. S. Taylor et al., 'Hepatitis B in Plasma Fractionation Workers,' *Journal of the American Medical Association*, vol. 230, no. 6 (1974), 850–53.

Dana Kuhn, one of Tom and Lorraine's clients . . . et seq. Author interview with Dana Kuhn, November 18, 2023, and Dana Kuhn, 'The Trail of AIDS in the Hemophilia Community,' unpublished manuscript, September 9, 1994, shared with the author.

Ricky had been diagnosed . . . Fox News, 'The Ray Brothers: Kelly Ring Talks with Florida Family Years After Children's Deaths from AIDS,' www.fox13news.com/news/the-ray-brothers-florida-family-recalls-childrens-aids-deaths-after-transfusions.

By 1992 Brad Cross . . . et seq. Author interview with Gary and Karen Cross, November 1, 2022, and Cross, *Vial 023.*

'They slowly waste away . . .' Author interview with Tom and Lorraine Mull, July 12, 2021.

At that point, at least eleven . . . Weinberg and Shaw, *Blood on Their Hands.*

Over a thousand cases . . . Krever Report, Part IV.

The National Hemophilia Foundation warned . . . National Hemophilia Foundation, 'AIDS update,' Hemophilia Information Exchange, no. 83, May 24, 1989, courtesy of Tom and Lorraine Mull.

Lorraine still believed the facts . . . Author interviews with Tom and Lorraine Mull, July 12, 2021, October 29, 2022 and April 5, 2023.

Gary secured their trial . . . et seq. Author interview with Gary and Karen Cross, November 1, 2022.

'I grew up with all these . . .' Author interview with Jennifer Cross, April 10, 2023.

Tom and Lorraine's case . . . et seq. Cross v. Cutter trial transcript, courtesy of Tom and Lorraine Mull.

'This was a tragedy . . .' Starr, *Blood.*

But Cutter's lawyers said . . . Court Listener, *Cross v. Cutter Biological.*

accuse them of 'contributory negligence' . . . Cross, *Vial 023.*

Dr Aledort had been a hero . . . et seq. Michael McLeod, 'Bad Blood: Every Day a Hemophiliac Dies of AIDS. It Didn't Have to Happen,' *Orlando Sentinel*, December 19, 1993.

was on a 'shame list' . . . Author interview with Gary and Karen Cross, November 1, 2022.

Dr Rosenberg from California . . . Starr, *Blood.*

the doctor had earnt hundreds of thousands . . . Ken Dixon v. Alpha, Armour, Cutter, Baxter, Tulane Educational Fund, Tulane School of Medicine, and Dr Abe Andes, February 3, 1999, trial transcript courtesy of Tom and Lorraine Mull hereafter Dixon trial.

In the trial, Dr Aledort testified . . . et seq. Court Listener, *Cross v. Cutter Biological.*

Chapter 9: Poisoned Lines

'We were supplying the world with plasma' . . . Author interview with Douglas Starr, September 14, 2021, and Starr, *Blood.*

As the AIDS crisis developed . . . Weinberg and Shaw, *Blood on Their Hands.*

'It was a giant money-making industry,' . . . et seq. Author interviews with Tom Mull, July 12, 2021, October 29, 2022 and April 5, 2023.

Plasma donation was popular among the inmates . . . et seq. Prison Insight, 'Louisiana State Penitentiary,' https://prisoninsight.com/correctional-facilities/state/louisiana/louisiana

-state-penitentiary/, and ACLU, 'Captive Labor: Exploitation of Incarcerated Workers,' www.aclu.org/report/captive-labor-exploitation-incarcerated-workers.

'Dear Sir,' wrote David Grillette . . . et seq. Letter from David Grillette to Tom Mull, January 12, 1997, courtesy of Jennifer Cross.

'I'm writing on behalf of . . .' et seq. Letter from Richard Vincent to Tom Mull, February 15, 1998, courtesy of Tom and Lorraine Mull.

The center was in a concrete building . . . Weinberg and Shaw, *Blood on Their Hands.*

Richard went through the rigmarole . . . Richard Vincent deposition, August 4, 1998, courtesy of Jennifer Cross.

For this work, they were . . . Sophia Chase, 'The Bloody Truth: Examining America's Blood Industry and its Tort,' *William & Mary Business Law Review*, vol. 3, no. 2 (2012).

The process was uncomfortable . . . Author interview with Douglas Starr, September 14, 2021.

'It wasn't nothing to see . . .' Richard Vincent deposition, August 4, 1998, courtesy of Tom and Lorraine Mull.

'honeymoon suite' . . . Weinberg and Shaw, *Blood on Their Hands.*

Tom quizzed the guards . . . et seq. Author interviews with Tom and Lorraine Mull, October 29, 2022 and April 5, 2023, Richard Vincent deposition, August 4, 1998, courtesy of Tom and Lorraine Mull.

Louisiana Biologics, which turned over . . . Weinberg and Shaw, *Blood on Their Hands*, and Chase, 'The Bloody Truth.'

There were FDA-licensed plasma centers . . . Krever Report, 'The Risk in Factor Concentrates.'

Bayer's Cutter paid the state . . . Court document from August 3, 1998, courtesy of Tom and Lorraine Mull.

In Arkansas, a blood banking company . . . Encyclopedia of Arkansas, 'Arkansas Prison Blood Scandal,' https://encyclopediaofarkansas.net/entries/arkansas-prison-blood-scandal-3732/.

In 1995, the FDA formally recommended . . . Weinberg and Shaw, *Blood on Their Hands.*

In France, where blood . . . Sharon Waxman, 'Transfusion of Death.'

As Tom learnt more . . . et seq. Author interviews with Tom and Lorraine Mull, July 12, 2021, October 29, 2022 and April 5, 2023, and Cross, *Vial 023.*

Life expectancy for people with hemophilia . . . Terence L. Chorba et al., 'Effects of HIV Infection on Age and Cause of Death for Persons with Hemophilia A in the United States,' *American Journal of Hematology*, 66 (2001), 229–40.

Mull & Mull was being held together . . . Author interviews with Tom and Lorraine Mull, July 12, 2021, October 29, 2022 and April 5, 2023.

Michael Baum might have won . . . et seq. Author interview with Michael Baum, August 12, 2021.

Court documents had shown . . . Weinberg and Shaw, *Blood on Their Hands.*

'We need a few good arms! . . .' et seq. Advertisements in various magazines, www.wisnerbaum.com/documents/hemophilia/exhibits/Exhibit-10-FNC.pdf.

an internal Cutter letter . . . Memo from John Hink to Lee Hershberger, August 30, 1982, www.wisnerbaum.com/documents/hemophilia/exhibits/Exhibit-8-FNC.pdf.

In another internal memo . . . Memo from Steven Ojala to Cutter employees, December 21, 1982, www.wisnerbaum.com/documents/hemophilia/exhibits/Exhibit-9-FNC.pdf.

'strong evidence to suggest . . .' Cutter letter to warden of Arizona State Prison, January 19, 1983, www.wisnerbaum.com/documents/hemophilia/exhibits/Exhibit-11-FNC.pdf.

By March, Cutter had paused . . . Letter from John Hink, March 3, 1983, courtesy of Tom and Lorraine Mull.

'That was the big "Aha!" moment . . .' Author interview with Tom and Lorraine Mull, July 12, 2021.

Dr Kay Noel struggled to remember . . . et seq. Author interview with Dr Jeanne Kay Noel, September 2, 2021, and Dr Jeanne Kay Noel deposition, August 12, 1998, courtesy of Tom and Lorraine Mull.

From the mid-1970s, hemophilia doctors . . . Leonard B. Seeff, 'The History of the "Natural History" of Hepatitis C (1968–2009),' *Liver International*, vol. 29, no. s1 (2009).

In New Jersey, a lawyer . . . et seq. Weinberg and Shaw, *Blood on Their Hands*.

Captain Emanuel Rappaport from the US Army . . . Emanuel M. Rappaport, 'Hepatitis Following Blood or Plasma Transfusions: Observations in Thirty-Three Cases,' *Journal of the American Medical Association*, vol. 128, no. 13 (1945), 932–39.

'deeply concerned . . .' Letter from Sam T. Gibson to John W. Palmer, July 19, 1968, courtesy of Donna Shaw.

'We do not understand the concern . . .' Letter from John W. Palmer to Sam T. Gibson, July 23, 1968, courtesy of Donna Shaw.

Dr Joseph Garrott Allen . . . McLeod, 'Bad Blood.'

Dr Shanbrom wrote to the higher-ups . . . et seq. Weinberg and Shaw, *Blood on Their Hands*, and Institute of Medicine, *HIV and the Blood Supply*.

In 1972 Cutter ran heat . . . Research by Dr Frank Putnam for legal case, courtesy of Tom and Lorraine Mull.

Within four months, Dr Charles Heldebrant . . . Dr Charles Heldebrant deposition, June 1, 1993, courtesy of Tom and Lorraine Mull.

Bayer waged a campaign against it . . . Wisner Baum, 'Background Plaintiffs Position,' www.wisnerbaum.com/hemophilia-aids/background-plaintiffs-position.

'AIDS has become the center . . .' Letter from Merrill T. Boyce to Rainer Froitzheim, June 6, 1983, www.wisnerbaum.com/documents/hemophilia/exhibits/Exhibit-64-FNC.pdf, and Walt Bogdanich and Eric Koli, '2 Paths of Bayer Drug in 80's: Riskier One Steered Overseas,' *New York Times*, May 22, 2003.

It continued to manufacture . . . Letter from Steven Ojala to Dr Elaine Esber, August 9,1985, https://www.wisnerbaum.com/documents/hemophilia/exhibits/Exhibit-18-FNC.pdf.

some forty thousand people . . . Starr, *Blood*.

In autumn 1984 the CDC . . . et seq. Krever Report, Part IV.

Rather than revoking the four . . . David Kessler, FDA commissioner, testified in 1993 that it had erred in its relationship which was 'emblematic of our collegial approach to regulated industry at that time. Those days are behind us.'

'did not want any attention . . .' et seq. Memo from Steven Ojala to Cutter employees, May 30, 1985, www.wisnerbaum.com/documents/hemophilia/exhibits/Exhibit-25-FNC.pdf.

The companies conceded . . . Letter from Steven Ojala to Dr Elaine Esber, August 9, 1985, www.wisnerbaum.com/documents/hemophilia/exhibits/Exhibit-18-FNC.pdf.

Professor Jean-Pierre Allain is on one side . . . Author interview with Professor Jean-Pierre Allain, July 21, 2022.

But Dr Francis from the CDC . . . Dr Don Francis deposition, August 3, 1993, courtesy of Tom and Lorraine Mull.

As lawyer Eric Weinberg developed . . . et seq. Weinberg and Shaw, *Blood on Their Hands*.

'The issue is not one of regulation . . .' et seq. Minutes of the 7th meeting of the Recombinant DNA Steering Committee at Revlon Healthcare, October 15, 1985, courtesy of Donna Shaw.

In the years Donna Shaw reported . . . Author interview with Donna Shaw, June 14, 2021.

Douglas Starr interviewed . . . Author interview with Douglas Starr, September 14, 2021.

'It was clear to anyone . . .' *Congressional Record*, vol. 140, no. 36 (March 25, 1994).

'They were very cold . . .' *et seq.* Author interviews with Dr Jeanne Kay Noel, September 2, 2021 and May 3, 2023.

Chapter 10: The Trial

Allain's fellow inmates fascinated . . . *et seq.* Author interview with Professor Jean-Pierre Allain, July 21, 2022.

'The Outside observer . . .' Brahams, 'Trial and Tribulations of J-P Allain.'

Fifteen hundred doctors and researchers . . . Alan Riding, 'Scandal Over Tainted Blood Widens in France,' *New York Times*, February 13, 1994.

more than three hundred people . . . David Crary, 'Health Experts Urge Pardon for Defendants in French AIDS Scandal,' AP News, January 19, 1994.

'The circumstances of this case . . .' *et seq.* Steve Connor, 'HIV Blood Professor Was Paid in Jail,' *Independent*, November 2, 1994, and Paul Webster and Chris Mihill, 'HIV Blood Doctor Begins Jail Term,' *Guardian*, July 14, 1993.

The ministers were accused . . . Krever Report, Part IV.

Abbott Laboratories had applied . . . Riding, 'Scandal Over Tainted Blood Widens.'

'Young physicians are reluctant . . .' 'Haemophilia: Recent History of Clinical Management,' Wellcome Institute for the History of Medicine, London, on February 10, 1998, https://discovery.ucl.ac.uk/id/eprint/2076/1/wit4.pdf.

'He was really taken to the cleaners . . .' Author interview with Professor Edward Tuddenham, July 26, 2022.

Allain's phone rang . . . *et seq.* Author interviews with Professor Jean-Pierre Allain and Dr Helen Lee, July 21, 2022.

Dr Garretta, finding his reputation . . . Starr, *Blood* and Eric Favereau, 'Sang contaminé.'

Dufoix had given a statement . . . www.bfmtv.com/politique/le-sang-contamine-chemin-de-croix-de-laurent-fabius_AN-202008180001.html.

'hurl the industry into bankruptcy . . .' Author interview with Tom Mull, April 4, 2023.

they would pay $640 million . . . Krever Report, Part IV.

'I knew they were plumb guilty . . .' Author interview with Dana Kuhn, January 23, 2023.

At the end of a day's campaigning . . . Author interview with Gary and Karen Cross, November 1, 2022.

'The federal government did not . . .' Weinberg and Shaw, *Blood on Their Hands.*

Congress would provide compassionate payments . . . Federal Register, Ricky Ray Hemophilia Relief Fund Program, www.federalregister.gov/documents/2000/05/31/00-13418/ricky-ray-hemophilia-relief-fund-program.

By then, more than . . . Dr Bruce Evatt et al., 'Effects of HIV Infection on Age and Cause of Death for Persons with Haemophilia A in the United States,' *American Journal of Hematology*, vol. 66 (2001), 229–40.

Leo Dixon had taken . . . *et seq.* Author interview with Leo Dixon, January 27, 2023, and Cross, *Vial 023.*

In Missouri, a jury . . . Weinberg and Shaw, *Blood on Their Hands.*

'This is a vial of Factor VIII . . .' *et seq. Dixon trial*, November 4, 1998.

one of his star witnesses . . . Author interview with Dr Jeanne Kay Noel, September 2, 2021.

The continuous objections . . . et seq. Author interviews with Tom and Lorraine Mull, July 12, 2021 and April 4, 2023, Gary and Karen Cross, November 1, 2022, and Michael Baum, August 12, 2021.

As Tom questioned Dr Aledort . . . Author interview with Leo Dixon, January 27, 2023.

'I took care of these people . . .' et seq. Dixon trial, February 3, 1999.

'No, I don't think that would . . .' Dixon trial, January 15, 1999.

Michael revealed the thousands . . . Dixon trial, March 9, 1999.

Tom was utterly exasperated . . . Author interview with Tom and Lorraine Mull, April 4, 2023.

Gary Cross could at last . . . et seq. Author interviews with Gary and Karen Cross, November 2022, Tom and Lorraine Mull, July 12, 2021 and April 4, 2023, and Dana Kuhn, January 23, 2023, Gary and Karen Cross, November 1, 2022, Cross, *Vial 023.*

Michael Baum had time to decompress . . . et seq. Author interview with Michael Baum, August 12, 2021.

Bayer said it would not . . . Cutter, Far East marketing memo, 1984, www.wisnerbaum.com /documents/hemophilia/exhibits/Exhibit-22-FNC.pdf.

The marketing team said the 'luster' . . . Cutter, Far East Region marketing memo, 1985, www.wisnerbaum.com/documents/hemophilia/exhibits/Exhibit-23-FNC.pdf.

Bayer later said it didn't . . . et seq. Bogdanich and Koli, '2 Paths of Bayer Drug in 80's.'

Bayer's marketing manager for . . . et seq. Telex from Cutter to Hong Kong supplier, May 6, 1985, www.wisnerbaum.com/documents/hemophilia/exhibits/Exhibit-24-FNC.pdf.

'expect to sell substantial quantities . . .' et seq. Bogdanich and Koli, '2 Paths of Bayer Drug in 80's,' and Telex from Cutter to Taiwan supplier, September 20, 1985, www.wisnerbaum .com/documents/hemophilia/exhibits/Exhibit-32-FNC.pdf.

The hemophilia population was . . . et seq. World Federation of Hemophilia, 'Report on the Annual Global Survey 2020,' and Krever Report, Part IV.

Canada's response was comprehensive . . . Krever Report, Part I: 'Introduction.'

survivors pushed for a public inquiry . . . Weinberg and Shaw, *Blood on Their Hands.*

'an important tenet in the philosophy . . .' Kumanan Wilson, 'The Krever Commission – 10 Years Later,' *Canadian Medical Association Journal,* vol. 177, no. 11 (2007), 1387–89.

'There was no conduct that showed . . .' Cameron French, 'Doctors Acquitted in Canada Tainted-Blood Trial,' Reuters, October 2, 2007.

Germany's pharma laws . . . Krever Report, Part IV.

'Each day I can watch . . .' et seq. Starr, *Blood.*

Japanese government agreed to settle . . . Kevin Sullivan and Mary Jordan, 'Japan to Compensate for Tainted Blood,' *Washington Post,* March 16, 1996.

'Lives were at stake!' . . . et seq. Starr, *Blood.*

Saddam Hussein's regime in Iraq . . . Paul von Zielbauer, 'Bad Blood: HIV-Infected Iraqi Survivors File Suit,' – *New York Times,* September 4, 2006.

In 2003 some three hundred . . . Author interviews with Joe, July 27, 2021 and July 7, 2022, and Frankie, July 20, 2021 and July 12, 2022.

Chapter 11: 'We Accuse'

Joe was standing outside . . . et seq. Author interviews with Joe, July 27, 2021 and July 7, 2022.

In 1993 an angry faction . . . Infected Blood Inquiry, Paul Thomas Bullen, written evidence, WITN3114004.

In Newcastle, one group . . . et seq. Infected Blood Inquiry, Carol Grayson, oral evidence, June 8, 2022, and Carol Grayson, written evidence, WITN1055001.

Many had similar experiences . . . Infected Blood Inquiry, Susan Douglas, oral evidence, September 15, 2022.

In a letter from 11 January 1983 . . . Letter from Professor Arthur Bloom and Dr Charles Rizza to hemophilia center directors, January 11, 1983, courtesy of Tainted Blood. The letter is dated 1982 but is possibly misdated, in the opinion of the Infected Blood Inquiry.

Peter and Carol went to the police . . . et seq. Infected Blood Inquiry, Carol Grayson, oral evidence, June 8, 2022, and Carol Grayson written evidence, WITN1055004.

'the worst treatment disaster . . .' House of Lords Hansard Debates for April 23, 2009, vol. 709, https://hansard.parliament.uk/lords/2009-04-23/debates/09042350000686/HealthContaminatedBloodProducts.

'The government does not accept . . .' Infected Blood Inquiry, Carol Grayson, oral evidence, June 8, 2022.

'preoccupied with preventing . . .' Kamran Abbasi, 'BSE Inquiry Plays Down Errors,' *British Medical Journal*, vol. 321 (2000).

'I am now satisfied . . .' et seq. Letter from David Owen to Sir Michael Buckley, March 22, 2002, courtesy of Carol Grayson.

Lord Owen hoped that . . . James Meikle, 'Owen Demands Inquiry into Infected Blood Scandal,' *Guardian*, August 19, 2002.

Unfortunately, none of the key . . . et seq. Infected Blood Inquiry, Lord David Owen, oral evidence, September 22, 2020.

the most senior civil servant . . . et seq. Infected Blood Inquiry, Lord Nigel Crisp, written evidence, WITN3996001.

'There are many of us who think . . .' *Panorama*, 'Contaminated Blood: The Search for the Truth,' BBC TV, July 13, 2017.

The Skipton Fund would pay . . . Infected Blood Inquiry, Presentation note on the Skipton Fund (2003–2017), March 22, 2021, INQY0000245.

It cost around 10 cents . . . Author interview with Professor Edward Tuddenham, May 28, 2023.

After a five-year battle . . . James Meikle, 'Victory for Haemophilia Patients,' *Guardian*, February 13, 2003.

'For some of us, it has literally . . .' *Bed of Lies*, *Telegraph* podcast.

'The government of the day . . .' 'Widow Is to Learn How Husband Got Killer Transfusion,' *Evening Chronicle*, December 22, 2005.

Clair wanted to move . . . et seq. *Bed of Lies*, *Telegraph* podcast, McGoogan, 'The Tainted Blood Scandal,' and Infected Blood Inquiry, Clair, oral evidence, May 2, 2019, and Clair, written evidence, WITN1589001.

'It is irritating that somebody . . .' et seq. Infected Blood Inquiry, Peter Stevens, oral evidence, February 24, 2021.

The manifesto opened . . . et seq. Tainted Blood, 'Accusations Document,' https://archercbbp.files.wordpress.com/2017/03/taintedbloodaccuse.pdf.

Chapter 12: Breakthrough

Andy Burnham was in the garden . . . et seq. Author interview with Andy Burnham, January 31, 2023; Infected Blood Inquiry, Andy Burnham, oral evidence, July 15, 2022, and Andy Burnham, written evidence, WITN7060001.

'a horrific human tragedy' . . . et seq. Lord Peter Archer of Sandwell, Archer Inquiry, https://archercbbp.wordpress.com/.

The government would double . . . House of Commons Hansard Debates for July 1, 2007, Archer Inquiry, https://hansard.parliament.uk/Commons/2009-07-01/debates /09070156000004/ArcherInquiry.

One of the protestors was David Tonkin . . . Infected Blood Inquiry, David Tonkin, written evidence, WITN1567008.

'There is no evidence that individuals . . .' Infected Blood Inquiry, Andy Burnham, oral evidence, July 15, 2022.

Fred had cirrhosis of the liver . . . House of Commons Hansard Debates for October 14, 2010, Contaminated Blood and Blood Products, https://hansard.parliament.uk/commons /2010-10-14/debates/10101429000001/ContaminatedBloodAndBloodProducts.

'has been, and remains, infected by error . . .' England and Wales High Court Decisions, Andrew March and the Secretary of State for Health, April 16, 2010, www.bailii.org/ ew/cases/EWHC/Admin/2010/765.html.

Scotland's deputy first minister Nicola Sturgeon . . . et seq. Penrose Inquiry, Final report, and STV Regional News, 'The Penrose Inquiry,' March 25, 2015, www.youtube.com /watch?v=eont3tS-raY.

From 2019 to 2023, 110 people . . . Infected Blood Inquiry, Beatrice Morgan, oral evidence, January 31, 2023.

people stood up and shouted 'whitewash'. . . Sandra Dick, 'Report Burned Amid Blood Probe "Whitewash,"' *Edinburgh News*, March 25, 2015.

'It is difficult to imagine . . .' 'Britain's Cameron Apologizes Over Infected Blood in 70s, 80s,' Reuters, March 25, 2015.

'They have just been biding . . .' Author interview with Richard Warwick, June 24, 2021.

Jason was a twenty-six-year-old . . . et seq. Multiple author interviews with Jason Evans, 2021, 2022 and 2023, and Infected Blood Inquiry, Jason Evans, written evidence, WITN1210001.

a government memo from 1987 . . . Department of Health memo, 'Use of Factor VIII by Haemophiliacs,' October 20, 1987, courtesy of Jason Evans.

That week, his research was printed . . . Caroline Wheeler, 'Fresh "Cover-Up" Evidence Found in Contaminated Blood Scandal,' *Express*, May 28, 2017.

'147 will die . . .' Department of Health memo, February 1991, courtesy of Jason Evans.

'It is difficult to see what more . . .' House of Commons Hansard Debates for November 24, 2016, Contaminated Blood and Blood Products, https://hansard.parliament.uk /commons/2016-11-24/debates/9369C591-D01B-4479-B78A-E74243142B88 /ContaminatedBloodAndBloodProducts.

When Des Collins agreed . . . et seq. Author interview with Des Collins, July 5, 2021.

'NHS Tainted Blood Shame . . .' et seq. Ben Spencer, Richard Marsden and Xantha Leatham, 'NHS Tainted Blood Shame,' *Daily Mail*, July 3, 2017.

Andy Burnham was preparing . . . Author interview with Andy Burnham, January 31, 2023, and Hansard, Contaminated Blood debate, https://hansard.parliament.uk/commons/2017 -04-25/debates/3AE7573D-7990-4A16-B375-A1AB786F90AE/ContaminatedBlood.

Chapter 13: Inquiry

at least 1,553 people . . . Infected Blood Inquiry, Expert report to the Infected Blood Inquiry: Statistics.

He wanted to convey as much . . . et seq. Infected Blood Inquiry, Derek Martindale, Carole Hill, Perry Evans, oral evidence, April 30, 2019.

Clair's turn to take the stand . . . et seq. McGoogan, 'The Tainted Blood Scandal,' and *Bed of Lies, Telegraph* podcast.

On Frankie's day to give evidence . . . Author interview with Frankie, July 20, 2021, and Infected Blood Inquiry, Frankie, oral evidence, October 16, 2019.

Joe relived some of the worst . . . Author interview with Joe, July 27, 2021.

On a Friday afternoon in late June . . . et seq. Infected Blood Inquiry, Presentation about Treloar's, June 25, 2021.

Treloar's formed a key part . . . Infected Blood Inquiry, Presentation note on Treloar's, June 2021, INQY0000281.

'There was nothing consensual . . .' Infected Blood Inquiry, Nicholas Sainsbury, John Peach, Gary Bennett, oral evidence, June 22, 2021.

A mother whose son died . . . Infected Blood Inquiry, Sheila Squires, written evidence, September 30, 2020.

Gary Webster had requested . . . Author interview with Gary Webster, July 14, 2022.

Dr Kirk's research didn't stop there . . . Infected Blood Inquiry, Presentation note on Treloar's, June 2021, INQY0000281.

About the 'close investigation' . . . Infected Blood Inquiry, Letter from William d'Auvergne Maycock to Dr John Craske, February 20, 1978, BPLL0002271_002.

'It seems likely that . . .' Dr John Craske, 'The Epidemiology of Factor VIII and IX Associated Hepatitis in the UK,' presentation at a symposium in Glasgow, September 1980, courtesy of Jason Evans.

'The British market will accept . . .' Infected Blood Inquiry, Presentations on the licensing of blood products and pharmaceutical companies involved in blood products: Hyland, Travenol and Immuno, September 23, 2021.

'We'll monitor you . . .' Infected Blood Inquiry, Clair, oral evidence, May 2, 2019.

At Treloar's, prophylaxis . . . et seq. Infected Blood Inquiry, Presentation note on Treloar's, June 2021, INQY0000281.

Gary sued Treloar's for negligence . . . At the time of writing, their court case had been postponed until after the inquiry reported. Also pending until after Sir Brian's report was the original claim against the Department of Health for misfeasance in public office.

Dr Liakat Parapia was certain . . . et seq. Author interviews with Dr Liakat Parapia, July 21, 2021 and April 24, 2023.

'embarrassingly large supply' . . . Infected Blood Inquiry, Dr Huw Lloyd, oral evidence, February 8, 2022.

Three-quarters of Dr Jones's patients . . . Berridge, *AIDS in the UK.*

Alder Hey had continued . . . Infected Blood Inquiry, Panel about the experiences of parents whose children were infected at Alder Hey Children's Hospital, September 29, 2022.

Day after day, doctors . . . et seq. Infected Blood Inquiry, Steven Snowden KC and Andrew Bragg, oral evidence, January 17, 2023.

Professor Tuddenham was willing . . . Author interview with Professor Edward Tuddenham, August 6, 2021, and Infected Blood Inquiry, Professor Edward Tuddenham, oral evidence, October 22, 2020.

The proportion of people . . . Infected Blood Inquiry, Expert report to the Infected Blood Inquiry: Statistics.

Birchgrove member Alan Burgess . . . Author interview with Alan Burgess, July 27, 2021.

Lord Fowler told Sir Brian . . . Haroon Siddique, 'Norman Fowler: Contaminated Blood Compensation Was Doomed to Failure,' *Guardian*, September 22, 2021.

Lord Clarke quickly made it clear . . . et seq. Infected Blood Inquiry, Lord Kenneth Clarke, oral evidence, July 27, 2021 and July 29, 2021.

said he had lacked the full picture . . . Infected Blood Inquiry, Lord John Patten, oral evidence, May 20, 2022.

'go away and stop rocking the boat . . . ' Infected Blood Inquiry, Professor Richard Tedder, oral evidence, October 13, 2022.

'It sounds most unlike me' . . . Infected Blood Inquiry, Dr Diana Walford, oral evidence (continued), July 20, 2021.

'extremely seriously and diligently' . . . Infected Blood Inquiry, Lord Simon Glenarthur, oral evidence (continued), July 23, 2021.

'What had happened was incredibly bad luck' . . . Infected Blood Inquiry, Sir John Major, oral evidence, June 27, 2022.

'We should be humble enough . . .' Infected Blood Inquiry, Lord David Owen, oral evidence, September 22, 2020.

'the depressingly familiar pattern . . .' et seq. Author interview with Andy Burnham, January 31, 2023, and Infected Blood Inquiry, Andy Burnham, oral evidence, July 15, 2022.

his constituent Mike Dorricott . . . et seq. Infected Blood Inquiry, Jeremy Hunt, written evidence, WITN3499001, and Jeremy Hunt, oral evidence, July 27, 2022.

payments of no less than £100,000 . . . Author interview with Des Collins, July 5, 2021, Haroon Siddique, 'Infected Blood Scandal Payments Could Run into Billions, Report Suggests,' *Guardian*, June 7, 2022. At the time of writing, the compensation process was yet to begin.

'My conclusion is that wrongs were done . . .' Infected Blood Inquiry, Sir Brian Langstaff interim compensation report.

Richard ruminated about moving . . . Author interview with Richard Warwick, December 2, 2022.

'morally, ethically and criminally wrong' . . . et seq. Infected Blood Inquiry, Submission of Milners, December 16, 2022, SUBS0000055.

'This was a brutal, unacceptable . . .' Infected Blood Inquiry, Steven Snowden KC and Andrew Bragg, oral evidence, January 17, 2023.

upwards of £100 million by March 2022 . . . Infected Blood Inquiry Finance Report, April 2021 to March 2022.

Richards outlined the issues . . . et seq. Infected Blood Inquiry, Sam Stein KC and Jenni Richards KC, oral evidence, February 3, 2023.

Chapter 14: Living

Clair was in the garden . . . Bed of Lies, *Telegraph* podcast.

Jason saw one of those . . . Author interview with Jason Evans, April 13, 2023.

'The villains in this story . . .' et seq. Author interview with Des Collins, July 5, 2021.

'I'm very proud of the fact . . .' Infected Blood Inquiry, Christopher Bishop, oral evidence November 4, 2021.

Today, none of the four companies . . . et seq. Infected Blood Inquiry, Rajinder Bassi, written evidence on behalf of Revlon, Inc., WITN6391001; author interviews with Analidis Ochoa, July 29, 2021 and May 12, 2023; Starr, *Blood*, Thomas Burton, 'Baxter Confirms Pact to Acquire Immuno,' *Wall Street Journal*, August 30, 1996.

Green Cross sold Alpha . . . Grifols, *When a Dream Comes True: An Illustrated History of 75 Years of Grifols* (DAU, 2015).

The industry is prospering . . . 'Global Blood Plasma Derivatives Market Report 2022,' www.globenewswire.com/en/news-release/2022/12/02/2566488/28124/en/Global -Blood-Plasma-Derivatives-Market-Report-2022-Featuring-Bayer-Takeda -Pharmaceutical-Grifols-Biotest-More.html.

Wolfgang Marguerre started his business career . . . 'Wolfgang Marguerre & Family,' *Forbes* profile, accessed May 2023.

'They gave the most lavish parties . . .' Author interview with Professor Edward Tuddenham, April 28, 2023.

'New donors can earn over $800 . . .' www.octapharmaplasma.com.

CSL Plasma, meanwhile . . . Josh Carter, 'Companies Want Your Plasma, and They're Willing to Pay Big Bucks to Get It,' WLOX, March 29, 2022.

Between $20 and $50 per donation . . . Author interview with Analidis Ochoa, May 12, 2023.

In destitute districts . . . *Blood Business: How the Plasma Industry Works*, *ENDEVR*, 2017.

Companies say the short-term . . . www.grifolsplasma.com/en/first-donation/faqs and www .cslplasma.com/start-donating.

an investigation by ProPublica . . . Stephanie Dodt, 'Judge Lifts US Ban on Mexicans Entering Country to Sell Blood Plasma,' *ProPublica*, September 20, 2022.

The HIV and hepatitis C disasters . . . Starr, *Blood*, and Weinberg and Shaw, *Blood on Their Hands*.

In 2012, the Association of . . . www.abpi.org.uk/reputation/disclosure-uk/about-disclosure -uk/history/.

'I'm glad that has been . . .' Author interview with Professor Edward Tuddenham, August 6, 2021.

In 2016, pharma companies . . . Owen Amos, 'Why Opioids Are Such an American Problem,' BBC News, October 25, 2017.

Already, there are diseases . . . Weinberg and Shaw, *Blood on Their Hands*.

Other blood-borne diseases . . . www.cdc.gov/parasites/babesiosis/disease.html, and www .cdc.gov/zika/transmission/blood-tissue-safety.html.

'It absolutely could happen again . . .' Author interview with Donna Shaw, June 14, 2021.

'Do I think the corporate world . . .' Author interview with Dr Jeanne Kay Noel, September 2, 2021.

Companies including Purdue Pharma . . . American Bar Association, 'Opioid Lawsuits Generate Payouts, Controversy,' September 2019, www.americanbar.org/news /abanews/aba-news-archives/2019/09/opioid-lawsuits-generate-payouts-controversy.

'It's very similar because . . .' Author interview with Gerald Posner, September 17, 2021, and Gerald Posner, *Pharma: Greed, Lies, and the Poisoning of America* (Avid Reader Press/ Simon & Schuster, 2020).

'But,' he says, 'that doesn't . . .' Author interview with Des Collins, July 5, 2021.

In 2021 1.6 million people . . . www.who.int/groups/global-prep-network/global-state-of -prep.

The NHS, meanwhile, said . . . www.england.nhs.uk/2022/12/nhs-set-to-eliminate -hepatitis-c-ahead-of-rest-of-the-world.

Gene therapy could fix the defect . . . James Gallagher, 'Transformational Therapy Cures Haemophilia B,' BBC News, July 21, 2022, and Sky News, 'Gene Therapy Cuts Risk of Bleeding in Haemophilia B Patients, Study Finds,' July 21, 2022.

In late 2022, the FDA approved . . . Miryam Naddaf, 'Researchers Welcome $3.5-Million Haemophilia Gene Therapy – but Questions Remain,' *Nature*, December 6, 2022.

'Even now their take . . .' et seq. Author interviews with Professor Edward Tuddenham, August 6, 2021 and April 28, 2023, and Caroline Peachey, 'Europe Approves First Gene Therapy for Treatment of Haemophilia A,' *European Pharmaceutical Review*, August 30, 2022.

'As a Christian, I look . . .' Author interview with Professor Edward Tuddenham, August 6, 2021.

'It's just inhuman . . .' Author interview with Tom and Lorraine Mull, October 29, 2022.

'Brad made us stronger . . .' Author interview with Gary and Karen Cross, November 1, 2022.

Many of those who made it . . . et seq. Author interviews with Ade Goodyear, Richard Warwick, Frankie and Joe.

Terry Tottenham, the lawyer . . . et seq. Author interview with Tom and Lorraine Mull, October 29, 2022, March 22 and April 5, 2023.

Index